The Psycho-Analysis of Children

The Writings of Melanie Klein

THE PSYCHO-ANALYSIS OF CHILDREN

NARRATIVE OF A CHILD ANALYSIS

LOVE, GUILT AND REPARATION
AND OTHER WORKS

ENVY AND GRATITUDE AND OTHER WORKS

MELANIE KLEIN

The Psycho-Analysis of Children

**Authorized Translation by
ALIX STRACHEY**

**Revised in Collaboration with
ALIX STRACHEY by H. A. THORNER**

DELACORTE PRESS / SEYMOUR LAWRENCE

To the memory of
KARL ABRAHAM
in gratitude and admiration

CONTENTS

NOTE TO THE REVISED TRANSLATION

THE first English translation of Melanie Klein's *Die Psychoanalyse des Kindes* by Alix Strachey appeared at almost the same time as the German edition of the book (1932). Mrs Strachey discussed her translation in detail with Mrs Klein, whose agreement made it the authentic English text. It also became the basis for translations into other languages, including French.

Nevertheless there are a number of differences between the two versions:

(1) Some otherwise inexplicable variations possibly reflect late alterations made by Mrs Klein in the German text after the translation had been made from it.

(2) Apart from these, certain passages in the German text were deliberately not included in the first translation. The most important omissions were the case of Mr A in Chapter XII and parts of the case history of Mr B. These were left out for reasons of discretion which were valid at the time of publication. The case of Mr A was, however, included in the later French translation, and in this edition it is newly translated from the German.

(3) The German text bears the character and style of the spoken word. It was apparently the basis, if not the actual text, of the lectures which Mrs Klein gave in London. This would explain the many repetitions which are natural when speaking, and the frequent, detailed and lengthy footnotes which contain material unsuited to a lecture. The original translation excluded many repetitions in the interest of easier reading. They are however included in the present edition for the sake of accuracy. When the German text uses the first person singular as a speaker would, the original translation generally gave the plural 'we' instead of 'I'. The revised translation has reverted to the singular in order to maintain the style of the spoken word.

In general the new edition attempts to remain as faithful as possible to the German printed text even at the expense of sacrificing a claim to literary style.

The paragraphing of the original translation has been adopted for this edition as it follows the English usage, according to which a new paragraph introduces a fresh thought, while the German usage often introduces a new thought at the end of the previous paragraph. In this revised edition all quotations from Freud follow the text of the *Standard Edition*.

NOTE TO THE REVISED TRANSLATION

With regard to terminology, a few changes have been made. For example, 'Wisstrieb', originally translated as 'epistemological instinct', has now been rendered as 'instinct (or desire) for knowledge'. 'Phase der Höchstblüte des Sadismus' which was originally given as 'phase of maximal sadism' is now translated as 'phase when sadism is at its height' except in the Preface to the Third Edition which was written by Melanie Klein in English. 'Gegenständlich', earlier translated as 'concrete', is now rendered as 'presentational' in order to distinguish it from the use of 'concrete' as in 'concrete thinking'.

Following the practice of the *Standard Edition* of Freud's works, square brackets have been used to indicate all additions to the text. The footnotes are numbered as in the German edition but those which I have added are indicated by an additional letter, as for example in Chapter III I have added footnotes 1a and 1b.

H. A. THORNER

London, April 1974

PREFACE TO THE FIRST EDITION

THIS book is based on the observations I have been able to make in the course of my psycho-analytic work with children. My original plan was to devote the first part of it to a description of the technique I have worked out and the second to a statement of the theoretical conclusions to which my practical work has gradually brought me, and which now seem to be suited to serve as a basis for my technique. But in the course of writing this book—a task which has extended over several years—the second part has outgrown its limits. In addition to my experience in child analysis, the observations I have made in analysing adults have led me to apply my views concerning the earliest developmental stages of the child to the psychology of the adult as well, and I have come to certain conclusions which I shall bring forward in these pages as a contribution to the general psycho-analytic theory of the earliest stages of the development of the individual.

That contribution is in every respect based on the body of knowledge which we owe to Freud. It was by applying his findings that I gained access to the minds of small children and could analyse and cure them. In doing this, moreover, I was able to make those direct observations of early developmental processes which have led me to my present theoretical conclusions. Those conclusions confirm fully the discoveries that Freud has made in the analysis of adults, and are an endeavour to extend our knowledge in one or two directions.

If this endeavour should in any way be successful, and if this book should really add a few more stones to the growing edifice of psycho-analytic knowledge, my thanks in the first instance would be due to Freud himself, who has not only raised that edifice and placed it on foundations that permit its further extension, but who has always directed our attention to those points from which the new work should proceed.

I should next like to mention the part which my two teachers, Dr Sandor Ferenczi and Dr Karl Abraham, have played in the development of my psycho-analytic work and its results. Ferenczi was the first to make me acquainted with psycho-analysis. He also made me understand its real essence and meaning. His strong and direct feeling for the unconscious and for symbolism, and the remarkable *rapport* he had with the minds of children, have had a lasting influence on my understanding of the psychology of the small child. He also drew my attention to my capacity for child analysis, in which he took a great personal interest, and encouraged me to devote myself to this field of psycho-analytic therapy, then still very little explored. He furthermore did all he could to help me along this path and gave me much support in my first efforts. It is to him that I owe the foundations from which my work as an analyst developed.

In Dr Karl Abraham I had the great good fortune to find a second teacher with the faculty of inspiring his pupils to put out their best energies in the service of psycho-analysis. In Abraham's opinion, the progress of psycho-analysis depended upon each individual analyst—upon the value of his work, the quality of his character and the level of his scientific attainments. These high standards have been before my mind, when, in this book on psychoanalysis, I have tried to repay some part of the great debt I owe to that science. Abraham clearly understood the great practical and theoretic potentialities of child analysis. At the First Conference of German Psycho-Analysts at Würzburg in 1924, in connection with a paper I had read upon an obsessional neurosis in a child,[1] he said, in words that I shall never forget: 'The future of psycho-analysis lies in play technique.' The study of the mind of the small child taught me certain facts which seemed strange at first sight. But Abraham's confidence in my work encouraged me at that time to follow the path on which I had started. My theoretical conclusions are a natural development of his own discoveries, as I hope this book will show.

In the last few years my work has received generous and wholehearted support from Dr Ernest Jones. At a time when child analysis was still in its first stages, he foresaw the part it was destined to play in the future. It was at his invitation that I gave my first course of lectures in London in 1925 as a guest of the British Psycho-Analytical Society; and these lectures have given rise to the first part of my present book. The second part is based on another course of lectures, entitled 'Adult Psychology in the light of Child Analysis', given in London in 1927. The deep conviction with which Dr Jones has made himself an advocate of child analysis has opened the way for this field of work in England. He himself has made important contributions to the problem of early anxiety-situations, the significance of aggressiveness for the sense of guilt, and the earliest stages of the sexual development of women. The results of his studies are in close touch with my own in all essential points.

I should like in this place to thank my other English fellow-workers for the sympathetic understanding and cordial support they have given to my work. Miss M. Nina Searl, whose collaboration with me was based on common conviction and personal friendship,

[1] This report forms the basis of Chapter III of this book.

has done lasting service towards the advancement of child analysis in England, both from a practical and a theoretical point of view, and towards the training of child analysts. The help I received from Mr and Mrs James Strachey was of great significance. They too have done a great deal for this book, which they have not only translated most ably, but have also influenced the writing of, by their valuable and stimulating suggestions. My thanks are due next to Dr Edward Glover for the warm and unfailing interest he has shown in my work, and for the way in which he has assisted me by his sympathetic criticism. He has been of special service in pointing out the respects in which my conclusions agree with the already existing and accepted theories of psycho-analysis. I also owe a deep debt of gratitude to my friend Mrs Joan Riviere, who has given such active support to my work and has always been ready to help me in every way.

Last but not least, let me very heartily thank my daughter, Dr Melitta Schmideberg, for the devoted and valuable help which she has given me in the preparation of this book.

London, July 1932   MELANIE KLEIN

PREFACE TO THE THIRD EDITION[1]

In the years which have elapsed since this book first appeared, I have arrived at further conclusions—mainly relating to the first year of infancy—and these have led to an elaboration of certain essential hypotheses here presented. The purpose of this Preface is to give some idea of the nature of these modifications. The hypotheses I have in mind in this connection are as follows: in the first few months of life, infants pass through states of persecutory anxiety which are bound up with the 'phase of maximal sadism'; the young infant also experiences feelings of guilt about his destructive impulses and phantasies which are directed against his primary object—his mother, and first of all her breast. These feelings of guilt give rise to the tendency to make reparation to the injured object.

In endeavouring to fill in the picture of this period in greater detail, I found that certain shifts of emphasis and time relations were inevitable. Thus I have come to differentiate between two main phases in the first six to eight months of life, and I described them as the 'paranoid position' and the 'depressive position'. (The term 'position' was chosen because—though the phenomena involved occur in the first place during early stages of development—they are not confined to these stages but represent specific groupings of anxieties and defences which appear and re-appear during the first years of childhood.)

The paranoid position is the stage when destructive impulses and persecutory anxieties predominate and extends from birth until about three, four or even five months of life. This necessitates an alteration in dating the phase when sadism is at its height but does not involve a change of view regarding the close interaction between sadism and persecutory anxiety at their height.

The depressive position, which follows on this stage and is bound up with important steps in ego development, is established about the middle of the first year of life. At this stage sadistic impulses and phantasies, as well as persecutory anxiety, diminish in power. The infant introjects the object as a whole, and simultaneously he becomes in some measure able to synthesize the various aspects of the object as well as his emotions towards it. Love and hatred come closer together in his mind, and this leads to anxiety lest the object, internal and external, be harmed or destroyed. Depressive feelings

[1][This preface was written for the third English edition and was not published in German. See Note to the Revised Translation.]

xiii

and guilt give rise to the urge to preserve or revive the loved object, and thus to make reparation for destructive impulses and phantasies.

The concept of the depressive position not only entails an alteration in dating early phases of development, it also adds to our knowledge of the emotional life of young infants and therefore vitally influences our understanding of the whole development of the child.

This concept throws new light, too, on the early stages of the Oedipus complex. I still believe that these begin roughly in the middle of the first year. But since I no longer hold that sadism is at its height at this period, I place a different emphasis on the beginning of the emotional and sexual relation to both parents. Therefore, while in some passages (see Chapter VIII) I suggested that the Oedipus complex starts under the dominance of sadism and hatred, I would now say that the infant turns to the second object, the father, with feelings both of love and of hatred. (In Chapters IX, X and XII, however, these issues were considered from another angle, and there I came close to the view I now hold.) I see in the depressive feelings derived from the fear of losing the loved mother—as an external and internal object—an important impetus towards early Oedipus desires. This means that I now correlate the early stages of the Oedipus complex with the depressive position.

There are also a number of statements in this book which, in keeping with my work over the last sixteen years, I might wish to reformulate. Such reformulation, however, would not entail any essential alteration in the conclusions here put forward. For this book as it stands, represents fundamentally the views I hold today. Moreover, the more recent development of my work derives organically from the hypotheses here presented: e.g. processes of introjection and projection operating from the beginning of life; internalized objects from which, in the course of years, the super-ego in all its aspects develops; the relation to external and internal objects interacting from earliest infancy and vitally influencing both the super-ego development and object relations; the early onset of the Oedipus complex; infantile anxieties of a psychotic nature providing the fixation points for the psychosis. Furthermore, play technique—which I first evolved in 1922 and 1923 and which I presented in this book—still stands in all essentials; it has been elaborated but not altered by the further development of my work.

London, May 1948   M. K.

INTRODUCTION

THE beginnings of child analysis go back more than two decades, to the time when Freud himself carried out his analysis of 'Little Hans'.[1] The great theoretical significance of this first analysis of a child lay in two directions. Its success in the case of a child of under five showed that psycho-analytic methods could be applied to small children; and, perhaps more important still, the analysis could establish, beyond doubt, the existence of the hitherto much-questioned infantile instinctual trends in the child himself which Freud had discovered in the adult. In addition, the results obtained from it held out the hope that further analyses of small children would give us a deeper and more accurate knowledge of the working of their minds than analysis of adults had done, and would thus be able to make important and fundamental contributions to the theory of psycho-analysis. But this hope remained unrealized for a long time. For many years child analysis continued to be a relatively unexplored region within psycho-analysis, both as a science and a therapy. Although several analysts particularly Dr H. v. Hug-Hellmuth[2] have since undertaken analyses of children, no fixed rules as regards its technique or application have been worked out. This is doubtless the reason why the great practical and theoretical potentialities of child analysis have not yet been generally appreciated, and why those fundamental principles and aspects of psycho-analysis which have long since been adopted in the case of adults have still to be clarified and proved where children are concerned.

It is only within the last ten years or so that more work has been done in the field of child analysis. In the main, two methods have emerged—one represented by Anna Freud and the other by myself.

Anna Freud has been led by her findings in regard to the ego of the child to modify the classical technique, and has worked out her method of analysing children in the latency period independently of my technique. Her theoretical conclusions are in certain respects different from mine. In her opinion children do not develop a transference-neurosis,[3] so that a fundamental condition for analytical

[1] 'Analysis of a Phobia in a Five-Year-Old Boy' (1909). (*S.E.* **10**, p. 3 ff.)
[2] 'On the Technique of Child Analysis' (1921).
[3] 'The child is not, like the adult, prepared to produce a new edition of its love-relationships because, as one might say, the old edition is not yet exhausted. Its original objects, the parents, are still real and present as love-objects—not only in fantasy as with the adult neurotic;' And again, 'But there is no necessity for the child to exchange the parents for him' (the analyst)

treatment is absent. Moreover, she thinks that a method similar to the one employed for adults should not be applied to children, because their infantile ego-ideal is still too weak.[1] These views differ from mine. My observations have taught me that children, too, develop a transference-neurosis analogous to that of grown-up persons, so long as we employ a method which is the equivalent of adult analysis, i.e., which avoids all educational measures and which fully analyses the negative impulses directed towards the analyst. They have also taught me that in children of all ages, it is very hard even for deep analysis to mitigate the severity of the super-ego. Moreover, in so far as it does so without having recourse to any educational influence, analysis not only does not harm the child's ego, but actually strengthens it.

It would be an interesting task, no doubt, to make a detailed comparison of these two methods on the basis of factual data and to evaluate them from a theoretical point of view. But I must content myself in these pages with giving an account of my technique and of the theoretical conclusions which it has enabled me to come to. So relatively little is known at present about the analysis of children that our first task must be to throw light on the problems of child analysis from various angles and to gather together the results so far obtained.

'since compared to them he has not got the advantages which the adult finds when he can exchange his phantasy-objects for a real person.' (*The Psycho-Analytical Treatment of Children*, p. 34.)

[1] She mentions the following reasons (p. 49): 'The fact that a child's ego-ideal is weak; that its demands and neurosis are dependent on the outer world; that it is unable to control the emancipated instincts; and that the analyst himself must guide them.' Further, on page 31: 'But with a child, negative impulses towards the analyst—however revealing they may be in many respects—are essentially inconvenient, and should be dealt with as soon as possible. The really fruitful work always takes place with a positive attachment.'

Part I

THE TECHNIQUE OF CHILD ANALYSIS

Chapter I

THE PSYCHOLOGICAL FOUNDATIONS
OF CHILD ANALYSIS[1]

PSYCHO-ANALYSIS has led to the creation of a new child psychology. Psycho-analytic observations have taught us that even in their earliest years, children experience not only sexual impulses and anxiety, but also great disappointments. Along with the belief in the asexuality of the child has gone the belief in the 'Paradise of Childhood'. These are the conclusions which were gained from both analysis of adults and direct observation of children, and which are confirmed and supplemented by the analysis of small children.

Let me begin, with the help of examples, by sketching a picture of the mind of the young child as I have learnt to know it from these early analyses. My patient Rita, who at the beginning of her treatment was two and three-quarter years old, had a preference for her mother till the end of her first year. After that she showed a markedly greater fondness for her father, together with a good deal of jealousy of her mother. For instance, when she was fifteen months old she used repeatedly to express a desire to be left alone in the room with her father and to sit on his knee and look at books with him. At the age of eighteen months her attitude changed once more and her mother was re-installed as the favourite. At the same time she began to suffer from night-terrors and fear of animals. She grew more and more strongly fixated upon her mother and developed an intense dislike of her father. At the beginning of her third year she became increasingly ambivalent and difficult to manage, until at last, at the age of two and three-quarters, she was brought to me to be analysed. At that time she had a very marked obsessional neurosis. She exhibited obsessive ceremonials and alternated between 'goody-goodiness' mixed with feelings of remorse, and uncontrollable 'naughtiness'. She had attacks of moodiness which showed all the signs of a melancholic depression; and in addition she suffered from severe anxiety, an extensive inhibition in play, a total inability to tolerate any kind of frustration, and an excessive woefulness. These difficulties made the child almost impossible to manage.[2]

[1] This chapter is an expanded version of my paper, 'The Psychological Principles of Early Analysis' (1926) *Writings*, I.

[2] Rita had shared her parents' bedroom until she was nearly two, and in her analysis she showed the consequences of having witnessed the primal scene.

Rita's case clearly showed that the *pavor nocturnus* which appeared at the age of eighteen months was a neurotic working over of her Oedipus conflict.[1] Her attacks of anxiety and rage, which turned out to be a repetition of her night terrors, and her other difficulties as well, were very closely connected with strong feelings of guilt arising from that early Oedipus conflict.

I will now turn to consider the content and the causes of these early feelings of guilt by reference to another case. Trude, aged three years and nine months,[2] repeatedly played 'make believe' in her analysis that it was night-time and that we were both asleep. She then used to come softly over to me from the opposite corner of the room (which was supposed to be her own bedroom) and threaten me in various ways, such as that she was going to stab me in the throat, throw me out of the window, burn me up, take me to the police, etc. She would want to tie up my hands and feet, or she would lift up the rug on the sofa and say she was doing 'Po—Kaki—Kuki'. This, it turned out, meant that she wanted to look inside her

---

When she was two years old her brother was born, and this event led to the outbreak of her neurosis in its full force. Her analysis lasted for eighty-three sessions and was left unfinished, as her parents went to live abroad. In all important points it resulted in a quite considerable improvement. The child's anxiety was lessened and her obsessive ceremonials disappeared. Her depressive symptoms, together with her inability to tolerate frustrations, were a good deal moderated. At the same time as analysis lessened her ambivalence towards her mother and improved her relations to her father and brother, it reduced the difficulties of her upbringing to a normal level. I was able to convince myself at first hand of the lasting nature of the results of her analysis some years after its termination. I found then that she had entered upon the latency period in a satisfactory manner, and that her intellectual and characterological development were satisfactory. Nevertheless, when I saw her again I got the impression that it would have been advisable to have continued her analysis somewhat further. Her whole character and nature showed unmistakable traces of an obsessional disposition. In this connection it must be remarked that her mother suffered from a severe obsessional neurosis and had had an ambivalent relation towards the child from the first. One result of the changes for the better which analysis had effected in Rita was that her mother's attitude towards her had also greatly improved; but even so it remained a severe handicap in the child's development. There is no doubt that if her analysis had been carried through to the end and her obsessional traits still further cleared up, she would have gained a more effective counterbalance against the neurotic and neurosis-inducing environment in which she lived. Seven years after the end of her treatment I heard from her mother that she continued to develop satisfactorily.

[1] In Chapter VIII I shall give fuller reasons for assuming that in these emotions the early stages of the Oedipus conflict were already finding utterance.

[2] Here, as elsewhere, the age given denotes the age at which the child started analysis.

4

mother's bottom for the 'Kakis' (faeces), which signified children to her. On another occasion she wanted to hit me in the stomach and declared that she was taking out my 'A—A's' (stool) and was making me poor. She then seized the cushions, which she repeatedly called children, and hid herself with them behind the sofa. There she crouched in the corner with an intense expression of fear, covered herself up, sucked her fingers and wetted herself. She used to repeat this whole process whenever she had made an attack on me. It corresponded in every detail with the way she had behaved in bed when, at a time when she was not yet two, she started to have very severe night terrors. At that time, too, she had run into her parents' bedroom again and again at night without being able to say what it was she wanted. By analysing her wetting and dirtying herself which stood for attacks upon her parents copulating with each other, these symptoms were removed. Trude had wanted to rob her pregnant mother of her children, to kill her and to take her place in coitus with her father. She was two years old when her sister was born. It was those impulses of hatred and aggression which, in her second year, had given rise to an increasingly strong fixation upon her mother and to a severe anxiety and sense of guilt which found expression, among other things, in her night terrors. I conclude from this that the small child's early anxiety and feelings of guilt have their origin in aggressive trends connected with the Oedipus conflict.[1] At the time when Trude was most clearly exhibiting the behaviour I have described in the analysis, she used to manage to hurt herself in some way almost every time before she came for her

[1] In the paper upon which this chapter is based ('The Psychological Principles of Early Analysis', 1926) I had already put forward the view that hatred and aggressive trends are the deepest cause and foundation of feelings of guilt; and since then I have brought fresh evidence in support of that opinion in a number of other writings. In my paper 'The Importance of Symbol-Formation in the Development of the Ego', read at the Oxford Congress in 1929, I was able to give a more extended formulation of it. I said: 'It is only in the later stages of the Oedipus conflict that the defence against the libidinal impulses makes its appearance; in the earlier stages it is against the accompanying *destructive* impulses that the defence is directed'. This statement agrees in some points, I think, with the conclusions Freud has reached in his recent book, *Civilization and its Discontents* (1930), in which he says: 'But if this is so, it is after all only the aggressiveness which is transformed into a sense of guilt, by being suppressed and made over to the super-ego. I am convinced that many processes will admit of a simpler and clearer explanation if the findings of psychoanalysis with regard to the derivation of the sense of guilt are restricted to the aggressive instincts' (*S.E.* **21**, p. 138). And on the next page: 'It now seems plausible to formulate the following proposition. When an instinctual trend undergoes repression, its libidinal elements are turned into symptoms and its aggressive components into a sense of guilt.'

analytic session. It turned out that the objects against which she had hurt herself—a table, a cupboard, a fireplace, etc.—signified, in keeping with the primitive and infantile identification, her mother or her father, who were punishing her.[1]

Returning to our first case, we find that before she was two years old, Rita became conspicuous for the remorse she used to feel at every small wrongdoing, and for her over-sensitiveness to reproach. For instance, she once burst into tears when her father laughingly uttered a threat against a bear in her picture-book. What determined her identification with the bear was her fear of her real father's displeasure. Her inhibition in play originated from her sense of guilt. When she was only two years and three months old she used to play with her doll—a game which gave her little pleasure—and would repeatedly declare that she was not the doll's mother. Analysis showed that she was not permitted to play at being its mother, because, among other things, the doll-child stood for her little brother whom she had wanted to steal from her mother during the latter's pregnancy. The prohibition, however, did not proceed from her real mother, but from an introjected one who treated her with far more severity and cruelty than the real one had ever done. Another symptom—an obsession—which Rita developed at the age of two was a bed-time ritual which took up a lot of time. The main point of it was that she had to be tightly tucked up in the bedclothes, otherwise a 'mouse or a Butzen' would get in through the window and bite off her own 'Butzen'.[2] Her doll had to be tucked up too, and this double ceremonial became more and more elaborate and long-drawn-out and was performed with every sign of that compulsive attitude which pervaded her whole mind. On one occasion during her analytic session she put a toy elephant to her doll's bed so as to prevent it from getting up and going into her parents' bedroom and 'doing something to them or taking something away from them'. The elephant was taking over the role of her internalized parents whose prohibiting influence she felt ever since, between the ages of one year and three months and two years, she had wished to take her mother's place with her father, rob her of the child inside her, and injure and castrate both parents. The meaning of the ceremonial now became clear: being tucked up in bed was to prevent

[1] A certain plaintiveness of disposition and a tendency to fall down or get hurt, things so especially common in small children, are, according to my experience, effects of the sense of guilt.

[2] Rita's castration complex was manifested in a whole series of symptoms and also in her characterological development. Her play, too, clearly showed the strength of her identification with her father and her fear—arising from her castration complex—of failing in the masculine role.

her from getting up and carrying out her aggressive wishes against her parents. Since, however, she expected to be punished for those wishes by a similar attack on herself by her parents, being tucked up also served as a defence against such attacks. The attacks were to be made, for instance, by the '*Butzen*' (her father's penis), which would injure her genitals and bite off her own '*Butzen*' as a punishment for wanting to castrate him. In these games she used to punish her doll and then give way to an outburst of rage and fear, thus showing that she was playing both parts herself—that of the powers which inflict punishment and that of the punished child itself.

These games also proved that this anxiety referred not only to the child's real parents, but also, and more especially, to its excessively stern introjected parents. What we meet with here corresponds to what we call the super-ego in adults.[1] The typical signs, which are most pronounced when the Oedipus complex has reached its height and which precede its decline, are themselves only the final stage of a process which has been going on for years. Early analysis shows that the Oedipus conflict sets in as early as the second half of the first year of life and that at the same time the child begins to build up its super-ego.

Finding then, as we do, that even quite young children are under pressure of feelings of guilt, we have at least one fundamental precondition for the analysis of the small child. And yet many conditions for their successful treatment seem to be missing. Their relation to reality is a weak one; there is apparently no inducement to them to undergo the trials of an analysis, since they do not as a rule feel ill; and lastly, and most important of all, they cannot as yet give, or cannot give in a sufficient degree, those associations of speech which are the principal instrument of an analytic treatment of adults.

Let us take this last objection first. The very differences between the infantile mind and the grown-up one showed me, in the first instance, the way to get at the associations of the child and to understand its unconscious. These special characteristics of the child's psychology have furnished the basis of the technique of play analysis which I have been able to work out. The child expresses its phantasies, its wishes and its actual experiences in a symbolic way through play and games. In doing so, it makes use of the same archaic and phylogenetically-acquired mode of expression, the same language, as it were, that we are familiar with in dreams; and we can only fully understand this language if we approach it in the way Freud has taught us to approach the language of dreams. Symbolism is only a part of it. If we wish to understand the child's play correctly

[1] In my opinion the child's earliest identifications already deserve to be called 'super-ego'. The reasons for this view will be given in Chapter VIII.

THE PSYCHO-ANALYSIS OF CHILDREN

in relation to its whole behaviour during the analytic session we must not be content to pick out the meaning of the separate symbols in the play, striking as they often are, but must take into consideration all the mechanisms and methods of representation employed by the dream-work, never losing sight of the relation of each factor to the situation as a whole. Early analysis of children has shown again and again how many different meanings a single toy or a single bit of play can have, and that we can only infer and interpret their meaning when we consider their wider connections and the whole analytic situation in which they are set. Rita's doll, for instance, would sometimes stand for a penis, sometimes a child she had stolen from her mother, and sometimes her own self. Full analytic impact can only be obtained if we bring these play-elements into their true relation with the child's sense of guilt by interpreting them down to the smallest detail. The whole kaleidoscopic picture, often to all appearances quite meaningless, which children present to us in a single analytic session, how they pass from playing with a toy to impersonating something with their own person, and then again return to playing with water, to cutting out in paper or drawing, how the child does this or that, why it changes its game and what means it chooses to express the content of its games—all these things are seen to have method in them and will become meaningful if we interpret them as we do dreams. Very often children will express in their play the same things that they have just been telling us in a dream, or will bring associations to a dream in the play which succeeds it. For play is the child's most important medium of expression. If we make use of this play technique we soon find that the child brings as many associations to the separate elements of its play as adults do to the separate elements of their dreams. These separate play-elements are indications to the trained observer; and as it plays, the child talks as well, and says all sorts of things which have the value of genuine associations.

It is surprising how easily children will sometimes accept the interpretation and even show unmistakable pleasure in doing so. The reason probably is that in certain strata of their minds, communication between the conscious and the unconscious is as yet comparatively easy, so that the way back to the unconscious is much simpler to find. Interpretation often has rapid effects, even when it does not appear to have been taken in consciously. Such effects show themselves in the way in which they enable the child to resume a game it has broken off in consequence of the emergence of an inhibition, and to change and expand it, bringing deeper layers of the mind to view in it. And as anxiety is thus resolved and desire to play restored, analytic contact, too, becomes established once

8

more. As the interpretation releases the energy which the child had to expend on maintaining repression, fresh interest in play is generated. On the other hand, we sometimes encounter resistances which are very hard to overcome. This most usually means that we have come up against the child's anxiety and sense of guilt belonging to deeper layers of its mind.

The archaic and symbolic forms of representation which the child employs in its play are associated with another primitive mechanism. In its play, the child acts instead of speaking. It puts actions—which originally took the place of thoughts—in the place of words; that is to say, that 'acting out' is of utmost importance for it. In his 'From the History of an Infantile Neurosis', Freud writes: 'An analysis which is conducted upon a neurotic child itself must, as a matter of course, appear to be more trustworthy, but it cannot be very rich in material; too many words and thoughts have to be lent to the child, and even so the deepest strata may turn out to be impenetrable to consciousness.'[1] If we approach the child patient with the technique of adult analysis it is quite certain that we shall not penetrate to those deepest levels; and yet it is upon reaching these levels that, for the child no less than for the adult, the success and value of analysis depends. But if we take into consideration how the child's psychology differs from that of the adult—the fact that its unconscious is as yet in close contact with its conscious and that its most primitive impulses are at work alongside of highly complicated mental processes—and if we correctly grasp the child's mode of expression, then all these drawbacks and disadvantages vanish and we find that we may expect to make as deep and extensive an analysis of the child as of the adult. More so in fact. In child-analysis we are able to get back to experiences and fixations which, in the analysis of adults can often only be reconstructed, whereas the child shows them to us as immediate representations.[2]

In a paper read before the Salzburg Congress in 1924,[3] I put forward the thesis that behind every form of play-activity lies a process of discharge of masturbatory phantasies, operating in the form of a continuous motive for play; that this process, acting as a repetition-compulsion, constitutes a fundamental mechanism in children's play and in all their subsequent sublimations; and that

[1] *S.E.* **17**, p. 8.
[2] Early analysis offers one of the most fruitful fields for psycho-analytic therapy precisely because the child has the ability to represent its unconscious in a direct way, and is thus not only able to experience a far-reaching emotional abreaction but actually to live through the original situation in its analysis, so that with the help of interpretation its fixations can to a considerable extent be resolved.
[3] Not published.

inhibitions in play and work spring from an unduly strong repression of those phantasies, and with them, of the whole imaginative life of the child. Linked to these masturbatory phantasies of the child are its sexual experiences, which along with them, find representation and abreaction in its play. Among such re-enacted experiences, the primal scene plays a very important part and generally occupies the foreground of the picture in early analysis. It is, as a rule, only after a good deal of analysis has been done, and both the primal scene and the child's genital trends have been to some extent uncovered, that we reach representations of its pre-genital experiences and phantasies. For instance, Ruth, aged four years and three months, had, as an infant, suffered hunger for a considerable time because her mother had not had enough milk. When playing she used to call the water-tap the 'milk-tap'. She explained her game by saying that the milk was going into the 'mouths' (the holes of the waste pipe), but that only very little was going into them. She showed her unsatisfied oral desires in countless games and make-believes and in her whole attitude of mind. She would declare, for instance, that she was poor, that she had only one overcoat, that she didn't get enough to eat, etc. — all of which was quite untrue.

The case of Erna, a six-year-old obsessional patient, whose toilet training had been a considerable factor in her neurosis,[1] demonstrated those experiences to me in the greatest detail in her analysis. For instance, she sat a small doll down on a brick and made it defaecate in front of a row of other admiring dolls. She then repeated the same theme, but this time we had to play the parts ourselves. I had to be a baby which was dirtying itself and she was the mother. She admired and caressed the baby. Then she changed, became furious and suddenly played the part of a severe governess who was ill-treating the child. In this sense she was portraying to me what she had felt in her early childhood when her nursery training had begun and she had believed that she was losing the excessive love she had enjoyed as a baby.

In child analysis we cannot rate too highly the importance of acting-out and phantasies in the service of the repetition-compulsion. The small child, of course, uses acting-out most of all, but even the older one is constantly having recourse to this primitive mechanism. The pleasure gain he gets in this way provides an indispensable stimulus to continue his analysis, though it should never be more than a means to an end.

When the analysis has been started and a certain amount of anxiety has been resolved in the small patient by interpretation, the sense of relief he experiences as a consequence of it—often after

[1] A more detailed account of Erna's case will be given in Chapter III.

THE PSYCHOLOGICAL FOUNDATIONS

only the first few sessions—will help him to go on with the work. For, whereas he has hitherto had no incentive to be analysed, he has now got an insight into the use and value of the analytical work, which is as effective a motive for being analysed as is the adult's insight into his illness. The child's capacity for insight of this kind testifies to an essential amount of contact with reality which we would not expect in so small a child. This point, the child's relationship to reality, deserves further discussion.

In the course of analysis we can see that the child's relation to reality, at first so feeble, gradually gains in strength as the result of analytic work. The small patient will begin, for instance, to distinguish between his make-believe mother and his real one, or between his toy brother and his live one. He will insist that he only meant to do this or that to his toy brother, and that he loves his real brother very much. Only after very strong and obstinate resistances have been surmounted will he be able to see that his aggressive acts were aimed at the object in the real world. But when he has come to understand this, young as he is, he will have made a very important advance in his adaptation to reality. Trude, my three-years-and-nine-months-old patient, after having had only one analytic session with me, went abroad with her mother. Six months later her analysis was resumed. It took quite a long time before she mentioned anything of all the things she had seen and done during her travels and then only in connection with a dream: She and her mother were back in Italy in a certain restaurant she knew, and the waitress didn't give her any raspberry syrup because there wasn't any left. The interpretation of this dream showed, among other things,[1] that she had not got over the pain at the withdrawal of the mother's breast and her envy of her younger sister. Whereas she had reported to me all sorts of apparently unimportant daily events and had repeatedly alluded to small details out of her first analytic session six months earlier, the only reason for mentioning her travels was an incident of frustration connected with the frustration arising from the analytic situation. Her travels were otherwise of no interest to her.

Neurotic children do not tolerate reality well, because they cannot tolerate frustrations. They protect themselves from reality by denying it. What is fundamental and decisive for their future adaptability to reality is their greater or lesser capacity to tolerate those

[1] The dream was a punishment-dream. It proved to be based upon death-wishes derived from her oral frustration and her Oedipus situation and directed against her sister and mother, together with the sense of guilt resulting from those wishes. My analysis of very young children's dreams in general has shown me that in them, no less than in play, not only wishes but also counter-tendencies coming from the super-ego are always present, and that even in the simplest wish-dreams the sense of guilt is operative in a latent way.

frustrations that arise out of the Oedipus situation. In small children, too, an over-strong rejection of reality (often disguised under an apparent docility and adaptability) is, therefore, an indication of neurosis and only differs from the adult neurotic's flight from reality in its form of expression. For this reason one of the results of early analysis should be to enable the child to adapt itself to reality. If this has been successfully achieved, one sees in children, among other things, a lessening of educational difficulties as the child has become able to tolerate the frustrations entailed by reality.

We have now seen, I think, that in child analysis our angle of approach has to be somewhat different from what it is in the analysis of adults. Taking the shortest cut across the ego, we apply ourselves in the first instance to the child's unconscious and from there gradually get into touch with its ego as well. By means of lessening the excessive pressure of the super-ego which is much more heavy on the feeble ego of the small child than on that of the adult, we strengthen the ego and help it to develop.[1]

I have spoken of the rapid effect that interpretation has upon children and how this is observable in a great number of ways, such as the expansion of their play, the strengthening of their transference and decrease of their anxiety, etc. Nevertheless, they do not seem to work over such interpretations consciously for some time. This task, I found, was accomplished later on, and was bound up and in step with the development of their ego and the growth of their adaptation to reality. The process of sexual enlightenment follows an analogous course. For a long time, analysis does no more than bring out material connected with sexual theories and birth-phantasies. The sexual enlightenment follows gradually by removing the unconscious resistances which work against it. Full sexual enlightenment, therefore, like a full adaptation to reality, is one of the consequences of a completed analysis. Without it no analysis can be said to have reached a successful termination.

In the same way as the mode of expression is different in the child, so is the analytic situation as a whole. And yet in both child and adult the main principles of analysis are the same. Consistent interpretation, gradual resolution of the resistances, steady reference back of the transference, whether positive or negative, to earlier situations—these establish and maintain a correct analytic situation

[1] After the termination of its analysis the child cannot alter the circumstances of its life as the adult often can. But analysis will have helped it very greatly if it has enabled it to develop more freely and to feel better in its actual environment. Furthermore, the removal of the child's neurosis often has the effect of minimizing the difficulties of its milieu. It has been my experience that the mother will react in a much less neurotic way as soon as analysis has begun to effect favourable changes in her child.

with the child not less than with the adult. A necessary condition for this achievement is that the analyst should refrain, as he does with adult patients, from exerting any kind of non-analytic and educational influence upon the child. The transference should therefore be handled throughout in the same way as in adult analysis and, as a consequence, we will see symptoms and difficulties gathering round the analytic situation. This leads to a renewal of earlier symptoms or difficulties and 'naughtiness' which corresponds to them in the child. It will, for instance, begin to wet its bed once more; or, in certain situations which repeat an earlier one, it will, even if it is three or four years old, start talking like a small child of one or two.

As the newly-gained knowledge is at first mainly unconsciously worked over, the child is not confronted all at once with a situation that calls upon it to revise its relation to its parents; this development occurs at first emotionally. In my experience, this gradual working over of the knowledge brings nothing but relief to the child and a marked improvement in its relationship to its parents, together with a better social adaptation and easier up-bringing. The demands of its super-ego having been moderated by analysis, its ego, now less oppressed and consequently stronger, is able to carry them out more easily.

As analysis continues, children grow able to some extent to substitute for the processes of repression, those of critical rejection. This is seen when, in a later stage of their analysis, they become so detached from the sadistic impulses which once governed them, and to whose interpretation they opposed the strongest resistances, that they sometimes make fun of them.[1] I have heard quite small children joke, for instance, about the idea that they once really wanted to eat their Mummy up or cut her into pieces. The decrease of the sense of guilt which accompanies these changes also enables sadistic desires which were before entirely repressed to undergo sublimation. This comes out in the removal of inhibitions both in play and learning and the appearance of a number of fresh interests and activities.

In this chapter I have taken as my point of departure my technique of early analysis, because it is fundamental for analytic methods. Since in so far as the peculiarities of the minds of quite

---

[1] This observation, that when their super-ego becomes less harsh children develop a sense of humour, confirms, I think, Freud's theory of the nature of humour, which, according to him, is the effect of a friendly super-ego. In concluding his paper on 'Humour' (1928) (*S.E.* **21**, p. 166) he says: 'And finally, if the super-ego tries, by means of humour, to console the ego and protect it from suffering, this does not contradict its origin in the parental agency.'

small children often persist quite strongly in older ones, I have found this very technique indispensable in my work with older children as well. On the other hand, of course, the ego of the older child is more fully developed, so that that technique has to undergo some modification when it is applied to children in the latency period and at puberty. This subject will receive fuller attention later on and I shall therefore only dwell on it very briefly here. Whether such a modified technique will more nearly approximate to early analysis or to adult analysis depends not only upon the age of the child but upon the special character of the case.

Speaking generally, the following principles are fundamental to my technique for all age-groups. As children and young people suffer from a more acute degree of anxiety than do adults, we must gain access to their anxiety and to their unconscious sense of guilt and establish the analytic situation as rapidly as possible. In small children this anxiety usually finds an outlet in anxiety attacks; during the latency period it more often takes the form of distrustful rejection, while in the intensely emotional age of puberty it once more leads to an acute generation of anxiety which now, however, in conformity with the child's more developed ego, frequently finds expression in resistances of a defiant and violent nature, which may easily cause the analysis to be broken off. A certain amount of anxiety can quickly be resolved in children of all ages if the negative transference is, from the start, systematically treated and dissolved.

But in order to gain access to the child's phantasies and unconscious, let us be guided by those methods of indirect symbolic representation which the small as well as the older child employs. Once the child's phantasy has become more free as a consequence of its lessened anxiety, we have not only gained access to its unconscious but have also mobilized in an ever greater degree, the means at its command for expressing[1] its phantasies. And this holds good even in those cases where we have to start from material which appears to be completely devoid of phantasy.

In conclusion I should like to sum up briefly what has been said

---

[1] If we do this we shall succeed in making speech—as far as the child is already able to speak—an instrument of its analysis. The reason why we have to do without verbal associations for long periods of their analysis is not only because small children cannot speak with ease but because the acute anxiety they suffer from only permits them to employ a less direct form of representation. Since the primary archaic mode of representation by means of toys and of action is an essential medium of expression for the child, we could certainly never carry out a deep analysis of a child by means of speech alone. Nevertheless, I believe that no analysis of a child, whatever its age, can be said to be really terminated unless the child has employed speech in analysis to its full capacity, for language constitutes the bridge to reality.

in this chapter. The more primitive nature of the child's mind makes it necessary to find an analytic technique especially adapted to the child, and this we find in play analysis. By means of play analysis we gain access to the child's most deeply repressed experiences and fixations and are thus able to exert a radical influence on its development. The difference between this method of analysis and that of adult analysis, however, is purely one of technique and not of principle. The analysis of the transference-situation and of the resistance, the removal of the early infantile amnesia and of the effects of repression, as well as the uncovering of the primal scene—all these things play analysis does. It can be seen that all criteria of the psycho-analytic method apply to this technique too. Play analysis leads to the same results as the adult technique, with only one difference, namely, that the technical procedure is adapted to the mind of the child.

Chapter II

THE TECHNIQUE OF EARLY ANALYSIS

In the first chapter of this book I have tried to show, on the one hand, what special psychological mechanisms we find operative in the small child, as distinct from the adult, and, on the other, what parallels exist between the two. These differences and similarities which necessitate a special technique have led me to develop my method of play analysis.

On a low table in my analytic room there are laid out a number of small and simple toys—little wooden men and women, carts, carriages, motor-cars, trains, animals, bricks and houses, as well as paper, scissors and pencils. Even a child that is usually inhibited in its play will at least glance at the toys or touch them, and will soon give me a first glimpse into its complexes by the way in which it begins to play with them or lays them aside, or by its general attitude towards them.

I shall demonstrate the principles of play technique by examples from the analysis of a small child. Peter, aged three years and nine months, was very difficult to manage. He was strongly fixated upon his mother and very ambivalent. He was unable to tolerate frustrations, was totally inhibited in play and gave the impression of being an extremely timid, plaintive and unboyish child. At times his behaviour would be aggressive and sneering, and he got on badly with other children, especially with his younger brother. His analysis was intended to be chiefly a prophylactic measure, since there had been several cases of severe neurosis in the family. But in the course of it it became obvious that he was suffering from such a serious neurosis himself and from such a degree of inhibition that he would almost certainly not have been able to meet the demands of school life and would, sooner or later, have broken down.[1]

---

[1] I may add that at the end of his analysis, which took up 278 sessions, his difficulties had disappeared and there was an extensive change for the better in his whole character and disposition. He had lost not only his morbid fears but his general timidity, and had become a happy and lively child. He had overcome his inhibition in play and had begun to get on well with other children, in particular with his little brother. His development since has been excellent. According to the latest accounts of him, six years after the end of his analysis, he was doing well at school, was full of interest in things, learned

16

At the very beginning of his first session Peter took the toy carriages and cars and put them first one behind the other and then side by side, and alternated this arrangement several times. In between he took two horse-drawn carriages and bumped one into another, so that the horses' feet knocked together, and said: 'I've got a new little brother called Fritz.' I asked him what the carriages were doing. He answered: 'That's not nice,' and stopped bumping them together at once, but started again quite soon. Then he knocked two toy horses together in the same way. Upon which I said: 'Look here, the horses are two people bumping together.' At first he said: 'No, that's not nice,' but then, 'Yes, that's two people bumping together,' and added: 'The horses have bumped together too, and now they're going to sleep.' Then he covered them up with bricks and said: 'Now they're quite dead; I've buried them.' In his second session he at once arranged the cars and carts in the same two ways as before—in a long file and side by side; and at the same time he once again knocked two carriages together, and then two engines— just as in the first session. He next put two swings side by side and, showing me the inner and longish part that hung down and swung, said: 'Look how it dangles and bumps.' I then proceeded to interpret. Pointing to the 'dangling' swings, the engines, the carriages and the horses, I said that in each case they were two people—Daddy and Mummy—bumping their 'thingummies'[1] (his word for genitals) together. He objected, saying: 'no, that isn't nice', but went on knocking the carts together, and said: '*That's* how they bumped their thingummies together.' Immediately afterwards he spoke about his little brother again. As we have seen, in his first session, too, his knocking together of the two carriages and horses had been followed by his remarking that he had got a new little brother. So I continued my interpretation and said: 'You thought to yourself that Daddy and Mummy bumped their thingummies together and that is how your little brother Fritz came.' He now took another small cart and made all three collide together. I interpreted: 'That's your own thingummy. You wanted to bump your thingummy along with Daddy's and Mummy's thingummies.' He thereupon added a fourth cart and said: 'That's Fritz.' He next took two of the

---

well, and was good at games. He was easy to manage and able to meet all the social requirements of his age. It is, moreover, worth noting that both during his analysis and in the few years afterwards he had to undergo unnaturally great strains on account of various upheavals in his family life.

[1] I always find out beforehand from the child's mother what special words the child uses for the genitals, excremental processes, etc., and adopt them in speaking to it. For purposes of clearness, however, I shall not reproduce these special words in my reports on further cases.

smaller carts and put each on to an engine. He pointed to a carriage and horse and said: 'That's Daddy'—placing another at its side—'That's Mummy.' He pointed once more to the Daddy carriage and horse and said: 'That's me,' and to the Mummy one and said: 'That's me, too,' thus demonstrating his identification with both parents in coitus. After this he repeatedly hit the two small carts together and told me how he and his little brother let two chickens into their bedroom so that they could calm down, but that they had knocked about and spat in there. 'He and Fritz', he added, 'were not rude gutter boys and did not spit.' When I told him that the chickens were his and Fritz's thingummies bumping into one another and spitting—that is, masturbating—he agreed with me after a little resistance.

I can only refer briefly here to the way in which the child's phantasies, as set forth in his play, became more and more free in response to continual interpretation; how the inhibition in play lessened and the scope of his play gradually widened; and how certain details in it were repeated over and over again until they were clarified by interpretation, and then gave place to fresh details. Just as associations to dream-elements lead to the uncovering of the latent content of the dream, so do the elements of children's play, which correspond to those associations, afford a view of its latent content. And play analysis, no less than adult analysis, by systematically treating the actual situation as a transference-situation and establishing its connection with the originally experienced or phantasied one, gives children the possibility of completely living out and working through that original situation in phantasy. In doing this, and in uncovering their infantile experiences and the original cause of their sexual development, the analysis resolves fixations and corrects errors of development.

The next extract I shall give from Peter's case is intended to show that the interpretations made in the first sessions were confirmed by later analysis. One day, a few weeks later, when one of the toy men happened to fall over, Peter flew into a rage. Immediately afterwards he asked me how a toy motor-car was made and 'why it could stand up'. He next showed me a tiny toy deer falling over, and then said he wanted to urinate.[1] In the lavatory he said to me: 'I'm

---

[1] In Chapter I I have given my reasons for the view that with children, no less than with adults, the analytic situation can only be established and maintained so long as a purely analytic attitude is maintained towards the patient. But in dealing with children certain modifications of this principle become necessary, without, however, in any way departing from its essentials. For instance, if a very small patient wants to go to the lavatory, and is still unused to doing so alone at home, it is my practice to go with him. But I do the least

doing number one—I *have* got a thingummy.' When he was back in the room again he took a toy man, whom he called a boy, who was sitting in a little house, which he called the lavatory, and stood him in such a way that a dog which he placed beside him 'shouldn't see him and bite him'. But he placed a toy woman so that she could see him, and said: '*Only* his Daddy mustn't see him.' Thus it was evident that he identified the dog, which was in general an object of great fear to him, with his father, and the defaecating boy with himself. After this he kept on playing with the motor-car whose construction he had already admired, and made it move along again and again. Suddenly he asked angrily: 'Whenever is it going to stop?' and added that some of the toy men he had put up must not ride in it, knocked them over, and set them up again with their backs to the car, next to which he once more put a whole row of cars and carriages, side by side this time. He then suddenly expressed a desire to pass stool, but contented himself with asking the defaecating toy man (boy) whether he had finished. He again turned to the motor-car, admired it and began to alternate incessantly between admiration and rage at its continual movement, the desire to pass stool and asking the 'boy' if he had done.

In the analytic session just described, Peter had been depicting the following things: the toy man, the deer, etc., which kept falling down, represented his own penis and its inferiority in comparison

---

possible for him and thus remove from such assistance the character of an act of love which the unconscious of the child desires, or at least reduce it to the bare minimum; and thereby demonstrate, as on all other occasions, the attitude of friendly reserve which seems as necessary for the establishment and maintenance of the analytic situation in child analysis as it is in the analysis of adults. It is also essential to subject to analytic interpretation the satisfaction afforded to the patient by the analysis itself and the deeper motives that underlie his desire for such a satisfaction, and to connect them with the associations or play which immediately precede or follow them. In the case of Peter, for instance, after having made water and said: 'I'm doing number one—I *have* got a thingummy' he went on to play the game with the boy on the lavatory seat. The details of the game which followed his remarks, namely that the father-substitute (the dog) was *not* to see the boy in the lavatory, but the woman *was* to see him, revealed the reasons for Peter's desire to urinate immediately before and his wish that I should be present while he did it. In the same way I always analyse very thoroughly the reasons why a child assigns this or that role to me in its games of make-believe, or requires this or that bit of help for itself or its dolls or animals. How far we can establish the analytic situation in treating children can be seen, for instance, from the fact that it is the exception for even the youngest ones to carry out exhibitionist actions in reality, and that even during periods of the strongest positive transference it very seldom happens that a child will climb on to my lap or kiss and hug me. Incontinence is also a rare event in the analytic hour, even with very small children.

THE PSYCHO-ANALYSIS OF CHILDREN

to his father's erect member. His going to pass water immediately after was done to prove the contrary to himself and to me. The motor-car which would not stop moving and which aroused both his admiration and anger was his father's penis that was performing coitus all the time. After feeling admiration for it he became enraged and wanted to defaecate. This was a repetition of his passing stool at the time when he had witnessed the primal scene. He had done this so as to disturb his parents while they were copulating and, in phantasy, to harm them with his excrements. In addition, the lump of stool appeared to the boy as a substitute for his inferior penis.

We must now try to link this material with Peter's first analytic session. In putting the motor-cars end to end during his very first session, he was making reference to his father's powerful penis; in putting them side by side he was symbolising the frequent repetition of coitus—that is, his father's potency—and he did this again later by means of the car that kept on moving. The rage he had felt at witnessing his parents' coitus was already expressed in his first session by his wanting the two horses who were going to sleep to be 'dead and buried', and in the effect which accompanied that wish. That these pictures of the primal scene with which he began his analysis were related to actual repressed experiences of his infancy, was proved by his parents' own account to me. According to this, the child had only shared their bedroom during one period, when he was eighteen months old and they were away on their summer holidays. During that period he had become especially hard to manage, slept badly and began to be dirty again, although he had become almost clean in his habits several months before. It appeared that though the railings of his cot did not prevent him from seeing his parents have sexual intercourse, they made it more difficult, and this was symbolized by the toy men who were knocked over and then placed with their backs to the row of vehicles. The falling over of the toys also represented his own feelings of impotence. Up to that period the patient used to play with his toys exceedingly well, but after it he could do nothing with them except break them. As early as in his first analytic session he demonstrated the connection between the destruction of his toys and his observations of coitus. Once, when he had put the motor-cars, which symbolized his father's penis, in a row side by side and had made them run along, he lost his temper and threw them all about the room, saying: 'We always smash our Christmas presents straight away; we don't want any.' Smashing his toys thus stood in his unconscious for smashing his father's genitals. This pleasure in destruction and inhibition in play, which he brought into his analysis, were gradually overcome

20

and disappeared together with his other difficulties during the course of it.

In uncovering bit by bit the primal scene I was able to gain access to Peter's very strong passive homosexual attitude. After having depicted his parents' coitus he had phantasies of coitus between three people. They aroused severe anxiety in him and were followed by other phantasies in which he was being copulated with by his father; in terms of his play in which the toy dog or motor-car or engine—all signifying his father—climbed on to a cart or a man, which stood for himself. In this process the cart would be damaged or the man would have something bitten off; and then Peter would show much fear of, or great aggressiveness towards, the toy which represented his father.

I shall now discuss some of the more important aspects of my technique in the light of the above extracts from an actual analysis. As soon as the small patient has given me some sort of insight into his complexes—whether through his play or his drawings or phantasies, or merely by his general behaviour—interpretations can and should begin. This does not contradict the well-tried rule that the analyst should wait till the transference is established before he begins interpreting, because with children the transference takes place immediately, and the analyst will often be given evidence straight away of its positive nature. But should the child show shyness, anxiety or even only lack of trust, such behaviour is to be taken as a sign of a negative transference, and this makes it still more imperative that interpretation should begin as soon as possible. For interpretation reduces the patient's negative transference by tracing the negative affects involved back to their original objects and situations. For instance, when Rita,[1] who was a very ambivalent child, felt a resistance she at once wanted to leave the room, and I had to make an interpretation immediately so as to resolve this resistance. As soon as I had clarified for her the cause of her resistance—always carrying it back to its original object and situation—it was resolved, and she would become friendly and trustful again and continue playing, supplying in its various details a confirmation of the interpretation I had just given.

In another instance I was able to see with impressive clearness the necessity of immediate interpretation. This was in the case of Trude, who, it will be remembered, came to me for a single session when she was three years and nine months old,[2] and then had to have her treatment postponed owing to external circumstances. This child was very neurotic and unusually strongly fixated upon her mother. She came into my room unwillingly and full of anxiety, and I was

[1] See Chapter I.   [2] *ibid.*

21

obliged to analyse her in a low voice with the door open. But soon she had given me an idea of the nature of her complexes. She insisted upon the flowers in a vase being removed; she threw a little toy man out of a cart into which she had previously put him and heaped abuse on him; she wanted a certain man with a high hat that figured in a picture-book she had brought with her to be taken out of it; and she declared that the cushions in the room had been thrown into disorder by a dog. My immediate interpretation of these utterances in the sense that she desired to do away with her father's penis,[1] because it was playing havoc with her mother, (as represented by the vase, the cart, the picture-book and the cushion) at once diminished her anxiety and she left me in a much more trustful mood than she had come, and said at home that she would like to come to me again. When, six months later, I was able to resume this little girl's analysis again, it appeared that she had remembered details of her single hour of analysis and that my interpretations had effected a certain amount of positive transference, or rather, some lessening of the negative transference in her.

Another fundamental principle of play technique is that the interpretation—so far as depth is concerned—must be adequate to reach the mental layer which is being activated. For instance, in his second session, Peter, after letting the cars roll along, laid a toy man on a bench, which he called a bed, and then threw him down and said that he was dead and done for. He next did the same thing with two little men, choosing for the purpose two toys that were already damaged. At that time, in conformity with the current material, I interpreted that the first toy man was his father, whom he wanted to throw out of his mother's bed and kill, and that the second man was himself to whom his father would do the same.[2] In connection with the clarification of the primal scene which had now been completed in all details Peter returned in various forms to the theme of the two broken men. It now appeared that this theme was determined by the fear, which also followed from the primal scene, of the mother as a castrating figure. In his phantasy she had taken his father's penis

[1] Trude's uncommonly strong castration complex played a very conspicuous part and dominated the picture for some time in her analysis. From beneath that complex, analysis brought to light a further anxiety which proved a more fundamental one — that of being attacked by her mother, robbed of the contents of her body and her children and severely injured internally. (See Chapter I.)

[2] I may mention that this interpretation — like all interpretations of death-wishes in the analyses of children — aroused very violent resistances in Peter. But he brought a confirmation of it in his next session when he suddenly asked: 'And if *I* were a Daddy and someone wanted to throw me down behind the bed and make me dead and done for, what would *I* think of it?'

inside herself and had not given it back to him; and she thus became an object of anxiety for the boy, because she now carried his father's terrifying penis (= his father) inside herself.[1]

Here is another example taken from the same case. In Peter's second session my interpretation of the material he had brought had been that he and his brother practised mutual masturbation. Seven months later, when he was four years and four months old, he brought forward a long dream, rich in associative material, from which the following is an extract. 'Two pigs were in a pig-sty and in my bed. They ate together in the pig-sty. There were also two boys in my bed in a boat; but they were quite big, like Uncle G— (a grown-up brother of his mother's) and E— (an older girl friend whom he thought almost grown-up).' Most of the associations I got from this dream were verbal ones. They showed that the pigs represented himself and his brother and that their eating meant mutual *fellatio*. But they also stood for his parents copulating together. It turned out that his sexual relations with his brother were based on an identification with his father and mother, in which Peter took the role of each in turn. After I had interpreted this material Peter started his next session by playing round the wash-basin. He put two pencils on a sponge and said: 'This is the boat that Fritz (his younger brother) and I got in.' He then put on a deep voice—as he often did when his super-ego came into action—and shouted at the two pencils: 'You're not to go about together all the time and do piggish things.' This scolding on the part of his super-ego at his brother and himself was also aimed at his parents (as represented by his Uncle G— and his grown-up friend E—)[2] and set free in him affects of the same kind as he had felt towards them when he had witnessed the primal scene. These were the affects which, among other things, he had already given vent to as early as in his second session, when he wanted the horses that had bumped together to be dead and buried. And yet, after seven months, the analysis of that material had not been completed. It is clear then, that my deep-going interpretations, given so early in the analysis, had in no way hindered the elucidation of the connections between the experience and the child's whole sexual development (and in particular of the way in which it determined the course of his relations with his brother), nor prevented a working through of the material involved.

[1] See Chapter VIII.
[2] He had selected two long pencils out of a collection of all sizes, thus once more expressing the fact, already elicited by his associations on the day before, that the two culprits—the pigs—were not only himself and his brother but his parents too, and that in his mutual masturbation he was identifying himself and his brother with them.

I have brought forward the above examples in order to support my view, based on empiric observation, that the analyst should not shy away from making a deep interpretation even at the start of the analysis, since the material belonging to a deeper layer of the mind will come back again later and be worked through. As I have said before, the function of deep-going interpretation is simply to open the door to the unconscious, to diminish the anxiety that has been stirred up and thus to prepare the way for analytic work.

I have repeatedly laid emphasis upon the child's capacity for making a spontaneous transference. This is to some extent due to the much more acute anxiety which the small child feels in comparison with the adult and to its greater readiness to react with anxiety. One of the greatest, if not *the* greatest psychological task which the child has to achieve, and which takes up the larger part of its mental energy, is the mastering of anxiety. In its unconscious, therefore, it primarily evaluates its objects with reference to whether they allay or arouse anxiety, and accordingly the child will turn towards them with a positive or a negative transference. Small children whose readiness for anxiety is great, often express their negative transference at once as undisguised fear, whereas in older ones, especially those in the latency period, the negative transference more often takes the form of distrustful reserve or simply dislike. In its struggle against its fear of the objects that are closest to it, the child is inclined to attach that fear to more distant objects (since displacement is one way of dealing with anxiety) and to see in them an embodiment of its 'bad' mother or 'bad' father. For this reason the strongly neurotic child who feels threatened most of the time, and who therefore is always on the look-out for its 'bad' mother or father will react to every stranger with anxiety.

We must never lose sight of the small children's readiness for anxiety and this appears also, to some degree, in older children. Even if they begin their analysis by exhibiting a positive attitude, we must be prepared to come upon a negative transference very soon, namely as soon as the analysis touches on any material accentuated by complexes. Immediately the analyst detects signs of that negative transference he should ensure the continuance of analytic work and establish the analytic situation by relating it to himself, at the same time tracing it back, with the help of interpretation, to its original objects and situations, and in this way resolve a certain amount of anxiety. His interpretation should intervene at some point of urgency in the unconscious material and so open a way to the child's unconscious mind. Where that point is will be shown by the multiplicity and frequent repetition, often in varied forms, of representations of the same 'play thought' (in Peter's case, for instance, we had in his first analytical session the arrangement of vehicles alternating between one behind or at the side of another, and the continual knocking together of the toy horses, carriages, engines, etc.) and also by the intensity with which these games are played, for this is a measure of the affect belonging to their content. If the analyst overlooks the urgency which is expressed in this way in the material, the child will usually break off its game and exhibit strong resistance or even open anxiety and not infrequently show a desire to run away. Thus by making a timely interpretation—that is to say as soon as the material permits—the analyst can cut short the child's anxiety, or rather regulate it. This applies also to those cases where the analysis has started with a positive transference. I have already given my reasons in detail why it is absolutely necessary to give interpretations as soon as anxiety and resistances become manifest or in those cases where analysis starts with a negative transference.

It follows from what has been said that not only a timely inter-pretation but a deep-going one is essential. If we are impressed by the urgency of the material presented, we have to trace not only the representational content but also the anxiety and sense of guilt associated with it right down to that layer of the mind which is being activated. But if we take the principles of adult analysis as a model and proceed first of all to get into contact with the superficial strata of the mind—those which are nearest to the ego and to reality—we shall fail with children in our object of establishing the analytical situation and reducing their anxiety. Repeated experience has convinced me of this. The same is true of the mere translation of symbols, of interpretations which only deal with the *symbolic* re-presentation of the material and do not concern themselves with the anxiety and sense of guilt that are associated with it. An interpre-tation which does not descend to those depths which are being activated by the material and the anxiety concerned, which does not, that is, touch the place where the strongest latent resistance is and endeavour in the first place to reduce anxiety where it is most violent and most in evidence, will have no effect whatever on the child, or will only serve to arouse stronger resistances in it without being able to resolve them again. But, as I have just tried to make clear in my extracts from Peter's analysis, these interpretations [just mentioned] by no means completely resolve the anxiety in the deeper layers of the mind, nor will the interpretations, which so soon penetrate to the deeper layers, in any way restrict the analytic work in the upper layers—that is to say, the analysis of the child's ego and its relation to reality. The establishment of the child's relations to reality as well as the stronger emergence of its ego take place in the analysis of children only step by step in connection with progress in

25

THE PSYCHO-ANALYSIS OF CHILDREN

ego development. They are a result, not a precondition, of the analytic work.

So far, we have been concerned in the main with discussing and illustrating the typical initiation and course of an early analysis. I should now like to consider certain unusual difficulties which I have met with and which have obliged me to adopt special technical methods. The case of Trude,[1] who was so apprehensive at her very first entering my flat, had already taught me that in such patients prompt interpretation was the only means of lessening anxiety and setting the analysis in motion. My little patient Ruth, aged four years and three months, was one of those children whose ambivalence shows itself in an over-strong fixation upon the mother and certain other women, while they dislike others, usually strangers. Already at a very early age, for instance, she had not been able to get used to a new nurse-maid; nor could she make friends at all easily with other children. She not only suffered from a great deal of undisguised anxiety which often led to anxiety-attacks and from various other neurotic symptoms, but also from apprehensiveness in general. In her first analytic session she absolutely refused to remain in the room with me alone. I therefore decided to ask her elder sister to be present during the analysis.[2] My intention was to establish a positive transference to achieve the eventual possibility of working alone with her; but all my attempts, such as simply playing with her, encouraging her to talk, etc., were in vain. In playing with her toys she would turn only to her sister (although the latter remained quite unresponsive) and would ignore me completely. The sister herself told me that my efforts were hopeless and that I had no chance of gaining the child's confidence even if I were to spend weeks on end with her instead of single hours. I therefore found myself forced to take other measures—measures which once more gave striking proof of the efficacy of interpretation in reducing the patient's anxiety and negative transference. One day while Ruth was once again devoting her attention exclusively to her sister, she drew a picture of a tumbler with some small round balls inside and a kind of lid on top. I asked her what the lid was for, but she would not answer me. On her sister repeating the question, she said it was 'to prevent the balls from rolling out'. Before this, she had gone through her sister's bag and

[1] See Chapter I.
[2] Actually her stepsister. She was about twenty years Ruth's senior, and a very intelligent girl who had herself been analysed. I have had another case in which I was obliged to reconcile myself to having a third person present. In both cases the arrangement was carried out under exceptionally favourable circumstances; but I may say that, for a number of reasons, I should never recommend such a procedure except in the last resort.

26

then shut it tightly 'so that nothing should fall out of it'. She had done the same with the purse inside the bag so as to keep the coins safely shut up. Furthermore, the material she was now bringing had been quite clear to me even in her previous sessions.[1] I now made a venture and told Ruth that the balls in the tumbler, the coins in the purse and the contents of the bag all meant children in her Mummy's inside, and that she wanted to keep them safely shut up so as not to have any more brothers and sisters. The effect of my interpretation was astonishing. For the first time Ruth turned her attention to me and began to play in a different, less constrained, way.[2]

Nevertheless, it was still not possible for her to be alone with me, as she reacted to that situation with anxiety-attacks. Since I saw the analysis was steadily diminishing her negative transference in favour of a positive one, I decided to go on having her sister in the room. After three weeks the latter suddenly fell ill and I found myself faced with the alternative of stopping the analysis or risking an anxiety-attack. With her parents' consent I took the second course. The nurse handed the little girl over to me outside my room and went away in spite of her tears and screams. In this very painful situation I again began by trying to soothe the child in a non-analytical, motherly way, as any ordinary person would. I tried to comfort her and cheer her up and make her play with me, but in vain. When she saw herself alone with me, she just managed to follow me into my room, but once there I could do nothing with her. She went quite white, and screamed, and showed all the signs of a severe attack of anxiety. Meanwhile I sat down at the toy-table and began to play by myself,[3] all the while describing what I was doing to the terrified child, who was now sitting in a corner. Following a sudden inspiration, I took as the subject of my game the material which she herself had produced in the previous session. At the end of it she had played round the wash-basin and had fed her dolls and given them

[1] In this analysis the child's desire to rob her mother's body, and her consequent feelings of anxiety and guilt, dominated the picture from the very beginning. The outbreak of her neurosis, moreover, had followed upon her mother's pregnancy and the birth of her younger sister.

[2] As has already been said, interpretation has the effect of changing the character of the child's play and enabling the representation of its material to become clearer.

[3] In especially difficult cases I use this technical device to get the analysis started. I have found that when children show their latent anxiety by being entirely inaccessible it often helps if I throw out a stimulus-word, as it were, by beginning to play myself. I apply this method within the narrowest possible limits. For instance, I may build some seats out of bricks and set some little figures near them. One child will call them a school and continue the game upon that basis; another will look upon them as a theatre and make the figures act accordingly, and so on.

27

huge jugfuls of milk, etc. I now did the same kind of thing. I put a doll to sleep and told Ruth I was going to give it something to eat and asked her what it should be. She interrupted her screams to answer 'milk', and I noticed that she made a movement towards her mouth with her two fingers (which she had a habit of sucking before going to sleep) but quickly took them away. I asked her whether she wanted to suck them and she said: 'Yes, but properly.' I recognized that she wanted to reconstitute the situation as it happened at home every evening, so I laid her down on the sofa and, at her request, put a rug over her. Thereupon she began to suck her fingers. She was still very pale and her eyes were shut, but she was visibly calmer and had stopped crying. Meanwhile I went on playing with the dolls, repeating her game of the session before. As I was putting a wet sponge beside one of them, as she had done, she burst out crying again and screamed, 'No, she mustn't have the *big* sponge, that's not for children, that's for grown-ups!' I may remark that in her two pre-vious sessions she had brought up a lot of material concerning her envy of her mother. I now interpreted this material in connection with her protest against the big sponge which represented her father's penis. I showed her in every detail how she envied and hated her mother because the latter had incorporated her father's penis during coitus, and how she wanted to steal his penis and the children out of her mother's inside and kill her mother. I explained to her that this was why she was frightened and believed that she had killed her mother or would be deserted by her. I gave these interpretations in this instance in the following way. All the while I began by applying my interpretations to the doll—showing her as I played with it that it was afraid and screaming, and telling her the reason—and then I proceeded to repeat the interpretations which I had given for the doll by applying them to her own person. In this way I established the analytical situation in its entirety. While I was doing this Ruth grew visibly quieter, opened her eyes and let me bring the table on which I was playing to the sofa and continue my game and my interpretations close beside her. Gradually she sat up and watched the course of the play with growing interest, and even began to take an active part in it herself. When the session was over and the nurse came to fetch the child away, she was surprised to find her happy and cheerful and to see her say goodbye to me in a friendly and even affectionate way. At the beginning of her next session, when her nurse left her, she again showed some anxiety, it is true, but she did not have a regular anxiety-attack nor burst into tears. On the other hand she immediately took refuge on the sofa and spontaneously took up the same position as she had done the day before, shutting her eyes and sucking her fingers. I was able to sit down beside her and continue my game of the previous hour straight away. The whole sequence of events of the day before was recapitulated, but in a shortened and mitigated form. And after a few sessions we had progressed so far that we experienced only faint traces of an anxiety-attack at the beginning of the session.

Analysis of Ruth's anxiety-attacks brought out the fact that they were a repetition of *pavor nocturnus*,[1] from which she had suffered very severely at the age of two. At that time her mother had been pregnant, and the little girl's wish to steal the new baby out of her mother's body and to hurt and kill her by various means had brought on a strong reaction against these wishes which manifested itself as a sense of guilt in the child, in consequence of which she had become unusually strongly fixated upon her mother. Saying good-night before she went to sleep meant saying goodbye for ever.[2] For, as a result of her desires to rob and kill her mother, she was afraid of being abandoned by her for ever or of never seeing her alive again, or of finding, in the place of the kind and tender mother who was saying good-night to her, a 'bad' mother who would attack her in the night. These were the reasons, too, why she could not bear to be left by herself. Being left alone with me meant being abandoned by her 'good' mother; and her whole terror of the 'bad' punishing mother was now transferred to me. By analysing this situation and bringing it to light I succeeded, as we have seen, in dispelling her anxiety-attacks and in making it possible for normal analytic work to begin.[3]

The technique which I employed in analysing Ruth's anxiety-attacks proved very effective in another case. During Trude's analysis her mother fell ill and had to be taken to hospital. This occurred just when the little girl's sadistic phantasies of attack upon

[1] See Chapter I.
[2] In her paper, 'The Genesis of Agoraphobia' (1928), Helene Deutsch points out that fear of the mother's death, based upon various hostile wishes against her, is one of the commonest forms of infantile neurosis and is closely connected with a fear of being separated from her and with home-sickness.
[3] Ruth's treatment remained unfinished, for her family had to return to their home abroad. Her neurosis, in consequence, was not completely removed. But in the 190 sessions she had I was able to effect the following improvements which, since I last heard of her two years after the termination of her analysis, have been maintained: her anxiety was greatly lessened, and also, more particularly, the various forms of timidity from which she suffered. As a result of this she got on better with other children and with adults and was able to adapt herself entirely to the requirements of her home and school life. Her fixation upon her mother was diminished and her attitude to her father improved. There was also a very decided change for the better in her relations to her brother and sisters. Her whole development, especially in respect of educability, social adaptation and capacity for sublimation, has since been a favourable one

her mother dominated the picture. I have already described in what detail this child of three years and nine months demonstrated these scenes of aggression before me, and how, overcome by the anxiety which followed upon them, she used to hide herself with the cushions behind the couch. But this never led to an actual anxiety-attack. When she came back after the interval caused by her mother's illness, however, she did have definite anxiety-attacks for several days in succession. The attacks only brought out her reaction to her aggressive impulses, i.e., the fear that she felt on account of them. During these attacks Trude, like Ruth, would assume a particular position—the position she used to get into at night when she began to have anxiety. She would creep into a corner, clasping closely to her the cushions which she often called her children, and would suck her fingers and wet herself. Here again interpretation of her anxiety led to the cessation of her anxiety-attacks.[1]

My own subsequent experiences, as well as those of Miss M. N. Searl and other child analysts, have borne out the effectiveness of these technical measures in other cases also. In the years of work which have elapsed since the treatment of these two cases, it has become quite clear to me that the essential prerequisite for conducting an early analysis—and, indeed, a deep-going analysis of older children—is certainty in grasping the material presented. A correct and rapid estimation of the significance of the material as it is presented at the time, both as regards the light it throws on the structure of the case and its relation to the patient's affective state at the moment, and above all a quick perception of the latent anxiety and sense of guilt it contains—these are the primary conditions for giving a right interpretation, i.e. an interpretation which will come at the right time and will penetrate to that level of the mind which is being activated by anxiety. The occurrence of anxiety-attacks in analysis can be reduced to a minimum if this technique is consistently adhered to. Should anxiety-attacks occur at the beginning of treatment, however—as may happen with neurotic children who are

[1] Trude's neurosis showed itself in severe night-terrors, in anxiety during the daytime when she was left alone, in bed-wetting, general timidity, an over-strong fixation on her mother and dislike of her father, great jealousy of her sisters and in various difficulties in her upbringing. Her analysis, which comprised eighty-two hours in seven months, resulted in a cessation of bed-wetting, and a great diminution of anxiety and timidity in various respects, and in a very favourable change in her relations to her parents and to her brothers and sisters. She had also suffered from colds which proved in analysis to be determined psychogenically to a great extent, and these, too, decreased in frequency and strength. In spite of this improvement her neurosis was not yet fully resolved when, for external reasons, her analysis had to come to an end.

subject to such attacks in ordinary life—a firm handling of this technique will usually succeed in quickly reducing them to such proportions that it becomes possible to conduct a normal analysis. The results obtained from analysing anxiety-attacks are also, I think, evidence of the general validity of some of the principles underlying play technique. I would refer to Trude's case in which, to begin with, I analysed the same kind of material without anxiety-attacks occurring, although intense anxiety was evidently connected with it. Owing to continuous and deep-going interpretations I succeeded in reducing the anxiety step by step and was able to let it come out in small doses. During the interruption of the analysis, on account of her mother's illness and absence from home, the anxiety increased to such an extent that it led to anxiety-attacks. After a few sessions these attacks once more ceased completely and gave way to a renewed appearance of 'dosed' [regulated] anxiety.

I should like to add a few remarks of a theoretical nature in connection with these anxiety-attacks. I have spoken of them as a repetition of *pavor nocturnus*; and I have referred to the position taken up by the patient during such attacks, or rather in the attempt to master them, and pointed out that it was a repetition of the child's anxiety-situation in bed at night. But I have also mentioned a specific early anxiety-situation which seemed to underlie both *pavor nocturnus* and anxiety-attacks. My observation of the cases of Trude, Ruth and Rita, together with the knowledge I have gained in the last few years, have led me to recognize the existence of an anxiety, or rather anxiety-situation, which is specific for girls and the equivalent of the castration anxiety felt by boys. This anxiety-situation culminates in the girl's idea that her mother will destroy her body, abolish its contents and take the children out of it, and so on. I shall return to this subject more fully in the second part of this volume. I should merely like to draw the reader's attention here to certain points of agreement between the material I have been able to collect from my early analyses and one or two statements that Freud has made in his book *Inhibitions, Symptoms and Anxiety* (1926). In it he states that the counterpart in the small girl of the boy's castration fear is her fear of loss of love. The fear of being lonely, of being abandoned by her mother, is shown very clearly in the material of the analyses of small girls I have quoted. But that fear, I think, has a deeper origin. It is based upon the child's impulses of aggression against her mother and her desires, springing from the early stages of her Oedipus conflict, to kill her and steal from her. These impulses lead not only to anxiety or to a fear of being attacked by her mother, but to a fear that her mother will abandon her or die.

Let us now return to a consideration of technical questions. The

31

form in which an interpretation is given is also of great importance. As I tried to show in examples I endeavour to put the contents of the unconscious phantasies as clearly and distinctly as possible.[1] In doing so I take the way in which the children think and speak using their own images as my model.[2] Peter, it will be remembered, pointed to the swing and said: 'Look how it dangles and bumps.' And so when I answered: 'That's how Daddy's and Mummy's thing-ummies bumped together,' he took it in at once. To take another instance: Rita (aged two years and nine months) told me that the dolls had disturbed her in her sleep: they kept on saying to Hans, the underground train man (a male doll on wheels): 'Just go on driving your train up and down.' On another occasion she put a triangular brick on one side and said: 'That's a little woman'; she then took a 'little hammer', as she called another long-shaped brick, and hit the brick-box with it exactly in a place where it was only stuck together with paper, so that she made a hole in it. She said: 'When the hammer hit hard, the little woman was *so* frightened.' The male doll, running the underground train and hitting with the hammer, stood for coitus between her parents, which she had witnessed till she was nearly two years old. My interpretation, 'Your Daddy hit hard like that inside your Mummy with his little hammer, and you were so frightened', fitted in exactly with her way of thinking and speaking.

In describing my methods of analysis I have often spoken of the small toys which are put at the children's disposal. I should like to explain briefly why these toys afford such valuable assistance in the technique of play analysis. Their smallness, their number and their great variety give the child a very wide range of representational

[1] In his 'Fragment of an Analysis of a Case of Hysteria' (1905) (*S.E.* **9,** p. 48) Freud says: 'It is possible for a man to talk to girls and women upon sexual matters of every kind without doing them harm and without bringing suspicion upon himself, so long as, in the first place, he adopts a particular way of doing it, and, in the second place, can make them feel convinced that it is unavoidable . . . The best way of speaking about such things is to be dry and direct; and that is at the same time the method furthest removed from the prurience with which the same subjects are handled in "society" . . . J'appelle un chat un chat.' This attitude is, *mutatis mutandis*, the one I adopt in analysing children. I talk of sexual matters in the simple words best suited to their way of thought.

[2] It must further be remembered that children are still for the most part under the sway of the unconscious, whose language, as dreams and play show, is presentational and pictorial. As we have occasion to see over and over again, children have a quite different attitude from adults to words. They assess them above all according to their pictorial qualities—to the phantasies they evoke. If we want to gain access to the child's unconscious in analysis (which, of course, we have to do via the ego and through speech), we shall only succeed if we avoid circumlocution and use plain words.

play, while their very simplicity enables them to be put to the most varied uses. Thus toys like these are well suited for the expression of phantasies and experiences in all kinds of ways and in great detail. The child's various 'play thoughts', and the affects associated with them (which can partly be guessed at from the subject-matter of its games, and which are partly plainly expressed), are presented side by side and within a small space, so that we get a good survey of the general connections and dynamics of the mental processes that are being put before us, and also, since spatial contiguity often stands for temporal contiguity, of the time-order of the child's varous phantasies and experiences.

It may be thought from what has been said that all we have to do in order to analyse a child is to put toys in front of it, and that it will then immediately begin to play with them in an uninhibited and easy fashion. That is not at all what happens. Inhibition in play is, as I have repeatedly pointed out, very frequently met with to a greater or lesser degree in children and is an extremely common neurotic symptom. But it is precisely in such cases, where all other attempts to get into contact with the patient fail, that toys are so very useful as a means of starting analysis. It rarely happens that a child, however inhibited in its play, will not at least look at the toys or pick up one or other of them and do something with it. Even though it will soon stop playing—as Trude did—yet we shall have got some idea of its unconscious on which to base our analytic work from having noticed what sort of game it has started, at what point its resistance has set in, how it has behaved in connection with that resistance, what chance remark it may have dropped at the time, and so on. The reader has already seen how it is possible for analysis, with the help of interpretation, to make the child's play more and more free and its representational content increasingly rich and revealing, and gradually to effect a reduction of its inhibition in play.

Toys are not the only requisites for a play analysis. There has to be a quantity of illustrative material in the room. The most important of these is a wash-basin with running water. This is usually not much used until a fairly late stage in the analysis, but it then becomes of great importance. I have gone through a whole phase of analysis with a child playing round the wash-basin (where are also provided a sponge, a glass tumbler, one or two small vessels, some spoons and paper). These games with water afford us a deep insight into the fundamental pre-genital[1] impulses of the child, and are also a means of illustrating its sexual theories, giving us a knowledge of the relation between its sadistic phantasies and its reaction-forma-

[1] Cf. the case of Ruth. It was in playing at the wash-basin that she brought out most fully her unsatisfied oral desires.

tions[1] and showing the direct connection between its pre-genital and genital impulses.

In many analyses drawing or cutting out play a large part. In others—especially with girls—the child's time is mostly spent in making clothes and finery for itself, its dolls or its toy animals, or in decking itself with ribbons and other ornaments. Each child has within easy reach paper, coloured pencils, knives, scissors, needles and thread and bits of wood and string. Very frequently children bring their own toys with them. Nor does the mere enumeration of the actual articles at hand exhaust the possibilities. We gain a great deal of light from the various uses to which the child will put each one of them, or the way in which it will change from one game to another. All the ordinary furniture of the room as well, such as chairs, cushions, etc., are pressed into the service of its activities. In fact, the furniture of the child analyst's room has to be specially selected for this purpose. The phantasies and imaginative games which develop out of ordinary play with toys are of great significance. In its games of make-believe the child acts out in its own person what in another, usually an earlier, stage of its analysis it shows by means of its toys. In these games the analyst is usually assigned one or more roles, and my practice is to get the child itself to describe those roles to me in as great detail as possible.

Some children show a preference for games of make-believe, others for the more indirect form of representation by means of playthings. Typical games of pretence are playing at mother and child, at being at school, building or furnishing a house (with the help of chairs, pieces of furniture, cushions, etc.), going abroad, travelling in the train, going to the theatre, being a doctor, working in an office, keeping shop, etc. The value of such games of pretence from an analytic point of view lies in their direct method of represen- tation, and consequently in the greater wealth of verbal associations they furnish. For, as has already been said in the first chapters one of the necessary conditions of a successfully terminated treatment is that the child, however young, should make use of language in analysis to the full extent of its capacity.

No mere description, I feel, can do justice to the colour, life and complexity which fill the hours of play analysis, but I hope I have said enough to give the reader some idea of the accuracy and reliability of the results which we are able to attain by this means.

---

[1] These games with water have a very interesting counterpart in playing with fire. Very often a child will first play with water and then go and burn paper and matches in the fire, or vice versa. The connection between wetting and burning comes out clearly in such behaviour, as well as the great im- portance of urethral sadism. (See Chapter VIII.)

Chapter III

AN OBSESSIONAL NEUROSIS IN A SIX-YEAR-OLD GIRL[1]

In the last chapter I have dealt with the underlying principles of the technique of early analysis. In the present one, I shall compare that technique with the technique of analysis in the latency period, using a case-history as an illustration. This case-history will also give me an opportunity of discussing some theoretical questions concerning principles and also of describing the technique used in the analysis of obsessional neurosis in children—a technique which, I had to work out in the course of treating this unusually difficult and interesting case.

Erna, a child of six, had a number of severe symptoms. She suffered from sleeplessness, which was caused partly by anxiety (in particular by a fear of robbers and burglars) and partly by a series of obsessional activities. These consisted in lying on her face and banging her head on the pillow, in making a rocking movement, during which she sat or lay on her back, in obsessional thumb-sucking and in excessive and compulsive masturbation. All these obsessional activities which prevented her from sleeping at night, were carried on in the day-time as well. This was especially the case with masturbation which she practised even in the presence of strangers, and, for instance, almost continuously at her kindergarten. She suffered from severe depressions, which she would describe by saying 'There's something about life I don't like.' In her relations to her mother she was over-affectionate, but would at times veer round to a hostile attitude. She completely dominated her mother, left her no freedom of movement and plagued her continually with her love and hatred. As her mother put it: 'She swallows me up.' The child might, too, be fairly described as ineducable. Obsessive brooding and a curiously un-childlike nature were visible in the suffering look upon the little girl's face. Besides this she made a strange and sexually precocious impression. A symptom which first became obvious during the analysis was that she had a very severe inhibition in learning. She was

---

[1] This chapter is based on a paper which I read at Würzburg in October 1924, at the First Conference of German Psycho-Analysts.

sent to school a few months after her analysis began, and it was soon evident that she was quite incapable of learning, nor could she adapt herself to her school-fellows. The fact that she herself felt that she was ill—at the very beginning of her treatment she begged me to help her—was of great assistance to me in analysing her.

Erna began her play by taking a small carriage which stood on the little table among the other toys and letting it run towards me. She declared that she had come to fetch me. But she put a toy woman in the carriage instead and added a toy man. The two loved and kissed one another and drove up and down all the time. Next a toy man in another carriage collided with them, ran over them and killed them, and then roasted and ate them up. Another time the fight had a different ending and the attacking toy man was thrown down; but the woman helped him and comforted him. She got a divorce from her first husband and married the new one. This third person was given the most various parts to play in Erna's games. For instance, the original man and his wife were in a house which they were defending against a burglar; the third person was the burglar, and slipped in. The house burnt down, the man and woman burst and the third person was the only one left. Then again the third person was a brother who came on a visit; but while embracing the woman he bit her nose off. This little man, the third person, was Erna herself. In a series of similar games she represented her wish to oust her father from his position with her mother. On the other hand, in many other games she showed her direct Oedipus wish to get rid of her mother and to win her father. Thus she made a toy teacher give the children violin lessons by knocking his head[1] against the violin, or stand on his head as he was reading out of a book. She then made him throw down book or violin as the case might be and dance with his girl pupil. The two next kissed and embraced each other. At this point Erna asked me all at once if I would allow a marriage between teacher and pupil. Another time a teacher and a mistress—represented by a toy man and woman— were giving the children lessons in manners, teaching them how to bow and curtsey, etc. At first the children were obedient and polite (just as Erna herself always did her best to be good and behave nicely), then suddenly they attacked the teacher and mistress, trampled them underfoot and killed and roasted them. They had

---

[1] Here is another game which shows clearly that to Erna's unconscious the head had the meaning of a penis: a toy man wanted to get into a car and stuck his head into the window, whereupon the car said to him, 'Better come right inside!' The car stood for her mother inviting her father to have coitus with her. (Compare also her obsessional symptom of banging her head on the pillow.)

now become devils, and gloated over the torments of their victims. But all at once the teacher and mistress were in heaven and the former devils had turned into angels, who, according to Erna's account, knew nothing about ever having been devils—indeed 'they never *were* devils'. God the Father, the former teacher, began kissing and embracing the woman passionately, the angels worshipped them and all was well again—though before long the balance was sure to be disturbed again one way or another.

Erna used very often to play at being mother. I was to be the child, and one of my greatest faults was thumb-sucking. The first thing which I was supposed to put into my mouth was an engine. She had already much admired its gilded lamps, saying, 'They're so lovely, all red and burning', and at once put them into her mouth and sucked them. They stood to her for her mother's breast and her father's penis. These games were invariably followed by outbreaks of rage, envy and aggression against her mother, to be succeeded by remorse and by attempts to placate her. In playing with bricks, for instance, she would divide them between us so that she had more bricks than I; then she would make up for this by taking fewer herself, but would nevertheless always manage to keep more in the end. She asked me to build with my bricks, but only that she might prove how much more beautiful her building was than mine or so that she might knock mine down, apparently by accident. She would sometimes make a toy man be judge and decide that her house was better than mine. From the details of the game it was apparent that she was giving expression to a long-standing rivalry with her mother in this business about our respective houses. In a later part of her analysis she brought out her rivalry in a direct form.

Besides playing these games she also began cutting out paper and making paper patterns. While she was doing this she told me that it was 'minced meat' she was making and that blood was coming out of the paper; upon which she gave a shudder and said she felt sick all at once. On one occasion she talked about 'eye-salad', and on another she said that she was cutting 'fringes' in my nose. She was here repeating the wish to bite off my nose which she had expressed in her very first hour. (And indeed she made a number of attempts to carry out her wish.) By this means she also showed her identity with the 'third person', the toy man who broke in and set fire to the house, etc., and who bit off the woman's nose. In her analysis, as in that of other children, cutting out paper proved to be very variously determined. It gave outlet to sadistic and cannibalistic impulses but at the same time served reactive tendencies because it represented a creative activity too. The beautifully cut-out patterns, for instance representing a table cloth, stood for her parents' genitals or the body of her mother restored from the destruction which in phantasy she had previously inflicted on them.

From cutting out paper Erna went on to playing with water. A small piece of paper floating in the basin was a captain whose ship had gone down. He was able to save himself because—so Erna declared—he had something 'long and golden' which held him in the water. She then tore off his head and announced: 'His head's gone; now he's drowned'. These games with water led deep into the analysis of her oral-sadistic, urethral-sadistic and anal-sadistic phantasies. Thus, for instance, she played at being a washerwoman, and used some pieces of paper to represent a child's dirty linen. I was the child and had to dirty my underclothes over and over again. (Incidentally, Erna brought her coprophilic and cannibalistic impulses clearly to view by chewing up the pieces of paper, which represented excrements and children as well as dirty linen.) As a washerwoman Erna also had many opportunities of punishing and humiliating the child, and played the part of the cruel mother. But since she also identified herself with the maltreated child, she was gratifying her masochistic wishes as well. She would often pretend that the mother made the father punish the child and beat it on the bottom. This punishment was recommended by Erna, in her role of washerwoman, as a means of curing the child of its love of dirt. Once, instead of the father, a magician came along. He knocked one child on the anus and then on the head with a stick, and as he did so a yellowish fluid poured out of the magic wand. On another occasion the child—a quite little one this time—was given a powder to take, which was 'red and white' mixed together. This treatment made the little child clean, and it was suddenly able to talk, and became as clever as its mother.[1] The magician stood for the penis, and knocking with the stick meant coitus. The fluid and the powder represented urine, faeces, semen and blood, all of which, according to Erna's phantasies, her mother put inside herself in copulation through her mouth, anus and genitals.

Another time Erna suddenly changed herself from a washerwoman into a fishwife who began to cry her wares. In the course of this game she turned on the water-tap (which she used to call the 'whipped cream tap') after wrapping some paper round it. When the paper was soaked through and fell into the basin she tore it up and offered it for sale as fish. The compulsive greed with which Erna drank from the water-tap during this game and chewed up the imaginary fish pointed very clearly to the oral envy which she had felt during the primal scene and in her primal phantasies. This

[1] These phantasies relate to the penis in its 'good' and curative aspect. In Chapters XI and XII I shall deal with this point more fully.

envy had affected the development of her character very deeply, and was also a central feature in her neurosis.[1] The equation of the fish with her father's penis, as well as with faeces and children, became apparent in her associations. Erna had a variety of fish for sale, and amongst them some 'Kokelfish' or, as she suddenly called them, 'Kakelfish'.[1a] While she was cutting these up she had a sudden urge to defaecate, and this showed that the fish were equated with faeces, while cutting them up was equated with the act of defaecation. As the fishwife, Erna cheated me—as the customer—in several ways. She took large quantities of money from me and gave me no fish in return. I was helpless against her, because she was assisted by a policeman; and together they 'wurled'[1b] the money, equated with fish, which she had got from me. This policeman represented her father with whom she copulated and who was her ally against her mother. My part in the game was to look on while she 'wurled' the fish, with the policeman, and then I had to try to get possession of it secretly. In fact, I had to pretend to do what she herself had wanted to do to her mother when she had witnessed her mother and father having sexual intercourse. These sadistic impulses and phantasies were at the bottom of her severe anxiety in regard to her mother. She repeatedly expressed fear of a 'robber woman' who would 'take out everything inside her'.

Erna's analysis, too, demonstrated that theatre and performances of all kinds symbolized coitus between the parents.[2] The numerous performances in which Erna made her mother play the part of an actress or a dancer, admired by all the spectators, showed the immense admiration—an admiration mixed with envy—which she had for her. Often, too, in identification with her mother, she herself pretended to be a queen before whom everyone bowed down. In all these representations it was always the child who got the worst of it. Everything which Erna did in the role of her mother—the tenderness she showed to her husband, the way in which she dressed herself up and allowed herself to be admired—had one chief purpose, which was to arouse the child's envy and to wound its feelings. Thus, for instance, when she, as queen, had celebrated her marriage with the king, she lay down on the sofa and wanted me, as the king, to lie down beside her. As I refused to do this I had to sit on a little

[1] I shall discuss later the connection between Erna's observations of her parents' sexual intercourse and her own neurosis.

[1a] 'Kaki' are faeces in nursery German.

[1b] An invented word resembling the German word for whipping cream.

[2] In my paper, 'Early Analysis' (1923), I have considered in greater detail the universal symbolic significance of the theatre, performances, productions, etc., as representing intercourse between the parents. I may also refer to Rank, 'Das Schauspiel im Hamlet' (1919).

chair by her side instead and knock at the sofa with my fist. This she called 'churning', and it meant copulating. Immediately after this she announcxd that a child was creeping out of her, and she represented the scene in a quite realistic way, writhing about and groaning. Her imaginary child then shared its parents' bedroom and had to be a spectator of sexual intercourse between them. If it interrupted it was beaten, and the mother kept on complaining of it to the father. If she, as the mother, put the child to bed it was only in order to get rid of it and to be able to be united with the father all the sooner. The child was incessantly being maltreated and tormented. It was given semolina pudding to eat that was so nasty as to make it sick, while at the same time its mother and father were enjoying marvellous foods made of whipped cream or a special milk prepared by Dr Whippo or Whippour—a name compounded from 'whipping' and 'pouring out'. This special food, which was eaten by the father and mother alone, was used in endless variations to represent the exchange of substances during coition. Erna's phantasies that in coition her mother incorporated her father's penis and semen and her father incorporated her mother's breasts and milk formed the basis of her hatred and envy against her two parents.

In one of Erna's games a 'performance was given by a priest' who turned on the water-tap, and his partner, a woman dancer, drank from it. The child, called 'Cinderella', was only allowed to look on and had to remain absolutely quiet. A sudden tremendous outbreak of anger on Erna's part at this point showed with what feelings of hatred her phantasies were accompanied and how badly she had succeeded in dealing with those feelings. Her whole relationship to her mother had been distorted by them, as every educational measure, every act of nursery discipline, every unavoidable frustration, was felt by her as a purely sadistic act on the part of her mother, done with a view to humiliating and ill-treating her.

Nevertheless, in her make-believe of being a mother Erna did show affection to her imaginary child so long as it was still only a baby. Then she would nurse and wash it and be tender to it, and even forgive it when it was dirty. This was because, in her view, she herself had only been treated lovingly as long as she was an infant in arms. To her older 'child' she would be most cruel, and would let it be tortured by devils in a variety of ways and often killed it in the end.[1]

---

[1] Where the child's fury against its object (in this case against the imaginary child) is really excessive, the fundamental situation is that the super-ego has turned against the id. The ego escapes from this intolerable situation by means of a projection. It presents the object as an enemy in order that the id can destroy it in a sadistic way with the consent of the super-ego. If the ego can effect an alliance between the super-ego and the id by this means, it can

That the child in this role, however, was also the mother turned into a child, was made clear by the following phantasy. Erna played at being a child that had dirtied itself, and I, as the mother, had to scold her, whereupon she became scornful and out of defiance dirtied herself more and more. In order to annoy the mother still further she vomited up the bad food I had given her. The father was then called in by the mother, but he took the child's side. Next the mother was seized with an illness called 'God has spoken to her'; then the child in turn got an illness called 'mother's agitation' and died of it, and the mother was killed by the father as a punishment. The child then came to life again and was married to the father, who kept on praising it at the expense of the mother. The mother was then brought to life again, too, but, as a punishment, was turned into a child by the father's magic wand; and now she in turn had to suffer all the humiliation and ill-treatment to which the child herself had been subjected before. In her numerous phantasies of this kind about a mother and a child Erna was repeating what she felt her own experiences had been, while on the other hand she was also expressing what she would like to do to her mother in a sadistic way if the child-mother relationship was reversed.

Erna's mental life was dominated by anal-sadistic phantasies. At a later stage of her analysis, starting, once more, from games connected with water, she produced phantasies in which faeces 'baked on' to clothes were also used for cooking and eating. Again, she played that she was sitting in the lavatory and eating what she produced there, or that we were giving it to one another. Her phantasies about our continually dirtying each other with urine and faeces came out more and more clearly in the course of the analysis. In one game she demonstrated that her mother had dirtied herself over and over again and that everything in the room had been turned into faeces through her mother's fault. Her mother was accordingly thrown into prison and starved there. She herself then had the job of cleaning up after her mother, and in that connection called herself 'Mrs Dirt Parade'—that is, a person parading with dirt. Through her love of tidiness she won the admiration and recognition of her father, who set her high above her mother and married her. She did his cooking for him. The drinks and food which they gave one another were once more urine and faeces, but this time a good kind instead of a harmful one. The above will serve as an example of the numerous

---

for the time being send out the sadism of the super-ego that was directed against the id into the external world. In this way the primary sadistic impulses which are directed against the object are increased by the hatred originally directed against the id. (Cf. Chapter VIII and also my paper, 'Personification in the Play of Children', 1929, *Writings*, 1.

and extravagantly anal-sadistic phantasies which became conscious in the course of her analysis.

Erna, who was an only child, was much occupied in her imagination with the arrival of brothers and sisters. Her phantasies in this context deserve special attention, since, so far as my observations show, they have a general application. Judging from them and from those of other children similarly situated, it would appear that an only child suffers to a far greater extent than other children from the anxiety it feels in regard to the brother or sister whom it is forever expecting, and from the feelings of guilt it has towards them on account of its unconscious impulses of aggression against them in their assumed existence inside its mother's body, because it has no opportunity of developing a positive relation to them in reality. This fact often makes it more difficult for an only child to adapt itself to society. For a long time Erna used to have attacks of rage and anxiety at the beginning and end of her analytic session with me, and these were partly precipitated by her meeting the child who came to me for treatment immediately before or after her and who stood to her for the brother or sister whose arrival she was always awaiting.[1] On the other hand, although she did not get on with other children, she felt a great need for their society at times. Her occasional wish for a brother or sister was, I found, determined by a number of motives. (1) The brothers and sisters which she desired meant a child of her own. This wish, however, was soon disturbed by severe feelings of guilt, because it would have meant that she had stolen the child from her mother. (2) Their existence would have reassured her that the attacks she had made in her phantasy on the children which she supposed to be inside her mother had damaged neither them nor her mother, and that consequently the interior of her own body was unharmed. (3) They would afford her the sexual gratification which her father and mother had denied her. (4) Erna had the phantasy that she would unite with them against her parents in order to kill her mother and capture her father's penis. They would be her allies[2] in the fight against her terrifying parents.

But these phantasies of Erna's would quickly be followed by feelings of hatred against her imaginary brothers and sisters—for

[1] As Erna had no brothers or sisters in real life, her unconscious fear and jealousy of them which played such an important part in her mental life were only revealed and lived through in the analysis. This is once more an example of the importance of the transference-situation in child analyses.

[2] In my paper, 'Early Stages of the Oedipus Conflict' (1928, *Writings*, 1), I have pointed out that children, in their sexual relations with one another, especially if they are brothers and sisters, have phantasies of being in league together against their parents and often experience a diminution of their anxiety and sense of guilt from this belief.

they were, ultimately, only substitutes for her father and mother — and by very severe feelings of guilt on account of the destructive acts which she, together with them, had committed against her parents in her phantasies. And she would usually end by having an attack of depression.

These phantasies, too, had their share in making Erna incapable of getting on good terms with other children. She shrank from them because she identified them with her imaginary brothers and sisters, so that on the one hand she regarded them as accomplices in her attacks upon her parents, and on the other she feared them as enemies because of her own aggressive impulses towards those brothers and sisters.

Erna's case throws light on another factor which seems to me to be of general importance. In the first chapter I drew attention to the peculiar relationship that children have to reality. I pointed out that failure in making a correct adaptation to reality could, in analysis, be recognized in the play of quite small children, and that it was necessary in analysis gradually to bring even the youngest child into complete touch with reality. With Erna, even after a good deal of analysis had been done, I had not succeeded in obtaining any detailed information about her real life. I got plenty of material regarding her extravagant sadistic impulses against her mother, but I never heard the least complaint or criticism from her about her *real* mother and what she actually did. Although Erna acknowledged that her phantasies were directed against her real mother — a fact which she had denied at an earlier stage of analysis — and although it became clearer and clearer that she copied her mother in an exaggerated and invidious manner, yet it was difficult to establish the connection between her phantasies and reality. All my efforts to draw her actual life more fully into the analysis remained ineffective, until I succeeded at least partially in analysing her deepest reasons for wanting to cut herself off from reality. Erna's relationship to reality proved to be largely a pretence, and this to a far greater extent than her behaviour would have led one to expect. The truth was that she was trying by every means to maintain a dream world in existence and to protect it from reality.[1] For instance, she used to imagine that the toy carriages and coachmen were in her service, that they came at her command and brought her everything she wished, that the toy women were her servants, and so on. Even while these phantasies were in progress she would often be seized with rage and depression. She would then go to the lavatory and there phantasy aloud while she defaecated. When she came out of the

[1] Many children make only an *apparent* return to reality when their games are interrupted. Actually they are still occupied with their phantasies.

lavatory she would fling herself on to the couch and begin to suck her thumb passionately, to masturbate and to pick her nose. I succeeded in getting her to tell me the phantasies which accompanied this defaecation, thumb-sucking, masturbation and nose-picking. By means of these pleasurable satisfactions and the phantasies bound up with them she was trying forcibly to continue the same dream-state which she had been keeping up while playing. The depression, anger and anxiety which seized her during her play were due to a disturbance of her phantasies by some incursion of reality. She remembered, too, how greatly she was put out if anyone came near her bed in the morning while she was thumb-sucking or masturbating. The reason for this was not only that she was afraid of being caught, but that she wanted to ward off reality. A pseudologia, which appeared during her analysis and grew to fantastic proportions, served the purpose of re-shaping an intolerable reality according to her desires. I could see in her excessive fear of her parents, especially her mother, one reason for this extraordinary cutting-off of reality —to which end she also employed megalomanic phantasies. It was in order to lessen this fear that Erna was driven to imagine herself as a powerful and harsh mistress over her mother, and this led to a great intensification of her sadism.

Erna's phantasies of being cruelly persecuted by her mother began to show their paranoid character more distinctly. As I have already said, she looked upon every step taken in her education and upbringing, even down to the least details of her clothing, as an act of persecution on the part of her mother. Not only so, but every-thing else that her mother did—the way she behaved towards her father, the things she did for her own amusement, and so on—were felt by Erna as a persecution of herself. Moreover, she felt herself continually spied upon. One cause of her excessive fixation upon her mother was the compulsion of continually keeping watch over her. Analysis showed that Erna felt responsible for every illness that her mother had, and expected a corresponding punishment because of her own aggressive phantasies. The severe, punishing mother and the hating child, between whom she perpetually alternated in her play and phantasies, showed the action of an over-harsh super-ego in many details. It needed a very deep-going analysis to elucidate these phantasies, which corresponded to what, in adult paranoiacs, are known as delusions. The experience I have gained since I first wrote down this case-history has led me to the conclusion[1] that the peculiar character of Erna's anxiety, of her phantasies and of

---

[1] Fuller consideration is given to this subject in the second part of this volume.

her relation to reality, is typical of cases with strong paranoid traits.[1]

At this point I must draw attention to Erna's homosexual trends, which had been excessively strong from early childhood onwards. After a great amount of her hatred of her father, arising out of the Oedipus situation, had been analysed, those trends, though undoubtedly diminished, were still very strong and seemed at first incapable of being resolved any further. It was only after strong resistances had been overcome that the real character and full strength of her persecution phantasies and their relation to her homosexuality came to light. Anal love-desires now emerged much clearer in their positive form alternating with phantasies of persecution. Erna once more played at being a shopwoman and that what she sold was faeces became obvious from the fact that, among other things, right at the beginning of her play she felt a desire to defaecate. I was a customer and had to prefer her to all other shop assistants and think her wares particularly good. Then she was the customer and loved me, and in this way she represented an anal love relationship between her mother and herself. These anal phantasies were soon followed by fits of depression and hatred which she chiefly directed against me but which were actually aimed at her mother. In this connection Erna produced phantasies of a flea which was 'black and yellow mixed' and which she herself at once recognized as a bit of faeces—dangerous, poisoned faeces, it turned out. This flea, she said, came out of my anus and forced its way into hers and injured her.[2]

In Erna's case I was able to confirm beyond doubt the transformation of love for the parent of the same sex into hatred, which is known as the cause of delusions of persecution, together with a marked prominence of the mechanisms of projection. Beneath Erna's homosexual attachment, at an even deeper level, lay an extraordinarily intense feeling of hatred against her mother, derived from her earliest Oedipus situation and her oral sadism. This hatred had as its result an excessive anxiety which, in its turn, was a

[1] See Chapter IX.

[2] In his 'Short Study of the Development of the Libido' (1924) Abraham says: (p. 489) 'Both van Ophuijsen' (in his paper 'On the Origin of the Feeling of Persecution', 1920) 'and Stärcke' (in his paper, 'The Reversal of the Libido-Sign in Delusions of Persecution', 1919) 'discovered during the course of their psychoanalytic practice that in paranoia the "persecutor" can be traced back to the patient's unconscious image of the faeces in his intestines which he identifies with the penis of the "persecutor", i.e. the person of his own sex whom he originally loved. Thus in paranoia the patient represents his persecutor by a part of his body, and believes that he is carrying it within himself. He would like to get rid of that foreign body but cannot.'

determining factor in every detail of her phantasies of persecution. We now come to a fresh lot of sadistic phantasies which in the intensity of their sadism exceeded anything which I had as yet come across in Erna's analysis. This was the most difficult part of the work and taxed Erna's willingness to co-operate in it to the utmost, since it was accompanied by extreme anxiety. Her oral envy of the genital and oral gratifications which she supposed her parents to be enjoying during intercourse proved to be the deepest foundation of her hatred. She gave expression to that hatred over and over again in countless phantasies directed against her parents united in copulation. In these phantasies she attacked them, and especially her mother, by means of her excrements, among other things; and what most deeply underlay her fear of my faeces (the flea), which she thought of as being pushed into her, were phantasies of herself destroying her mother's inside with her own dangerous and poisoned faeces.[1]

After these sadistic phantasies and impulses belonging to a very early stage of development had been further analysed, Erna's homosexual fixation upon her mother was lessened and her hetero-sexual impulses grew stronger. Until now the essential determinant of her phantasies had been her attitude of hatred and love towards her mother. Her father had figured chiefly as a mere instrument for coitus; he seemed to derive his whole importance from the mother-daughter relationship. In her imagination every sign of affection her mother showed her father, and indeed her whole relationship to him, had served no other purpose than to rob her, Erna, make her jealous and set her father against her. In the same way, in those phantasies in which she deprived her mother of her father and married him, all the stress had been laid on her hatred of her mother and her wish to hurt her. If in games of this type Erna was affection-ate to her husband, it would soon appear that the tenderness was only a pretence, designed to hurt her rival's feelings and to draw her father to her side. At the same time as she made these important steps in her analysis she also moved forward in her relations to him and began to entertain genuine feelings for him of a positive nature. Now that the situation was not governed so completely by hate and fear, the direct Oedipus relationship could establish itself. At the same

[1] As I have later found in the course of my analytic work, the child's fears of poisoned and dangerous excrement increase its fixation at the pre-genital levels by being a constant incentive to it to convince itself that those excre-ments—both its own and those of its objects—are not dangerous but 'good' things (cf. Chapter VIII of this volume). This is why Erna pretended that we were giving one another 'good' anal presents and loved one another. But the states of depression which followed upon these games of supposed love showed that at bottom she was terrified and believed that we—that is, her mother and she—were persecuting and poisoning each other.

time Erna's fixation upon her mother was lessened and her relationship to her, which had hitherto been so ambivalent, was improved. This alteration in the girl's attitude to both her parents was also based upon great changes in her phantasy-life and instinctual behaviour. Her sadism was diminished, and her phantasies of persecution were far less in number and intensity. Important changes, too, occurred in her relationship to reality, and these made themselves felt, among other things, in an increased infiltration of reality into her phantasies.

In this period of her analysis, after having represented her ideas of persecution in play, Erna would often say with astonishment: 'But Mother can't *really* have meant to do that? She's very fond of me *really*.' But as her contact with reality became stronger and her unconscious hatred of her mother more conscious, she began to criticize her as a real person with ever greater frankness, and at the same time her relations with her improved. This was made possible as the unconscious hatred became more conscious. Hand in hand with this improvement of the relationship to her mother, there appeared genuinely motherly and tender feelings in her attitude towards her imaginary children. On one occasion, after having been very cruel to one of them, she asked in a deeply moved voice: 'Should I *really* have treated my child like that?' Thus the analysis of her ideas of persecution and the diminution of her anxiety had succeeded not only in strengthening her heterosexual attitude but in improving her relations to her mother and in enabling her to have more maternal feelings herself. I should like to say here that in my opinion the satisfactory regulation of these fundamental attitudes, which determine the child's later choice of a love-object and the whole nature of the adult's experiences, is one of the criteria of a successful child analysis.

Erna's neurosis had appeared very early in her life. Before she was quite a year old she showed marked signs of a neurosis together with an unusual precocity in her mental behaviour. From that time on her difficulties increased continually, so that by the time she was between two and three years old her upbringing had become an insoluble problem, her character was already abnormal, and she was suffering from a definite obsessional neurosis. Yet it was not until she was about four years old that the unusual nature of her masturbatory habits and thumb-sucking was recognized. It will be seen, then, that this six-year-old child's obsessional neurosis was already a chronic one. Pictures of her at the age of about three show her with the same neurotic, brooding look upon her face that she had when she was six.

I should like to stress the unusual severity of this case. The

47

obsessional symptoms, which amongst other things deprived the child almost entirely of sleep, the depressions and other signs of illness, and the abnormal development of her character, were only a weak reflection of the entirely abnormal, extravagant and un-curbed instinctual life which lay behind them. The future prospects of an obsessional neurosis which, like this one, had for years been of a progressive character could not be described as other than decidedly gloomy. It may safely be asserted that the only remedy in a case of this kind was a timely treatment of psycho-analysis.

I shall now enter into a discussion of the structure of the case in greater detail. Erna's training in habits of cleanliness had presented no difficulty and had been completed unusually early, by the time she was one year old. No severity had been necessary: the ambition of the precocious child had been a powerful incentive to the speedy attainment of the required standards of cleanliness.[1] But this out-ward success went along with a complete internal failure. Erna's tremendous anal-sadistic phantasies showed to what degree she remained fixated at that stage and how much hatred and ambival-ence flowed from it. One factor in this failure was a constitutionally strong oral- and anal-sadistic disposition; but an important part was played by another factor—one which has been pointed out by Freud[2] as having a share in the predisposition to obsessional neurosis, namely a too rapid development of the ego in comparison with the libido. Besides this, analysis showed that another critical factor in Erna's development had been attained with only apparent success. She had never got over her weaning. And there was yet a third privation which she underwent subsequently to this. When she was between six and nine months old her mother had noticed with what evident sexual pleasure she responded to the usual nursery care and especially to the cleansing of her genitals and of her anus. The over-excitability of her genital zone was unmistakable. Her mother therefore exercised greater discretion in washing those parts, and the older and the cleaner the child grew the easier, of course, it was to do so. But the child, who had looked upon the earlier and more elaborate attention as a form of seduction, felt this later reticence as a frustration. This feeling of being seduced, behind which there lay a *desire* to be seduced, was constantly being repeated all through her life. In every relationship, e.g. to her nurse and the other people who brought her up and also in her analysis, she tried to repeat the

[1] What some of the sources of Erna's early ambition in this line were can be inferred from the phantasies in which she outdid her mother in cleanliness and was called 'Mrs Dirt Parade' by her father and married by him on account of it, while her mother had to starve in prison.

[2] 'The Predisposition to Obsessional Neurosis' (1913).

situation of being seduced, alternating with the accusation that she was being seduced. By analysing this specific transference situation it was possible to trace her attitude through earlier situations back to the earliest—to the experience of being cared for when she was an infant.

In each of the three factors that led to the production of Erna's neurosis the part played by constitutional factors was unmistakable.[1]

It now remains to be seen in what way her experience of the primal scene combined with those constitutional factors and thus brought about the full development of her obsessional neurosis. At the age of two and a half, and again at three and a half,[2] she had shared her parents' bedroom during a summer holiday. At these times she had had an opportunity of watching coitus between them. Not only were the effects of this observable in her analysis, but they were definitely established by external evidence. In the summer during which she had made her first observations, a markedly unfavourable change had taken place in her. Analysis showed that the

---

[1] I have subsequently come to the view, which I shall more fully substantiate in Chapter VIII, that an excessive oral sadism brings on the development of the ego too rapidly and also hastens that of the libido. The constitutional factors in Erna's neurosis which have been referred to above, her over-strong sadism, the too rapid development of her ego and the premature activity of her genital impulses, are thus interconnected. Since dealing with this case I have been able to discover yet another constitutional factor in the production of a neurosis. This consists of the insufficient capacity of the ego to tolerate anxiety. In many cases, of which Erna was one, the child's sadism arouses a degree of anxiety very early on which the ego cannot adequately master. It must be said in general that the capacity of the ego to master even ordinary amounts of anxiety varies with the individual; and this is a factor that helps to determine the neuroses.

[2] We have here an interesting analogy to the case described in Freud's 'History of an Infantile Neurosis' (1918). When Erna was five years old, that is, eighteen months after the last occasion on which she had watched her parents copulate, she was with them on a visit to her grandmother, and for a short time during the visit shared their bedroom, but without having an opportunity for observing coitus. Nevertheless, one morning Erna astonished her grandmother by saying: 'Daddy got into bed with Mummy and wigglewoggled with her.' The child's story remained inexplicable until her analysis showed that she had taken in what she had seen when she was two and a half, and, though she had forgotten it, it had remained stored up in her mind. When she was three and a half these impressions had been revived, but once again forgotten. Finally, eighteen months later, a similar situation (sleeping in her parents' bedroom) had excited in her an unconscious expectation of seeing the same events and had stirred up her earlier experiences. In Erna's case, as in that of the Wolf Man, the primal scene had been completely repressed but had been subsequently re-activated and brought for a moment into consciousness.

observation of intercourse had brought on her neurosis in its full force. The sight of her parents copulating had enormously intensified her sense of frustration and envy in regard to her parents and had raised to an extreme pitch her sadistic phantasies and impulses against the sexual gratification they were obtaining.[1]

Erna's obsessional symptoms found an explanation as follows. The obsessive character of her thumb-sucking was caused by phantasies of sucking, biting and devouring her father's penis and her mother's breasts. The penis represented the whole father and the breasts the whole mother.[2] The analysis also uncovered the severe depressive features in the clinical picture which I only shortly mention at this point.[3] I gave several examples for the unconscious meaning of the head as penis as it was effective in Erna's case. Banging her head against the pillow was intended to represent her father's movements in coitus. She told me that at night she could curb her fear of robbers and burglars only by 'bumping' with her head. She was thus freeing herself from this fear by identifying herself with the object of her fear.

The structure of her obsessive masturbation was very complicated. She distinguished between various forms of it; a pressing together of her legs which she called 'ranking'; a rocking movement, already mentioned, called 'sculpting'; and a pulling at the clitoris, called 'the cupboard game', in which she 'wanted to pull out something very long'. Further, she used to cause a pressure on her vagina by pulling the corner of a sheet between her legs. Various identifications were operative in these different forms of masturbation, according to whether, in the accompanying phantasies, she was playing the active part of her father or the passive one of her mother, or both at once. These masturbation phantasies of Erna's, which were very

[1] In his *Inhibitions, Symptoms and Anxiety* (1926), (*S.E.* **20**, p. 154) Freud states that it is the quantity of anxiety present which determines the outbreak of a neurosis. In my opinion, anxiety is liberated by the destructive tendencies (cf. Chapters VIII and IX), so that the outbreak of a neurosis would, in fact, be a consequence of an excessive increase of those destructive tendencies. In Erna's case it was her hatred heightened by witnessing the primal scene that brought on anxiety, and led to her illness.

[2] Cf. Abraham, 'A Short Study of the Development of the Libido' (1924), Part II.

[3] In her analysis she used repeatedly to complain of a queer feeling that she often had. She would sometimes wonder, she said, whether she was an animal or not. This feeling proved to be determined by her sense of guilt over her cannibalistic impulses. Her depression, which she used to express in the words, 'There's something I don't like about life', was shown by the analysis to be a genuine *taedium vitae* and to be accompanied by suicidal ideas. It had its roots in the feelings of anxiety and guilt resulting from the oral-sadistic trends.

strongly sado-masochistic, showed a clear connection with the primal scene and with her primal phantasies. Her sadism was directed against her parents in intercourse, and as a reaction to it she had phantasies of a correspondingly masochistic character.

During a whole succession of analytic sessions Erna masturbated in these various ways. Owing to the well-established transference, however, it was also possible to induce her to describe her masturbation phantasies in between times. I was able in this way to discover the causes of her obsessive masturbation and thus to free her from it. The rocking movements which began in the second half of her first year sprang from her wish to be masturbated and went back to the manipulations connected with her toilet as an infant. There was a period of the analysis during which she depicted her parents copulating in the most various ways in her games and afterwards gave vent to her full fury over the frustration involved. In the course of these scenes she would never fail to produce a situation in which she rocked herself about in a half-lying or sitting posture, exhibited, and eventually even made open requests to me to touch her genitals or sometimes to smell them. At that time—at the age of six—she once astonished her mother by asking her after her bath to lift up one of her legs and pat or touch her underneath, at the same time taking up the position of a child having its genitals powdered—a position which she had not been in for years. The clarification of her rocking movements led to the complete cessation of the symptom.

Erna's most resistant symptom was her inhibition in learning. It was so severe that, inspite of all the efforts she made, she took two years to master what children ordinarily learn in a few months. This difficulty was more strongly affected by the later part of her analysis, and when I concluded the treatment it had been reduced, though not entirely removed.

I have already gone into the favourable change which took place in Erna's relationship to her parents and in her libido position in general as a result of analysis, and have emphasized how it was only thanks to it that she was able to take the first steps in the direction of social adaptation. Her obsessional symptoms (obsessive masturbation, thumb-sucking, rocking, etc.) which were so severe as to be partly responsible for her sleeplessness, were removed. With their cure and the material lessening of anxiety, her sleep became normal. Her attacks of depression also ceased.[1]

Notwithstanding these favourable results, I did not consider that the analysis was by any means complete when it was broken off for external reasons after 575 hours of treatment, having extended over

[1] When I last had news of her, two and a half years after the end of the analysis, these improvements had been maintained.

two and a half years. The extraordinary severity of the case, which was manifested not only in the child's symptoms but in the distorted development of her character and completely abnormal personality, demanded further analysis in order to remove the difficulties from which she still suffered. That she was still in an insufficiently stable condition was shown by the fact that in situations of stress she had a tendency to relapse into some of her old troubles, though such relapses were always less severe than originally. In these circumstances it was always possible that a severe strain, or even the onset of puberty, might give rise to a fresh illness or some other difficulties.

This opens up a question of principal importance, namely, the question of when a child analysis can be said to be completed. In children of the latency age I cannot consider even very good results, such as fully satisfy their environment, as sufficient evidence that the analysis has been completed. I have come to the conclusion that the fact that an analysis has brought about a fairly favourable development in the latency period—however important that may be—is not in itself a guarantee that the patient's further development will be completely successful.[1] The transition to puberty, and from it to maturity, seems to me to be the test of whether a child analysis has been carried far enough or not. In Chapter VI I shall go further into this question and I will only state here as a matter of experience that analysis ensures the future stability of the child in direct proportion as it is able to resolve anxiety in the deepest layers. In this, and in the character of the child's unconscious phantasies, or rather in the changes that have been brought about in them, a criterion is to be found which helps us to judge whether an analysis has been carried sufficiently far.

To return to Erna's case, on an earlier occasion I have already said that at the end of the analysis, her phantasies of persecution were greatly reduced both in quantity and intensity. In my opinion, however, her sadism and anxiety could and should have been further diminished in order to prevent the possibility of an illness overtaking her at puberty or when she became grown-up. But since a continuation of the analysis was not possible at the time, its completion was left over for a future period.

I shall now proceed to discuss certain questions of a general nature in connection with Erna's case-history which also partly arose out of her analysis. I found that the extensive occupation of her

[1] In Chapter V, in connection with the analysis of Ilse, a child in the age of puberty, I shall consider in greater detail what are the factors that determine a successful transition to the latency period and what are the factors that determine a further successful transition to puberty.

analysis with sexual questions and the freedom which was allowed her in her phantasies and games[1] led to a diminution rather than to an increase of sexual excitement and preoccupation with sexual matters. Erna was a child whose unusual sexual precocity was noticeable to all. Not only the type of phantasies she had but her behaviour and movements were those of a very sensual girl in her puberty. This was shown especially in her provocative behaviour towards men and boys. Her behaviour in this respect, too, was very much changed for the better during the analysis, and when it was ended she showed a more childlike nature. Further, the analysis of her masturbation phantasies put an end to her compulsive masturbation.[2]

Another analytic principal which I should like to emphasize is that it is indispensable to make conscious as far as possible the doubts and criticisms which the child harbours in its unconscious concerning its parents and especially their sexual life. Its attitude to its environment cannot but benefit from this, since, in being brought into consciousness, its unconscious grievances and adverse judgments etc. are tested against reality and thus lose their former virulence. At the same time, its relations to reality improve. Again, its capacity to criticize parents consciously is already, as we saw in Erna's case, a result of its improved relations to reality.[3]

[1] In the preceding chapter I pointed out that a child analysis, just as an adult one, must be carried through in abstinence; but as the child is different from the adult, a different criterion must be used. For instance, in taking part in the games and phantasies of the child the analyst gives it a much greater amount of satisfaction in reality than he does the adult patient; but this amount of satisfaction is seen to be less than it at first appears to be. For play is a form of expression natural to the child, so that the part the analyst takes in it does not differ in character from the attention with which he follows the verbal expressions of adult patients in describing their phantasies. Furthermore it must be remembered that the satisfaction which children obtain in their analysis is for the most part one of phantasy. Erna, it is true, did masturbate regularly in her analytic hour over a certain period of time. But she was an exception. We must not forget that in her case obsessional masturbation was present in such measure that she used to masturbate most of the day, sometimes even in the presence of other people. When her compulsion had been considerably lessened, the analytical situation led to a cessation of masturbation during the analytic hours in favour of a mere representation of the masturbation phantasies involved.

[2] I mean by this that her excessive masturbation and her masturbation done in the presence of other people, which had their roots in a compulsion, had stopped. I do not mean that she gave up masturbating altogether.

[3] So long as Erna was so much cut off from reality I was only able to analyse material connected with her phantasies; but I was continually on the look-out for any threads, however weak, that might connect those phantasies with reality. In this way, and by constantly diminishing her anxiety, I was able

Coming now to a question of technique; as I have said more than once, Erna often used to have outbursts of anger during the analytic session. Her fits of anger and her sadistic impulses would not seldom assume threatening forms towards me. It is a familiar fact that analysis releases strong affects in obsessional neurotics; and in children these find a much more direct and uncontrolled expression than in adults. From the very beginning I made Erna clearly understand that she must not attack me physically. But she was at liberty to abreact her affects in many other ways; and she used to break her toys or cut them up, knock down the little chairs, fling the cushions about, stamp her feet on the sofa, upset water, smudge paper, dirty the toys or the wash basin,[1] break out into abuse, and so on, without the slightest hindrance on my part. But at the same time I used to analyse her rage, and this always lessened it and sometimes cleared it up altogether. There are thus three factors which technically have to be considered in dealing with a child's outbursts of emotion during treatment: (1) the child has to keep part of its affect under control, but it should only be required to do so in so far as there is a necessity for it in reality; (2) it may give vent to its affects in abuse and in the other ways mentioned above; and (3) its affects are lessened or cleared up by continuous interpretation and by tracing back the present situation to the original one.

The extent to which each of these methods is employed will, of course, greatly vary. For instance, with Erna I was driven early on to devise the following plan. At one period she used to have an outbreak of rage whenever I told her that the session was at an end, and I used therefore to open both the double-doors of my room so as to check her, knowing that it would be extremely painful to her if the person who came to fetch her saw anything of her outbursts. At this period, I may remark, my room used to look like a battlefield after Erna had left it. Later in the analysis she would content herself with hurriedly throwing down the cushions before she went out; while later still she used to leave the room perfectly calmly. Here is another example, taken from the analysis of Peter (aged three years and nine months) who was also at one time subject to violent outbursts of rage. At a later period of his analysis he said

---

gradually to strengthen her relation to reality. In the next chapter I shall try to show more clearly that in the latency period the analyst has very often to occupy himself for the most part with such phantasy material for long stretches of time before he can gain access to the child's real life and ego-interests.

[1] I regard it as an absolute necessity in child analysis that the room in which treatment is given shall be furnished in such a way that the child can abreact very freely. Damage to the furniture, floor, etc., must to a certain limit be accepted.

quite spontaneously, pointing to a toy: 'I can just as easily *think* I've broken that.'[1]

But it is essential that the demands of the analyst for partial control of affects by the child are not to be regarded as a pedagogic measure—they are made for rational reasons and are unavoidable. Such demands founded on a rational necessity can be understood by a child even if it will not always be able to carry them out. In the same way there are occasions on which I do not actually carry out the whole of the actions which have been allotted to me in a game, on the ground that their complete realization would be too awkward or unpleasant for me. Nevertheless, even in such cases I follow out the child's ideas as far as I possibly can. It is very important, too, that the analyst should show the least possible emotion in the face of the emotional outbursts of the child.

I propose now to make use of the data obtained from this case to illustrate the theoretical views which I have since formed[2] and which will be advanced in the second part of this volume. The gilded lamps of the engine, which Erna thought were 'so lovely, all red and burning' and which she sucked, represented her father's penis (cf. also the 'something long and golden' which held the captain up in the water) and were equated with her mother's breasts as well. That she had an intense feeling of guilt about sucking at things was shown by the fact that when I was playing the part of the child she declared that 'sucking' was my greatest fault. This sense of guilt can be explained by the fact that sucking also represented biting off and devouring her mother's breasts and her father's penis. I may refer here to my thesis that it is the process of weaning which, together with the child's wish to incorporate its father's penis, and its feelings of envy and hatred towards its mother, sets the Oedipus conflict in motion. This envy is founded on the child's early sexual theory that in copulating with the father the mother incorporates and retains his penis.[3]

[1] The remarks of even quite small children prove that they have fully grasped the nature of the transference-situation and understand that the lessening of their affects is brought about by interpreting the original situation together with the affects belonging to it. In such cases, for instance, Peter used often to distinguish between myself, who 'was like his Mummy', and his 'real Mummy'. For instance, in running his motor car up and down he spat at me and wanted to beat me, and called me a 'naughty beast'. He contradicted my interpretation violently, but by and by he became quiet and affectionate again and asked: 'When Daddy's thingummy went into Mummy like that, did I want to say "Beast" to my *real* Mummy?'

[2] Cf. also my paper, 'Early Stages of the Oedipus Conflict' (1928).

[3] Cf. Chapter VIII.

55

This envy proved to be the central point of Erna's neurosis. The attacks which she made at the beginning of her analysis as the 'third person' on the house which was occupied only by a man and a woman turned out to be a portrayal of her aggressive impulses against her mother's body and her father's penis assumed to be inside it. These impulses, stimulated by the little girl's oral envy, found expression in her game in which she sank the ship (her mother) and tore away from the captain (her father) the 'long, golden thing' and his head that kept him afloat, i.e. castrated him symbolically as he was copulating with her mother. The details of her phantasies of assault show to what heights of sadistic ingenuity these attacks upon her mother's body went. She would, for instance, transform her excrements into dangerous and explosive substances so as to wreck it from within. This was depicted by the burning down and destruction of the house and the 'bursting' of the people inside it. The cutting-out of paper (making 'mincemeat' and 'eye-salad') represented a complete destruction of the parents in the act of coition. Erna's wish to bite off my nose and to make 'fringes' in it was at the same time an attack directed against her father's penis which I was supposed to have incorporated, as was proved by the material produced in other cases.[1]

That Erna, in her phantasy, made attacks on her mother's body with an eye to seizing and destroying the other things also contained therein (i.e. faeces and children) is shown by the variety of fish around which there revolved that desperate struggle, in which every resource was employed, between the 'fishwife' (her mother) and me as the child (herself). She furthermore imagined, as we saw, that I, after having to look on while she and the policeman 'wurled' money, or fish, together, tried to gain possession of the fish at all costs. The sight of her parents in sexual intercourse had therefore induced a desire to steal her father's penis and whatever else might be inside her mother's body. Erna's reaction against this intention of robbing and completely destroying her mother's body was expressed in the fear she had, after her struggles with the fishwife, that a robber woman would take out everything inside her. It is this fear that I have described as belonging to the earliest danger-situation of the girl and which I consider as an equivalent to the castration anxiety of boys.[2] I may mention here the connection

[1] In other analyses, too, I have found that attacks — whether phantasized or real — upon my nose, feet, head, etc., never referred simply to those parts of my body as such; they were also directed against them as symbolic representations of the father's penis, attached to, or incorporated by me, that is, the mother.

[2] See also my 'Early Stages of the Oedipus Conflict' (1928, *Writings*, 1) where the connection between the subject's inhibition in work and his sadistic identification with his mother is discussed.

between this early anxiety-situation of Erna's and her extraordinary inhibition in learning, a connection which I have since met with in other analyses.[1] I have already pointed out that in Erna it was only the analysis of the deepest layers of her sadism and of her earliest Oedipus situation that influenced that inhibition. Her extraordinary sadism, which was fused with Erna's intense desire for knowledge, led—as a defence against it—to a complete inhibition of a number of activities which were based upon her desire for knowledge. Arithmetic and writing symbolized violent sadistic attacks upon her mother's body and her father's penis.[2] In her unconscious, these activities were equated with tearing, cutting up or burning her mother's body, together with the children it contained, and castrating her father. Reading, too, in consequence of the symbolic equation of her mother's body with books, had come to mean a violent removal of substances, children, etc. from the inside of her mother.[3]

Finally, I shall make use of this case to bring up yet another point to which, as a result of further experience, I have come to ascribe general validity too. The character of Erna's phantasies and of her relation to reality is, in my experience, typical for those cases in which paranoid traits are strongly operative. Furthermore, the underlying determinants which I found in her case for the development of her paranoid traits and the homosexuality bound up with them, have also turned out to be general basic factors in the genesis of paranoia. In the second part of this book (Chapter IX) this question will receive further discussion. I will only point out briefly here that I have discovered strong paranoic features in a number of analyses of children, and have thus been led to the conviction that one important and promising task of child analysis is to uncover and clear up psychotic traits in the early life of the individual.

[1] Compare my report on Ilse in Chapter V.

[2] On this point see also my paper, 'The Role of the School in the Libidinal Development of the Child' (1923), *Writings*, 1.

[3] In his paper, 'Some Unconscious Factors in Reading' (1930), James Strachey has pointed out this unconscious significance of reading.

Chapter IV

THE TECHNIQUE OF ANALYSIS IN THE LATENCY PERIOD

THE analysis of children in the latency period presents special difficulties. Unlike the small child, whose lively imagination and acute anxiety enables us to gain access to and contact with its unconscious more easily, children in the latency period have a very limited imaginative life, in accordance with the strong tendency to repression which is characteristic of their age; while, in comparison with the grown-up person, their ego is still undeveloped, and they neither have insight into their illness nor a desire to be cured, so that they have no incentive to start analysis and no encouragement to go on with it. Added to this is the general attitude of reserve and distrust so typical of this period of life—an attitude which is in part an outcome of their intense preoccupation with the struggle against masturbation and thus makes them deeply averse to anything that savours of search and interrogation or touches on the impulses they just manage to keep under control.

These peculiarities have the effect that we do not find a clear access to their analysis because children of this age group do not play like small children nor give verbal associations like adults. Nevertheless I have found it possible to establish the analytic situation without delay if I approach their unconscious from a point of departure that corresponds to the nature of the older child. The small child is still under the immediate and powerful influence of its instinctual experiences and phantasies and puts them in front of us straight away; it is therefore appropriate, as I found in early analyses, to interpret, even in the first sessions, the small child's representations of coitus and its sadistic phantasies; whereas the child in the latency period has already desexualized those experiences and phantasies much more completely and worked them over in a different form.

The seven-year-old Grete, a very reserved and mentally restricted child, with marked schizoid traits, was quite inaccessible. She drew pictures, however, and produced rather primitive sketches of houses and trees which she repeated over and over again in an obsessional way, first the one, then the other. From certain continu-

58

ally recurring changes in the colour and size of the houses and trees and from the order in which they were drawn, I inferred that the houses represented herself and her mother and the trees her father and brother, and their relations to one another. At this point I began to interpret, and told her that what she was concerned with was the sex difference between her father and mother and between herself and her brother and also the difference between grown-ups and children. She agreed with me and reacted to the interpretation immediately by making alterations in her drawings, which had hitherto been quite monotonous. (Nevertheless, for some months the analysis still proceeded chiefly with the help of her drawings.) In the case of Inge, aged seven, I was unable for several hours to find any means of approach. I kept up a conversation about her school and kindred subjects with some difficulty, and her attitude towards me was very mistrustful and reserved. She only became more lively as she began telling me about a poem which she had read at school. She thought it remarkable that long words should have alternated in it with short ones. A little while earlier she had spoken about some birds that she had seen fly into a garden but not out again. These observations had followed upon a remark she let fall to the effect that she and her girl friend had done as well at some game as the boys. I explained to her that she was occupied by a wish to know where children (the birds) really came from and also to understand better the sex difference between boys and girls (long and short words—the comparative skill of boys and girls). In this case too, I could see that this interpretation had the same effect on Inge as it had had on Grete. Contact was established, the material she brought became richer, and the analysis was set going.

In these and other cases, the repressed desire for knowledge dominated the picture. If in analyses of the latency period we choose this point for making our first interpretations—by which, of course, I do not mean explanations in the intellectual sense, but only interpretations of the material as it emerges in the form of doubts and fears or unconscious knowledge or sexual theories[1] and

[1] Sexual interest serves in this way as a means of approach to the repressed material. As a result of my interpretation Inge and Grete, for example, asked for no further sexual enlightenment but brought up material which opened the way to their anxiety and sense of guilt. This effect was brought about by the removal of a piece of repression. Inge, it is true, was partly conscious of her interest in the origin of children, but not of her broodings over sex differences nor of her anxiety on the subject. Grete had repressed both. The effect my interpretations had on both children was due to the fact that I demonstrated their interest to them by means of the material they gave me and so established a connection between their sexual curiosity, latent anxiety and sense of guilt. Purely intellectual explanations not only usually fail to answer the questions

so on—we soon come up against feelings of guilt and anxiety in the child and have thus established the analytic situation.

The effect of interpretation depends on having removed a certain amount of repression and shows itself in several ways. (1) The analytical situation is established. (2) The child's imagination becomes freer. Its means of representation grow in richness and extent; its speech becomes more abundant and the stories it tells more full of phantasy. (3) The child not only experiences relief but gets a certain understanding of the purpose of analytic work, and this is analogous to the adult's insight into his illness.[1] In this way, interpretations lead gradually to the overcoming of the difficulties mentioned at the beginning of the chapter, which, owing to the developmental conditions of the latency period, stand in the way of the commencement and the course of the analysis.

During the latency period, in consonance with the more intense repression of its phantasy and with its more developed ego, the child's games are more adapted to reality and less phantastic than those of the small child. In its games with water, for instance, we do not find such direct representations of oral wishes or of wetting and dirtying as in smaller children; its occupations serve the reactive tendencies much more and take on rationalized forms like cooking, cleaning and so on. I consider that the great importance of the rational element in the play of children at this age is not only due to a more intense repression of their phantasy, but also due to an obsessional over-emphasis of reality which is part and parcel of the special developmental conditions of the latency period.

In dealing with typical cases of this period we see again and again how the older child's ego, which is still much weaker than that of the adult, endeavours to strengthen its position by placing all its energies in the service of the repressive tendencies and finds

---

that are uppermost in the child's mind but stir up repressed material without dissolving it. When this happens the child reacts with the aversion to the explanation. In my paper, 'The Child's Resistance to Analysis' [which appears as part of 'The Development of a Child'—1921, *Writings*, 1], I put forward the view that children can only accept sexual enlightenment in so far as their own anxiety and internal conflicts do not prevent them, and that therefore their resistance to such enlightenment should be regarded as a symptom. Since then this view seems to have been generally accepted (cf. 'Über Sexuelle Aufklärung', *Sonderheft der Zeitschrift für psychoanalytische Pädagogik*, 1927; and O. Fenichel, 'Some Infantile Theories not Hitherto Described', 1927). Whenever an intellectual explanation does give relief it has usually succeeded in resolving some piece of repression in the top levels of the mind. Frank explanations in answer to *spontaneous* questions on this subject are received by the child as a proof of confidence and love and help to alleviate his sense of guilt by bringing sexual questions into open discussion.

[1] As I pointed out in Chapter II, this is equally true of very small children.

support in this endeavour by reality. It is here that I see the reason why we cannot expect assistance from the ego for the analytic work which runs counter to all the child's ego trends, and why we should come as soon as possible to terms with the unconscious agencies in order to assure the co-operation of the ego by these means step by step.

In contrast to small children, who are usually more inclined to play with toys at the beginning of their analysis, children in the latency period very soon start acting parts. With children of five to ten years I have played games of this sort which have been continued from one hour to another over periods of weeks and months, and one game has only given place to another when all its details and connections have been clarified by analysis. The game which is then next started commonly displays the same complex-directed phantasies in another form and with new details which lead to deeper connections. The seven-year-old Inge, for instance, could be described as a normal child so far as her nature and behaviour was concerned, in spite of certain troubles whose full extent was only revealed by analysis.[1] For a considerable time she played an office game with me, in which she was the manager who gave orders of every sort and dictated letters and wrote them, in contrast to her own severe inhibitions in learning and writing. In this her desires to be a man were clearly recognizable. One day she gave up this game and began to play at school with me. It is to be noted that she not only found her lessons difficult and unpleasant but had a great dislike for school itself. She now played at school with me for

[1] Inge's analysis, which occupied 375 hours in all, was in the nature of a prophylactic treatment. Her main trouble was an inhibition in regard to school, which did not seem very marked when she first came to me but which, in the course of her analysis, was discovered to be very deep-seated. Inge was a lively and active child, with a good adaptation to society and throughout could be called a normal child. Nevertheless, her analysis effected some re-markable changes in her. It turned out that her liveliness was founded on an active homosexual attitude and her generally good relations to boys on an identification with them. Moreover, analysis first disclosed the severity of the depressions she was liable to, and it showed that behind her apparent self-confidence there was a severe sense of inferiority and a fear of failure which were responsible for her difficulties in regard to school life. After her analysis she had a much freer, happier amd more open nature, her relations to her mother were more affectionate and frank and her sublimations increased in number and stability. Inge succeeded in entering the age of puberty without difficulty and developed satisfactorily. A change in her sexual attitude, as a result of which her feminine components were able to come to the fore to a much greater extent, augured well for her future life. In the seven years that have elapsed since the end of her treatment, she has developed very satis-factorily and has successfully entered the age of puberty.

quite a long time, by taking the part of the mistress while I represented the pupil; the kind of mistakes she made me make gave me important clues to the reasons for her own failure at school. Inge, as a youngest child, had, in spite of all appearances to the contrary, found the superiority of her elder brothers and sisters very hard to put up with, and when she went to school she had felt that the old situation was being reproduced. As the details of the lessons which she gave in the role of a mistress revealed, in the last resort and at a very early age, her own desire for knowledge[1] had not been satisfied and was repressed; and this was what made the superiority of her brothers and sisters so unbearable and the lessons at school so distasteful.

We have seen how Inge first made an extensive identification with her father [as shown by the game in which she was the manager] and then with her mother as shown by the game in which, reversing the mother-daughter role, she was the mistress and I the pupil. In her next game she was a toy-shop woman and I had to buy all sorts of things for my children, [this demonstrating] what her mother should have given her. The objects which she sold to me were penis-symbols (fountain-pens, pencils, etc.) and the child to whom I was to give them would, thanks to them, become clever and nimble. The wish-fulfilment in this game, in which the little girl's homosexual attitude and castration complex were once more uppermost, was to the effect that her mother should give her her father's penis so that with its help she might supplant her father and win her mother's love. In the further course of the game, however, she preferred to sell me as her customer things to eat for my children, and it became evident that her father's penis and her mother's breast were the objects of her deepest oral desires and that it was her oral frustrations that were at the bottom of her troubles in general and her difficulty in regard to learning in particular.

Owing to the feelings of guilt bound up with the oral-sadistic introjection of her mother's breast, Inge had at a very early stage looked upon her oral frustration as a punishment.[2] Her impulses

---

[1] In Chapter X the view is put forward that *in general* the first and most fundamental beginnings of the desire for knowledge appear at a very early stage of development, before the child is able to speak. In my experience these early questionings (which apparently remain entirely or partly unconscious) set in at the same time as the earliest sexual theories and the increase of sadism, towards the middle of the first year of life. They belong, that is, to the period which in my view ushers in the Oedipus conflict.

[2] According to Ernest Jones the child always regards deprivations as deliberately imposed on it by the persons about it (cf. his 'Early Development of Female Sexuality', 1927; also Joan Riviere's contribution to 'A Symposium on Child-Analysis', 1928).

of aggression against her mother, which arose out of the Oedipus situation, and her wish to rob her of her children had strengthened these early feelings of guilt and led to a very deep, though concealed, fear of her mother. This was why she was unable to maintain the feminine position and tried to identify herself with her father. But she was also unable to accept the homosexual position, on account of an excessive fear of her father, whose penis she wanted to steal. To this was added her feeling of inability to *do* in consequence of her inability to *know* (i.e. the early frustration of her desire for knowledge) to which her position as youngest child had contributed. She therefore failed at school in the activities that answered to her masculine components; nor, since she could not maintain the feminine position, which involved the conception and bearing of children in phantasy, was she able to develop feminine sublimations derived from that position. Owing to her anxiety and feelings of guilt, moreover, she also failed in the relation of child to mother (e.g. in her relation to the school-mistress), since she unconsciously equated the absorption of knowledge with the gratification of oral-sadistic desires, and this involved the destruction of her mother's breast and her father's penis.

While Inge was a failure in reality, in imagination she played every role. Thus in the game I have described, in which she played the part of office-manager, she represented her successes in the role of father; as the school-mistress she had numerous children, and at the same time exchanged her role of the youngest child for that of the oldest and most intelligent; while in the game of being a seller of toys and food, admittedly by a double displacement of roles, she reversed the oral frustrations.

I have brought this case forward to show how, in order to classify the underlying psychological connections, we have to investigate not only all the details of a given game but the reason why one game is changed for another. I have often found that such a change of game allows us an insight into the causes of changes from one psychological position to another or of fluctuations between such positions, and hence into the dynamics of the interplay of the forces of the mind.

The next case gives an opportunity of demonstrating the application of a mixed technique. Kenneth, aged nine and a half, a very infantile boy for his age, was fearful, shy and seriously inhibited, and he suffered from severe anxiety. From an early age he had suffered to a marked degree from morbid brooding. He was a complete failure at his lessons, his knowledge of school subjects being that of a child of about seven. At home he was exceedingly aggressive, sneering and difficult to control. His unsublimated and apparently uninhibited interest in all sexual matters was unusual; he used obscene words by preference and exhibited himself and masturbated in an unusually shameless manner for a child of his age.[1]

I shall outline his history briefly. At a very early age Kenneth had been seduced by his nurse. His memory of it was quite conscious, and the event had later become known to his mother. According to her, the nurse, Mary, had been very devoted to the child but had been very strict in her insistence upon his cleanliness. Kenneth's memories of being seduced went back to the beginning of his fifth year, but it is certain that it actually took place very much earlier. He reported, apparently with pleasure and without inhibition, that his nurse used to take him with her when she went to have her bath and used to ask him to rub her genitals. Besides this, he had nothing but good to tell of her; he stated that she had loved him and for a long time denied that she had treated him severely. At the beginning of his analysis he reported a dream which he had dreamt repeatedly since his fifth year: *he was touching an unknown woman's genitals and masturbating her.*

His fear of me started in the first session. Shortly after the beginning of his analysis he had the following anxiety dream: *All of a sudden a man was sitting in my chair instead of me. I then undressed, and he was horrified to see that I had an unusually large male genital organ.* In connection with the interpretation of this dream, rich material came up in regard to his sexual theory of the 'mother with a penis', a mental image which, as analysis proved, was very definitely embodied for him in Mary. He had evidently been afraid of her when he was a small child, for she had beaten him severely, but he was still unable to admit this fact until a later dream made him alter his attitude.

Infantile as Kenneth was in many respects, he very soon gained a clear insight into the aim and necessity of his analysis. He used sometimes to give associations in the manner of older children and chose of his own accord to lie on the sofa while he did so. The greater part of his analysis, indeed, was carried out in this way. Soon, however, he began to supplement his verbal material with action. He picked up some pencils from the table and made them represent people. Another time he brought some clothes pegs with him and these in turn became people and fought with one another. He also made them represent projectiles and constructed buildings

---

[1] Kenneth's treatment occupied 225 hours and could not be carried any further owing to external circumstances. His neurosis, though not actually removed, had by then been materially reduced. As far as his practical life was concerned, the partial results obtained led to the diminution of a number of difficulties: among other things he was able to comply better with the requirements of his school life and of his upbringing in general.

out of them. All this took place on the sofa on which he lay. Finally he discovered a box of bricks on the window-sill, brought the little play-table up to the sofa and accompanied his associations with representations by means of the bricks.

Of Kenneth's second dream, which carried the analysis a long step further, I will now relate as much as is necessary for illustrating the technique employed. *He was in the bathroom and was urinating; a man came in and fired off a bullet at his ear which knocked it off.* While he was telling me this dream Kenneth carried out various operations with the bricks, which he explained to me in the following way. He himself, his father, his brother and the nurse Mary were each represented by a brick. All these people were lying asleep in different rooms (the walls of which were also indicated by bricks). Mary got up, took a big stick (another brick) and came towards him. She was going to do something to him because he had been misbehaving himself in some way. (It turned out that he had masturbated and wetted himself.) While she was beating him with the stick he began to masturbate her and she at once stopped beating him. When she began to beat him again he again masturbated her and she stopped; and this process was repeated again and again till at last, in spite of everything, she threatened to kill him with the stick. His brother then came to his rescue.

Kenneth was exceedingly surprised when he recognized at last from this game and its associations that he had really been afraid of Mary. At the same time, however, part of his fear of both parents had also become conscious. His associations showed clearly that behind his fear of Mary lurked the fear of a bad mother in league with a castrating father. The latter was represented in his dream by the man who shot his ear off in the bathroom—the very place in which he had often masturbated his nurse.

Kenneth's fear of his two parents united against him, who were perpetually copulating with each other in his phantasy, proved to be extremely important in his analysis. It was only after I had made many subsequent observations of the same kind, which I described in my paper 'Early Stages of the Oedipus Conflict' (1928) and which I shall discuss in the second part of this book in greater detail [Chapter VIII], that I realized the fact that the fear of the 'woman with a penis' is founded upon a sexual theory, formed at a very early stage of development, to the effect that the mother incorporates the father's penis in the act of coitus,[1] so that in the last resort the

---

[1] In his 'Homosexualität und Ödipuskomplex' (1926) Felix Boehm has pointed out that the idea of the concealed female penis receives its pathogenic value by having been brought into connection, in the unconscious, with the idea of the father's dreaded penis hidden inside the mother.

woman with a penis signifies the two parents, joined together. I will illustrate this from the material which has been described here. In his dream Kenneth was first attacked by a man, but afterwards it was Mary who attacked him. She represented, as his associations showed, the 'woman with a penis', who stood for his mother united with his father. His father, who had earlier appeared as a man, was in the later part of his dream represented by his penis alone, i.e., by the stick with which Mary struck him.

I may here point out a feature which the technique of early analysis has in common with the play technique as it is employed in some cases of older children. Kenneth had become conscious of an important part of his early history by means of acting rather than of speaking. As his analysis proceeded he used often to get severe anxiety and could then only communicate his associations to me if he supplemented them by representations with the bricks. Indeed it happened not infrequently that, when this anxiety came on, words quite failed him and all he could do was to play. After his anxiety had again been reduced as the result of interpretations, he was able to speak more freely once more.

Another example of modification in technique is provided by the method I adopted with Werner, a nine-year-old obsessional neurotic. This boy, who behaved in many respects like an adult obsessional and in whom morbid brooding was a marked symptom, also suffered from severe anxiety which was, however, chiefly exhibited in great irritability and in fits of rage.[1] A great part of this analysis was carried on by means of toys and with the help of drawing. I was obliged to sit beside him at the play-table and to play with him even to a greater extent than I usually have to with most small children. Sometimes I had even to carry out the actions involved in the game alone by myself under his direction. For instance, I had to build up the bricks, move the carts about and so on, while he merely supervised my actions. The reason he gave for this was that his hands

---

[1] Werner's case presented the following symptoms: anxiety and timidity, which showed themselves in various forms but especially in anxiety at school and in great and increasing difficulties in learning; obsessional ceremonials that were constantly becoming more elaborate and took up hours at a time; and a severely neurotic character which made his upbringing extremely difficult. His analysis, which comprised 210 hours of treatment, removed these difficulties to a great extent. The boy's general development at the present time (five years after the end of the treatment) is very favourable. The obsessional ceremonials have ceased, he is good at his work, enjoys going to school, gets on with his associates both at home and at school and is well adjusted socially. His relations both with his immediate and his remoter environment are good. Above all, however—and this was not the case before—he takes pleasure in the most varied sorts of activities and sport and feels well.

sometimes trembled very much, so that he could not put the toys in their places or might upset or damage them. This trembling was a sign of the onset of an anxiety attack. I could in most cases cut the attacks short by carrying out the game as he wanted it, at the same time interpreting, in connection with his anxiety, the meaning of the actions (in the game). His fear of his own aggressiveness and his disbelief in his capacity to love had made him lose all hope of restoring the parents and brothers and sisters, whom, in his phantasy, he had attacked. Hence his fear that he might accidentally knock down the bricks and things which had already been put up. This distrust of his own constructive tendencies and of his ability to make restitution was one of the causes of his severe inhibition in learning and playing.

After his anxiety had been resolved to a large extent, Werner played his games without assistance from me. He did a great many drawings and gave abundant associations to them. In the last part of his analysis he produced his material chiefly in the form of free associations. Lying on the couch—a position in which he, like Kenneth, preferred to give his associations—he would narrate continuous phantasies of adventure in which apparatus, mechanical contrivances and so on played a large part. In these stories the material that had before been represented in his drawings appeared again, but enriched in many details.

Werner's intense and acute anxiety was mainly expressed, as I have said, in the form of fits of rage and aggressiveness and in a sneering, defiant and fault-finding attitude. He had no insight into his illness and used to insist that there was no reason why he should be analysed; and for a long period, whenever his resistances came up, he used to behave to me in a contemptuous and angry way. At home, too, he was a difficult child to manage, and his family would hardly have been able to induce him to go on with his treatment, if I had not very soon succeeded in resolving his anxiety bit by bit until his resistance to analysis was almost entirely confined to the analytic hour.

We now come to a case which presented technical difficulties of a quite unusual kind. The nine-and-a-half-year-old Egon displayed no very definite symptoms, but his development as a whole made a disquieting impression. He was completely withdrawn even with regard to those nearest to him, said only what was absolutely neces-sary, had almost no emotional ties and no friends, and there was nothing that interested him or pleased him. He was, it is true, a good scholar, but, and as analysis showed, only on an obsessional basis. When asked whether he would like anything or not, his stereotyped answer would always be 'I don't mind'. The un-childlike, strained expression of his face and the stiffness of his movements were most striking. His withdrawal from reality went so far that he did not see what was going on around him and failed to recognize familiar friends when he met them. Analysis revealed the presence of strong psychotic features which were increasing and would, in all probability, have led to the onset of schizophrenia at the age of puberty.

Here is a short summary of the boy's history. When he was about four years old he had been repeatedly threatened by his father for masturbating and told that he must at any rate always confess when he did it. In connection with these threats, marked changes in his character occurred. Egon began to tell lies and to have frequent outbursts of rage. Later his aggressiveness receded into the background and instead his whole attitude became more and more one of affect-free defiance and of increasing withdrawal from the external world.

For several weeks I got Egon to lie on the couch (which he did not refuse to do and apparently preferred to playing games) and tried in various other ways to set the treatment going, till I was forced to recognize that my attempts along these lines were hopeless. It became clear to me that the child's difficulty in speaking was so deeply rooted that my first task must be to overcome it analytically. The boy's need to help himself out by acting became clear to me when I realized that the scanty material I had so far been able to get from him had mostly been inferred from the way in which he played with his fingers while he let fall an occasional word—not amounting to more than a few sentences in a session— and I accordingly asked him once more whether, after all, he was not interested in my little toys. He gave his usual reply, 'I don't mind'. Nevertheless, he looked at the things on the play-table and proceeded to occupy himself with the little carts, and with them alone. There now developed a monotonous game which occupied his whole hour for weeks on end. Egon made the carts run along the table and then threw them on to the ground in my direction; I gathered by a look from him that I was to pick them up and push them back to him. In order to get away from the role of the prying father, against whom his defiance was directed, I played with him for weeks in silence and made no interpretations, simply trying to establish rapport by playing with him. During all this time the details of the game remained absolutely the same, but, monotonous as it was (and incidentally extremely tiring for me), there were many small points to be noted in it. It appeared that in his case, as in all analyses of boys, making a cart move along meant masturbation and coitus, making carts hit together meant coitus, and comparison of a larger cart with a smaller meant rivalry with his father or his father's penis.

When, after some weeks, I clarified this material to Egon in connection with what was already understood[1] it had a far-reaching effect in two directions. At home his parents were struck by the much greater freedom of his behaviour; and in analysis he showed what I have found to be the typical reaction to the resolving effect of interpretation. He began to add new details to his monotonous game—details which, though at first only noticeable to close observation, became clearer and, as time went on, brought about a complete alteration of the game. From merely pushing carts along, Egon went on to a building game, and with increasing skill he began to pile the carts one upon another to a very great height and to compete with me over it. Only now did he proceed for the first time to use the bricks, and it soon became evident that the things he built up were, however skilfully the fact was concealed, always human beings—or genitals—of both sexes. From this kind of building, Egon went on to a quite peculiar form of drawing. Without looking at the paper, he would roll a pencil about between his two hands and in this way produce lines. Out of these scrawls he then himself deciphered shapes, and these always represented heads, among which he himself clearly distinguished the male from the female. In the details of these heads and their relations to one another the material that had occurred in the earlier games soon reappeared—namely his uncertainty about the difference between the sexes and about coitus between his parents, the questions that were connected in his mind with these subjects, the phantasies in which he as a third party played a part in the sexual intercourse of his parents, etc. But his hatred and his destructive impulses, too, became obvious in the cutting out and cutting to bits of these heads, which at one and the same time represented the children in his mother's body and his parents themselves. It was only now that we realized that his piling up of carts as high as possible represented his mother's pregnant body for which he had envied her and whose contents he wished to steal from her. He had strong feelings of rivalry with his mother and his wish to rob her of his father's penis

[1] Further analysis showed that it had been quite pointless to withhold interpretation of the material for so long. Only after fifteen months, shortly before the termination of the analysis was the inhibition in speech overcome. I have never yet in any analysis seen any advantage follow from such a policy of non-interpretation. In most cases in which I have tried the plan I have very soon had to abandon it because acute anxiety has developed and there has been a risk of the analysis being broken off. In Egon's case, where the anxiety was under such powerful restraint, it was possible to continue the experiment longer.

and of her children had led to an acute fear of her. These representations were afterwards supplemented by the cutting out that he did, in which he gradually acquired considerable skill. Just as in his building activities, the shapes which he cut out represented only human beings. The way in which he brought these shapes into contact with one another, their different sizes, whether they represented men or women, whether they had some parts missing or too many, when and how he began to cut them to pieces—all these considerations took us deep into both his inverted and his direct Oedipus complex. His rivalry with his mother, based on his strong passive homosexual attitude, and the anxiety he felt concerning it, both in regard to his father and his mother, became more and more evident. His hatred of his siblings and the destructive impulses he had had towards them when his mother was pregnant found expression in the cutting out of shapes which were meant to represent small and inferior human beings. Here, too, the order in which he played his games was important. After cutting out and cutting to pieces, he would start building as an act of restoration; and similarly, the figures he had cut up he proceeded to over-decorate, urged by reactive tendencies, and so on. In all these representations, however, there always reappeared the repressed questions and the repressed early intense desire for knowledge which also proved to be an important factor in his inability to speak, his withdrawn character and his lack of interests.

Egon's inhibition in play dated back to the age of four, and in part to an even earlier time. He had made buildings before he was three and had begun cutting out paper rather later, but had only kept it up for quite a short time and even at that time had only cut out heads. He had never drawn at all, and after the age of four he had taken no pleasure in any of these earlier pursuits. What appeared now, therefore, were sublimations rescued from profound repression, partly in the form of revivals and partly as new creations; and the childlike and quite primitive manner in which he set about each of these pursuits belonged really to the level of a three- or four-year-old child. It may be added that simultaneously with these changes the boy's whole character took a turn for the better.

Nevertheless, his inhibition in speech was for a long time only slightly relieved. It is true that he gradually began to answer the questions which I put to him during his games in a freer and fuller way, but on the other hand I was for a long time unable to get him to give free associations of the kind that are usual in older children. It was not until much later and during the last part of the treatment, which occupied 425 hours in all, that we fully recognized and explored the paranoid factors underlying his inhibition in speech, which was then completely removed.[1] As his anxiety substantially diminished he began of his own accord to give me single associations in writing. Later on he used to whisper them to me and asked me to answer him in a low voice. It became ever clearer that he was afraid of being overheard by someone in the room, and there were some parts of the room which he would not go near on any account. If, for instance, his ball had rolled under the couch or the cupboard or into a dark corner, I had to fetch it back for him; while, as his anxiety increased, he would once more assume the same rigid posture and fixed expression which had been so marked in him at the beginning of his analysis. It came out that he suspected the presence of hidden persecutors watching him from all these places and even from the ceiling, and that his ideas of persecution went back, in the last resort, to his fear of the many penises inside his mother's body and his own. This paranoic fear of the penis as a persecutor had been very greatly increased by his father's attitude in watching him and cross-questioning him in regard to masturbation and had made him turn away from his mother as well, she being in league with his father (the 'woman with a penis'). As his belief in a 'good' mother became stronger in the course of analysis, he came to treat me more and more as an ally and as a protector from persecutors who were threatening him from every quarter. It was not until his anxiety in this respect had lessened and with it his estimation of the number and dangerousness of his persecutors, that he was able to speak and move more freely.[2]

The last part of Egon's treatment was conducted almost exclusively by means of free associations. There is no doubt in my mind that I only succeeded in treating and curing this boy by being able to gain access to his unconscious with the assistance of the play technique used for small children. Whether it would have been still possible to do this at a later age seems to me doubtful.[3]

[1] I intend to go more fully into this case in Chapter IX.

[2] Melitta Schmideberg has discussed a similar case in her paper, 'A Contribution to the Psychology of Persecutory Ideas and Delusions' (1931). The patient was a boy of about sixteen who scarcely spoke at all in his analysis. Here again the inhibition in speech was caused by ideas of persecution, and the boy did not begin to associate at all freely until analysis had lessened his paranoic anxiety.

[3] In general, too, the result of Egon's analysis was completely satisfactory. His face was no longer like a mask and the rigidity of his movements passed away. He began so take pleasure in the games, pastimes and interests common to boys of his age. His relations with his family and the world became good and he grew happy and contented. When last I heard from him, three and a half years after his analysis was finished, this healthy development had continued and had not been disturbed by certain severe strains to which he had been subjected in the meanwhile.

Though it is true that in general we make great use of verbal associations in dealing with children in the latency period, yet in many cases we can do so only in a manner that differs from that employed with adults. With children like Kenneth, for example, who soon consciously recognized the help given him by psycho-analysis and realized his need for it, or even with the much younger Erna, whose wish to be cured was very strong, it was possible from the very beginning occasionally to ask: 'Well? What are you thinking of now?' But with many children of under nine or ten it would be useless to put such a question. The way in which a child is to be questioned follows from the way it plays or associates.

If we watch the play of a quite small child we shall soon observe that the bricks, the pieces of paper and, indeed, all the things around it represent something else. If we ask it 'What is that?' while it is occupied with these articles (it is true that as a rule before we do this a certain amount of analysis must have been done and a transference established) we shall find out quite a lot. We shall often be told, for instance, that the stones in the water are children who want to come on shore or that they are people fighting one another. The question 'What is that?' will lead on naturally to the further question 'Well, what are they doing?' or 'Where are they now?' and so on. We have to elicit the associations of older children in a similar, though modified, fashion; but this, as a rule, can only be achieved when the repression of phantasy and the mistrust, which are so much stronger in them, have been diminished by a certain amount of analysis and the analytic situation has been established.

To go back to the analysis of the seven-year-old Inge. When she was playing the part of office-manager, writing letters, distributing work and so on, I once asked her: 'What is there in this letter?' and she promptly replied: 'You'll find that out when you get it.' When I received it, however, I found that it contained nothing but scribbles.[1] So shortly afterwards I said: 'Mr. X—(who also figured in the game) has told me to ask you what there is in the letter, as he must know, and would be glad if you would read it all out to him over the telephone.' Whereupon she told me, without making any difficulty, the whole contents of the phantasy letter and at the same time gave a number of illuminating associations. Another time, I

[1] Inge, who, as I have already mentioned, suffered from a severe inhibition in writing, had a burning wish to write 'quickly and beautifully' like grown-ups. The compromise between this wish and her inhibition was scribbling, which represented in her phantasy beautiful and skilful handwriting. Her wish if possible to excel the grown-ups in writing and her very strong ambition and curiosity, existing as they did side by side with a deep feeling that she knew nothing and could do nothing, played a great part in her failure in real life.

had to pretend to be a doctor. When I asked her what was supposed to be the matter with her, she answered: 'Oh, that makes no difference.' I then began to have a proper consultation with her like a doctor, and said: 'Now, Mrs —, you really must tell me exactly where you feel the pain.' From this there arose further questions—why she had fallen ill, when the illness had begun, etc. Since she played the part of the patient several times in succession I obtained abundant and deeply-buried material in this way. And when the situation was reversed and she was the doctor and I the patient, the medical advice she gave me supplied me with further information.

I shall now summarize what has been said in this chapter. In dealing with children of the latency period, it is essential above all to establish contact with their unconscious phantasies, and this is done by interpreting the symbolic content of their material in relation to their anxiety and feelings of guilt. But since the repression of phantasy in this stage of development is much more severe than in earlier stages, we often have to find access to the unconscious through representations which are to all appearances entirely devoid of phantasy. We must also, in typical analyses of the latency period, be prepared to find that it is only possible to resolve the child's repressions step by step and with much labour. In some cases for weeks or even months at a time the associations we get do not seem to have any meaning, for instance, reports out of newspapers or accounts of the contents of books or monotonous school notes. Moreover, such activities as monotonous obsessive drawing, building, sewing or making things—especially when we obtain few associations to them—seem to offer no means of approach to the phantasy life. But we need only recall the examples of Grete and Egon, mentioned earlier in this chapter, to remind ourselves that even activities and talk so completely without phantasy as these do open the way to the unconscious if we do not merely regard them as expressions of resistance but treat them as true material. By paying enough attention to small indications and by taking as our starting-point for interpretation the connection between the symbolism, sense of guilt and anxiety that accompany those representations, I found that there is always an opportunity for beginning and carrying on the work of analysis.

But the fact that in child analysis we get into communication with the unconscious before a fruitful relation with the ego has been established, does not mean that the ego has somehow been excluded from participating in the analytic work. Any exclusion of this kind would be impossible, considering that the ego is so closely connected with the id and the super-ego and that we can only find access to the unconscious through it. Nevertheless, analysis does not apply itself to the ego as such (as educational methods do) but only seeks to open up a path to the unconscious agencies of the mind—those agencies which are decisive for the formation of the ego.

To return to our examples once more. As we have seen, the analysis of Grete (aged seven) was for a long time almost entirely carried on by means of her drawings. She used, it will be remembered, to draw houses and trees of various sizes which she alternated in an obsessive way. Now, starting from these unimaginative and obsessional pictures, I might have tried to stimulate her phantasy and link it up with other activities of her ego in the way in which a sympathetic teacher might do. I could have got her to want to decorate and beautify her houses or to put them and the trees into a town with streets and thus to have connected her activities with whatever artistic or topographical interests she might chance to possess. Or I could have gone on from her trees to make her interested in the difference between one kind of tree and another, and perhaps in this way have stimulated her curiosity about natural history. Had any attempt of this kind succeeded, we should expect her ego-interests to come more to the fore and the analyst to get into closer contact with her ego. But experience has shown that in many cases such a stimulation of the child's imagination fails in its attempts to effect a loosening of the repression and thus to find a foothold for the beginning of analytic work.[1] Moreover, such a procedure is very often not feasible, because the child suffers from so much latent anxiety that we are obliged to establish the analytic situation as quickly as possible and begin actual analytical work at once. And even where there is a chance of gaining access to the unconscious by making the ego our starting-point, we shall find that the results are small in comparison with the length of time taken to obtain them. For the increase in the wealth and significance of the material thus gained is only a seeming one; in reality we shall not be doing more than meeting the same unconscious material but in more striking forms. In Grete's case, for instance, we might have been able to stimulate her curiosity and thus, in favourable circumstances, have led her to become interested, say, in the entrances and exits of houses and in the differences between trees and the way they grew. But these expanded interests would only be a less disguised version of the material she had been showing us in the monotonous drawings quite early in her analysis. The big and small trees and the big and small houses which she kept on drawing in a compulsive manner represented her mother and father and herself and her brother, as was indicated by the

[1] Cf. the analysis of Egon and Grete described in this chapter.

difference in the sizes, shapes and colours of her drawings and by the order in which they were done. What underlay them was her repressed curiosity about the difference between the sexes and other allied problems; and by interpreting them in that sense I was able to get at her anxiety and sense of guilt and to get the analysis going.

Now if the material which underlies noticeable and complicated representations is no different from that which underlies meagre ones, it is irrevelant from the point of view of analysis which of the two kinds of representation is chosen as the point of departure for interpretation. For in child analysis it is interpretation alone, in my experience, which starts the analytic process and keeps it going. Therefore it is also possible to interpret with certainty monotonous associations lacking phantasy, provided that the analyst understands the material sufficiently and links it with the latent anxiety. If one proceeds in this manner, strong ego-interests and sublimations will originate side by side with the resolution of quantities of anxiety and the removal of repression. In this way, for instance, Ilse—whose case will be considered in greater detail in the following chapter— gradually evolved out of her monotonous and obsessive drawing a decided gift for handicraft and skill in drawing, without my having in any way suggested or encouraged such an activity.

Before I go on to the subject of analyses of puberty, however, there still remains one problem to discuss. It is not, strictly speaking, of a technical nature but it is of importance in the work of the child analyst. I refer to the analyst's dealings with the parents of his patients. In order for him to be able to do his work there must be a certain relation of confidence between himself and the child's parents. The child is dependent on them and so they are included in the field of the analysis; yet it is not they who are being analysed and they can therefore only be influenced by ordinary psychological means. The relationship of the parents to their child's analyst entails difficulties of a peculiar kind, since it touches closely upon their own complexes. Their child's neurosis weighs very heavily upon the parents' sense of guilt, and at the same time as they turn to analysis for help, they regard the necessity of it as a proof of their guilt with regard to their child's illness. It is, moreover, very trying for them to have the details of their family life revealed to the analyst. To this must be added, particularly in the case of the mother, jealousy of the confidence which is established between the child and its (woman) analyst. This jealousy, which is to a very large extent based upon the subject's rivalry with her own mother-imago,[1] is also very noticeable in governesses and nurses, who are

[1] In certain cases in which I have analysed a mother and child simultaneously it has emerged that in the mother's unconscious there was a fear of

often anything but friendly in their attitude towards analysis. These, and other factors, which remain for the most part unconscious, give rise to a more or less ambivalent attitude in the parents, especially the mother, towards the analyst, and this is not removed by the fact of their having conscious insight into their child's need for analytic treatment. Hence, even if the child's relatives are consciously well disposed to its analysis, we must expect that they will to some extent be a disturbing element in it. The degree of difficulty they will cause will, of course, depend on their unconscious attitude and on the amount of ambivalence they have. This is why I have met with no less hindrance where the parents were familiar with analysis than where they knew practically nothing about it. For the same reason, too, I consider any far-reaching theoretical explanations to the parents before the beginning of an analysis as not only unnecessary but out of place, since such explanations are liable to have an unfavourable effect upon their own complexes. I content myself with making a few general statements about the meaning and effect of analysis, mention the fact that, in the course of it, the child will be given information upon sexual subjects and prepare the parents for the possibility of other difficulties arising temporarily during the treatment. In every case I refuse absolutely to report any details of the analysis to them. The child who gives me its confidence has no less claim to my discretion than the adult.

What we should aim at in establishing relations with the parents is, in my judgment, in the first place to get them to assist in our work principally by refraining as much as possible from all interference, external as well as internal, such as encouraging the child, through questions or otherwise, to talk about its analysis or lending any kind of support to whatever resistances against the analysis it may give utterance to. But we do need their more active co-operation on those occasions when the child is overtaken by really acute anxiety and violent resistances. In such situations—I may here recall the cases of Ruth and Trude[1]—it devolves upon those in charge of the child to find ways and means of getting it to come in spite of its difficulties. As far as my experience goes, this has always been possible; for, in general, even when resistance is strong there is a positive transference to the analyst, as well; that is to say, the child's attitude to its analysis is ambivalent. The help given us by the child's environment must, however, never be allowed to

being robbed of her children. The child's analyst represented to her a stern mother who was demanding the restitution of the children she had stolen away and was at the same time discovering and punishing the aggressive impulses she had once entertained against her brothers and sisters.

[1] See Chapter II.

become an essential adjunct to analytic work. Periods of such intense resistance should only occur rarely and not last long. The work of analysis must either prevent it, or, if that cannot be done, rapidly resolve it.

If we can succeed in establishing a good relation with the child's parents and in being sure of their unconscious co-operation, we are occasionally in a position to obtain useful knowledge about the child's behaviour outside analysis, such as any changes, appearances or disappearances of its symptoms that may occur in connection with the analytic work. But if information on these points is only to be got from parents at the price of raising difficulties of another kind, then I prefer to do without it, since, although valuable, it is not indispensable. I always impress upon the parents the necessity of not giving the child occasion to believe that any steps they may take in its upbringing are due to my advice, and of keeping education and analysis completely separated. In this way the analysis remains, as it should, a purely personal matter between myself and my patient.

With children no less than with adults, I regard it as essential that anlysis should be carried on in the analyst's place of work and that a definite hour should be kept to. As a further means of avoiding displacement of the analytic situation, I have found it necessary not to let the person who brings the child to analysis wait in my house. She brings the child and takes it away again at the appointed time.

Unless the mistakes that are being made are too gross, I avoid interfering with the way in which the child is being brought up, for errors in this field usually depend so largely upon the parents' own complexes that advice generally proves not only useless but calculated to increase their anxiety and sense of guilt; and this will only put further obstacles in the path of the analysis and have an unfavourable effect on the parents' attitude towards their child.[1]

[1] I will take as an illustration the instance of a mother who was well acquainted with analysis and who had great faith in it as a result of the satisfactory progress that was being made by her ten-year-old daughter, then under treatment for a severe neurosis. In spite of this I found it difficult to dissuade her from supervising her daughter's home-work, although it was clear even to her that doing so only increased the child's difficulties with her lessons. When at last, however, she had given this up at my request, I discovered from the child's analysis that her mother always tried to get her to say how the analysis was getting on. Once more at my request she stopped doing this; but then began telling the child that she had dark rings under her eyes in the mornings — a remark with which she had formerly accompanied her prohibition against masturbation. When these comments, which interfered with the analysis, had in turn been put a stop to, the mother began to pay an exaggerated attention to the child's clothes and to comment on the fact that she spent a long time in the W.C., and in this way increased the refractoriness of the child. At this point I gave up all attempts at influencing the mother on

This situation improves greatly after an analysis is finished or when it is far advanced. The removal or lessening of a child's neurosis has a good effect upon its parents. As the mother's difficulties in dealing with her child diminish, her sense of guilt diminishes too, and this improves her attitude towards the child. She becomes more accessible to the analyst's advice in regard to the child's upbringing and—this is the important point—has less *internal* difficulty in following that advice. Nevertheless, I do not, in the light of my own experiences, put much faith in the possibility of affecting the child's environment. It is better to rely upon the results achieved in the child itself, for these will enable it to make a better adaptation even to a difficult environment and will put it in a better position to meet any strains which that environment may lay upon it. This capacity for meeting strains has its limits, of course. Where the child's environment is too unfavourable, we may not be completely successful in our efforts and may have to face the possibility of the recurrence of a neurosis. I have, however, repeatedly found in cases of this kind that the results achieved, even if they did not involve a complete disappearance of the neurosis, have given a great measure of relief to the child in its difficult situation and have led to an improvement in its development. It seems quite safe to assume, moreover, that if we have brought about fundamental changes at the deepest levels, the illness, if it recurs, will not be so severe. It also seems worth while noting that in some cases of this sort a diminution in the child's neurosis has had a favourable effect upon its neurotic environment.[1] It may also sometimes happen that after a successfully completed treatment, the child can be removed to other surroundings, for instance to a boarding-school, a thing which had previously not been possible owing to its neurosis and lack of adaptability.

---

matters of this kind and accepted her interference as part of the analytic material; and after a certain time, during which I made no remonstrance, the interruptions diminished. In this case I was able to establish the fact that they all had the same unconscious meaning for the child; they signified enquiries and reproaches about masturbation. That they also had an analogous origin in the mother's complexes was proved by the fact that her conscious desire to stop the educational mistakes that I objected to was quite unavailing. Indeed, it seemed as though my advice only increased her difficulties in regard to her child. I may remark that I have had similar experiences in a number of other cases.

[1] In the case of a fourteen-year-old boy, for instance, whose family life was extremely trying and unfortunate and who was brought to me for analysis on account of characterological difficulties, I learnt that the improvements brought about in him had had a very beneficial effect on the character of his sister, who was about a year older and had not been analysed, and that his mother's attitude to him had also changed for the better.

Whether it is advisable for the analyst to see the parents fairly frequently, or whether it is wiser to limit meetings with them as much as possible must depend upon the circumstances of each individual case. In a number of instances I have found the second alternative the best means of avoiding friction in my relations with the mother.

The ambivalence which parents have towards their child's analysis also helps to explain a fact which is at once surprising and painful to the inexperienced analyst—namely, that even the most successful treatment is not likely to receive much acknowledgement from the parents. Although I have, repeatedly, come across parents with plenty of insight, yet I have found in the majority of cases that the parents very easily forgot the symptoms which made them bring their child for analysis and overlooked the significance of any improvement that took place. In addition to this we must remember that they are not in a position to form a judgment upon one part and, for that matter, the most important part, of our results. The analysis of adults proclaims its value by removing difficulties which interfere with the patient's life. We ourselves know, though the parents as a rule do not, that in child analysis we are preventing the occurrence of difficulties of the same kind, or even of psychoses. A parent, while regarding serious symptoms in its child as an annoyance, does not as a rule recognize their full importance, for the very reason that they do not have as great an effect on the child's actual life as a neurotic illness has on the life of a grown-up person. And yet I think we shall be well content to forgo our full due of recognition from that quarter so long as we bear in mind that the foremost aim of our work is to secure the well-being of the child and not the gratitude of its mother and father.

Chapter V

THE TECHNIQUE OF ANALYSIS IN PUBERTY

Typical analyses at the age of puberty differ in many essentials from analyses in the latency period. The instinctual impulses of the child are more powerful, the activity of his phantasy greater, and his ego has other aims and a different relation to reality. On the other hand there are points of similarity with the analysis of the small child, owing to the fact that at the age of puberty, we once again meet with a greater dominance of the instinctual impulses and the unconscious, and a much richer phantasy life. Moreover, in puberty manifestations of anxiety and affect are very much more acute than in the latency period, and are a kind of recrudescence of anxiety which is so characteristic of small children.

Warding off and modifying anxiety, which is also an essential function of the ego in the case of the small child is, however, carried out with greater success by the more developed ego of the adolescent. For he has developed his various interests and activities (sports and so on) to a great extent with the object of mastering that anxiety, of over-compensating for it and of masking it from himself and from others. He achieves this in part by assuming the attitude of defiance and rebelliousness that is characteristic of puberty. This provides a great technical difficulty in analysis at puberty; for unless we very quickly gain access to the patient's affects—strong as they are at this age—which he principally manifests in a defiant transference, it may very well happen that the analysis will suddenly be broken off. I may say that in analysing boys of this age I have repeatedly found that they have anticipated violent physical attacks from me during their first sessions.

The fourteen-year-old Ludwig, for example, failed to come to his second session and was only with great difficulty persuaded by his mother to 'give the analysis one more chance'. During this third session I succeeded in showing him that he identified me with the dentist. He asserted, it is true, that he was not afraid of the dentist (of whom my appearance reminded him) but the interpretation of the material that he brought was sufficient to convince him that he was; for it showed him that he expected the dentist as well as myself not only to pull out a tooth but to cut his whole body in pieces. By lessening his anxiety in this respect I established the analytic situation. True, in the further course of his analysis it often happened that large quantities of anxiety were generated, but his resistance was in essence kept within the analytic situation and the continuance of the analysis was assured.

In other cases, too, where I have observed hidden signs of latent anxiety, I have set about interpreting them in the very first session of treatment, and thus at once begun to reduce the child's negative transference. But even in cases where the anxiety is not immediately recognizable it may suddenly break out if the analytic situation is not soon established by interpreting the unconscious material. The material of the adolescent closely resembles that presented by the small child. At the ages of puberty and pre-puberty boys busy themselves in their phantasy with people and things in the same way as small children play with toys. What Peter, aged three years and nine months, expressed by means of little carts and trains and motors, the fourteen-year-old Ludwig expressed in long discourses, lasting for months, on the constructional differences between various kinds of motors, bicycles, motor-cycles, and so on. Where Peter pushed along carts and compared them with one another, Ludwig would be passionately interested in the question of which cars and which drivers would win some race; and whereas Peter paid a tribute of admiration to the toy man's skill in driving and made him perform all sorts of feats, Ludwig for his part, was never tired of singing the praises of his idols of the sporting world.

The phantasy of the adolescent is, however, more adapted to reality and to his stronger ego-interests, and its phantasy content is therefore much less easily recognizable than in small children. Moreover, in keeping with the adolescent's greater activities and his stronger relations to reality, the character of his phantasies[1] undergoes an alteration. The impulse to prove his courage in the real world and the desire for competition with others become more prominent. This is one of the reasons why sport, which offers so much scope for rivalry with others no less than for admiration of their brilliant feats and which also provides a means of overcoming anxiety, plays so large a part in the adolescent's life and phantasies.

These phantasies, which give expression to his rivalry with his

[1] In many analyses of boys of the pre-pubertal period or sometimes even the latency period, most of the time is taken up with stories about Red Indians, or with detective stories, or with phantasies about travel, adventures and fighting, told in serial form and often associated with descriptions of imaginary technical inventions, such as special kinds of boats, machines, cars, contrivances used in warfare, and so on.

father for the possession of his mother and in respect of sexual potency, are accompanied, as in the small child, by feelings of hatred and aggression, in every form and are also often followed by anxiety and a sense of guilt. But the mechanisms peculiar to the age of puberty conceal these facts very much better than do the mechanisms of the small child. The boy at puberty takes as his models heroes, great men, and so on. He can the more easily maintain his identification with these objects since they are far removed from him; and he can also over-compensate for the negative feelings attaching to his father-imagos with greater persistence. In splitting his father-imago, he diverts his aggressive trends to other objects. If, therefore, we bring together his over-compensatory admiration for some objects and his excessive hatred and scorn for others, such as schoolmasters, relations, etc., which we uncover during analysis, we can also find our way in the case of the older boy to a complete analysis of his Oedipus complex and his affects.

In some instances repression has led to such an extreme limitation of personality that the adolescent has only one single definite interest left—say, a particular sport. A single interest of this sort is equivalent to an unvarying game played by a small child to the exclusion of all others. It has become the representative of all his repressed phantasies and in general has the character of an obsessional symptom rather than a sublimation. Monotonous reports about football or bicycling may for months form the only topic of conversation in his analysis. Out of these associations, barren as they may appear, we have to extract the contents of his repressed phantasies. If we follow a technique analogous to that of dream- and play-interpretation and take into account the mechanisms of displacement, condensation, symbolic representation and so on, and if we notice the connections between minute signs of anxiety in him and his general affective state we can get behind this façade of monotonous interest[1] and gradually penetrate into the deepest complexes of his mind. An analogy is to be found here with a certain extreme type of latency-period analysis. We may recall the seven-year-old Grete's[2] monotonous drawing, which was quite lacking in phantasy but which was almost all I had to go on for months in her analysis; or Egon's case, which was of a still more extreme type. These children showed to an excessive degree the limitation of phantasy and of means of representation that is normal in the latency period. I have come to the con-

---

[1] Abraham, as he himself told me, carried out an analysis of a boy of about twelve years old mainly in what he described as 'stamp-language', in which details like the torn corners of a stamp, for instance, would afford a means of approaching his castration complex.

[2] Cf. Chapter IV.

clusion that, on the one hand, where we find such a severe limitation of interests and means of expression at the age of puberty we are dealing with a protracted period of latency, and, on the other, where there is an extensive limitation of imaginative activities (as in inhibitions in play, etc.) in early childhood it is a case of premature onset of the latency period. In either case, whether latency begins too soon or ends too late, severe disturbances are not only noticeable by the time-shift, but also by the excessive measure of the phenomena which normally go with the latency period.

I shall now bring forward one or two examples to illustrate what seems to me the proper technique for analysis at the age of puberty. In the analysis of the fifteen-year-old Bill[1] his uninterrupted chain of associations about his bicycle and about particular parts of it—for example, his anxiety lest he should have damaged it by riding too fast—had provided abundant material concerning his castration complex and his sense of guilt about masturbation.[2] He told me about a bicycling tour he had made with his friend, in the course of which they had exchanged their bicycles and he had been afraid, for no reason, that his bicycle had been damaged. On the basis of this and other things of the same kind which he told me, I pointed out to him that his fear seemed to go back to sexual acts which had occurred in childhood. He agreed and remembered some details about such a relation with a boy. His sense of guilt about it and his consequent fear of having damaged his penis and his body were quite unconscious.

In the analysis of the fourteen-year-old Ludwig, the introductory phase of which I described above, I was able to discover, by the help of similar material, the reason for his strong feelings of guilt about his younger brother. When, for instance, Ludwig spoke about his steam-engine being in need of repair, he at once went on to give associations about his brother's engine which would never be any good again. His resistance in connection with this and his wish that the session would soon come to an end turned out to be caused by his fear of his mother, who might discover the sexual relations which had existed between him and his younger brother and which he partly remembered.

[1] Bill was nervous, inhibited and had various neurotic difficulties. The analysis lasted only three months (45 hours). Six years after the analysis I heard that he was developing very well.

[2] That riding a bicycle symbolizes masturbation and coitus has been shown over and over again. In my paper, 'Early Analysis' (1923), I have referred to the general symbolic significance of balls, footballs, bicycles, etc., as the penis, and have discussed more fully the libidinal phantasies connected with various sports in consequence of these symbolic equations; so that by dealing with the patient's stories about sports in their symbolic aspect and relating them to his general affective state, the analyst can arrive at his libidinal and aggressive phantasies and at the sense of guilt which they give rise to.

These relations had left behind them severe unconscious feelings of guilt in him, for he, as the elder and stronger, had at times forced his brother into them. Since then he had felt responsible for the defective development of his brother, who was seriously neurotic.[1]

In connection with certain associations about a steamer trip that he was going to make with a friend, it occurred to Ludwig that the boat might sink, and he suddenly drew his railway season-ticket out of his pocket and asked me if I could tell him when it expired. He did not know, he said, which numbers referred to the month and which to the day. The date of 'expiry' of his ticket meant the date of his own death; and the trip with his friend was the mutual masturbation which he had performed in early childhood (with his brother/friend)[1a] and

[1] Ludwig's analysis was intended as a prophylactic measure. He suffered, it is true, from depressions, but these were not of an abnormal character. He was not fond of company, rather inactive and withdrawn into himself and not on good terms with his brothers and sisters. But his social adaptation was normal; he was a good scholar and there was nothing definitely wrong with him. His analysis occupied 190 sessions. As a result of it—I last had news of him three years after its termination—this boy, who could certainly be called a normal child, underwent changes of such a nature that even people outside his immediate circle, who did not know he was being analysed, noticed them. It turned out, for instance, that his disinclination to go to the theatre or the cinema was connected with a severe inhibition of his desire for knowledge, although, as has been said, he did his lessons well. When this inhibition had been removed, his mental horizon became wider and he advanced intellectually. The analysis of his strongly passive attitude led to the development of a number of activities. His attitude to his brothers grew better, as did his powers of social adaptation. These and other changes made a much more free, well-balanced and mature person of him; and moreover these changes, though not in themselves perhaps very decisive, reflected some deeper changes which would almost certainly become of importance later on. For along with the removal of his inactive attitude in ordinary life there went a change in his sexual orientation. His heterosexual trends became very much stronger and he got rid of certain difficulties which are known to be the basis of disturbances of potency in later life. Furthermore, it turned out that his depressions were allied to thoughts of suicide and went deeper than appeared at first. And his withdrawal into himself and dislike of company were based on a very decided flight from reality. These, I may add, were only some of the difficulties from which the boy was suffering, as his deep-going analysis showed.

In this connection I should like to point out how severe the difficulties of even normal children are (cf. Inge's case, for instance). This fact of analytic experience is borne out by observations of everyday life; for it is surprising how often people who have hitherto seemed quite normal will break down with a neurosis or commit suicide for some quite slight cause. But even in those people who do not fall ill the extent of their intellectual and sexual inhibitions and lack of capacity for enjoyment cannot be gauged except by psycho-analysis, as the treatment of normal adults confirmed.

[1a] The translator has accepted the oblique stroke as in the German text in spite of its ambiguity. The author probably means the older friend mentioned later so that one can stand for the other.

which had given rise to feelings of guilt and fear of death in him. Ludwig went on to say that he had emptied his electric battery in order not to dirty the box in which it was packed. He next told me how he had played football with a ping-pong ball with his brother indoors, and said that the ping-pong balls were not dangerous and one was not liable to get one's head banged or to break the windows with them. Here he remembered an incident of his early childhood, when he had received a painful blow from a football and lost consciousness. He had suffered no injury, but his nose or his teeth might easily have been hurt, he said. The memory of this incident proved to be a screen memory for his relations with an older friend who had seduced him. The ping-pong balls represented his younger brother's comparatively small and harmless penis, and the football that of his older friend. But since in his relations to his brother he identified himself with the friend who had seduced him, those relations aroused a strong sense of guilt in him on account of the [supposed] damage he had done his brother. His emptying of the battery and his fear of dirtying the box were determined by his anxiety about the defilement and injury which he brought upon his brother by putting his penis into his mouth and forcing him to perform *fellatio* and which he himself experienced as a result of having done that act with his older friend. His fear that he had dirtied and injured his brother internally was founded on sadistic phantasies about his brother and led to a still deeper basis of his anxiety and guilt, namely, his sadistic masturbation phantasies directed against his parents. Thus, starting from his confession about his relations with his brother—a confession expressed in symbolic form in his associations about the steam-engine which needed repairing—we gained access not only to other experiences and events in his life but to the deepest levels of anxiety in him. I should also like to draw attention to the wealth of symbolic forms in which the material was put forward. This is typical of analyses at the age of puberty, and, as in analyses of early childhood, calls for a corresponding interpretation of the symbols employed.

I now turn to the analysis of girls at the age of puberty. The onset of menstruation arouses strong anxiety in the girl. In addition to the various other meanings which it has and with which we are familiar, it is, in the last resort, the outward and visible sign that the interior of her body and the children contained there have been totally destroyed. For this reason the development of a complete feminine attitude in the girl takes longer and is beset by more difficulties than is the case with the boy in establishing his masculine position. This greater difficulty in the woman's development results in a reinforcement of the masculine component of the girl at puberty. In other cases only a partial development, mostly on the intellectual side, sets in at that time, while her sexual life and personality remain in a protracted latency which in many cases may last beyond the age of puberty. In analysing the first, active, type of girl with an attitude of rivalry towards the male sex, we often start from material similar to that produced by the boy. Very soon, however, the differences in structure between the masculine and the feminine castration complexes make themselves felt, as we get down to deeper levels of her mind and meet with the anxiety and sense of guilt which are derived from her feelings of aggression against her mother and which have led her to reject the feminine role and influenced the formation of her castration complex.

We now discover that it is her fear of having her body destroyed by her mother which has caused her thus to refuse to adopt the position of woman and mother. In this stage of her analysis the ideas she produces are very similar to what we get in small girls. In the second type, the girl whose sexual life is strongly inhibited, analysis is at first usually occupied with subjects of the kind put forward in the latency period. Reports on her school, her wish to please her mistress and do her lessons well, her interest in needlework, etc., take up a great part of the time. In these cases, accordingly, we must use the methods appropriate to the latency period and by resolving her anxiety step by step, free the repressed activities of her phantasy. When we have succeeded in doing this—at least to some extent—the girl's fears and guilt feelings emerge more clearly. These fears and guilt feelings had stood in the way of the maintenance of her feminine role and had led to a general sexual inhibition while, in the first type of girl, they had led to an identification with the father. Even girls in whom the feminine position predominates have anxiety during puberty which is more severe and more acute in its expression than in the adult woman. A defiant and negative transference is characteristic of this age and necessitates prompt establishment of the analytic situation. Analysis will frequently show that the girl's feminine position is exaggerated and pushed into the foreground partly in order to conceal and camouflage the anxiety arising from her masculinity complex and, deeper still, from the fears derived from her earliest feminine attitude.[1]

I shall now give an excerpt from an analysis which, though not absolutely typical of that period, will illustrate my general remarks on the technique to be applied to the analysis of girls in pre-puberty and puberty, and will also help to demonstrate the difficulties attendant upon their treatment at that age.

Ilse, aged twelve, presented marked schizoid features and her personality was unusually stunted. Not only had she not reached the

[1] Cf. Joan Riviere, 'Womanliness as a Masquerade' (1929).

level of an eight- or nine-year-old child intellectually, but she did not even possess the interests normal to children of that age. She showed very strikingly a marked inhibition of any imaginative activity. She had never played in the true sense of the word and took no pleasure in any occupation whatever except a compulsive and unimaginative drawing, the character of which I shall discuss later. For instance, she did not care for the company of others, did not like walking in the streets and looking at things, and had an aversion to the theatre, cinema and any kind of entertainment. Her chief interest was in food, and disappointments in this respect always led to fits of rage and depression. She was very jealous of her brothers and sisters, but less on account of having to share her mother's love with them than for some imagined preference in what her mother gave them to eat. The hostile attitude towards her mother and her brothers and sisters went along with a poor social adaptation in general. Ilse had no friends and apparently no desire to be liked or thought well of. Her relations with her mother were especially bad. From time to time she had violent outbursts of rage against her, but she was at the same time more than usually fixated to her. A long separation from her home surroundings—she spent two years in a boarding-school run by nuns—had made no lasting change in her condition.

When Ilse was about eleven-and-a-half years old her mother discovered her having sexual intercourse with her older brother. This incident aroused recollections in the mother which told her that it was not the first of its kind. Analysis showed that her conviction was well founded and also that the relationship between Ilse and her brother was continued after its discovery.

It was only at the urgent desire of her mother that Ilse came to be analysed, impelled by that uncritical docility far behind her years, which, along with her attitude of hatred, characterized her fixation to her mother. At first I suggested to her to lie on the couch. Her scanty associations were concerned mainly with a comparison between the furniture in my room and in her home, especially her own room. She left in a state of great resistance, refused to come to analysis next day and was only with great difficulty persuaded by her mother to do so after all. Now in cases of this kind it is necessary, in my experience, to establish the analytic situation quickly, for the support given by the child's family will not last long. Even in the first session I noticed the movements which Ilse had made with her fingers. She had constantly been smoothing the folds of her skirt as she made a few remarks about my furniture and compared it with that of her room at home. During the second hour, on her comparing a teapot I had in my room with one at home that was like it but not so beautiful, I started giving interpretations. I explained that the objects she compared really meant people; she was comparing me or her mother with herself to her own disadvantage because she felt guilty about having masturbated and believed it had damaged her body. I said that her continual smoothing out of the folds of her skirt meant both masturbation and an attempt to repair her genitals.[1] She denied this strongly; yet I could see the effect the interpretation had on her from the increase in the material she produced. Also, she did not refuse to come for the following session. Nevertheless, in view of her marked infantility and her difficulty in expressing herself in words and the acute anxiety from which she appeared to suffer, I thought it advisable to change over to play technique.

During the months that followed, Ilse's associations consisted in the main, of drawing—apparently without any phantasy—done with compasses, according to exact measurements. These measurements and calculations of parts of things was the main activity, and the compulsive nature of this occupation became increasingly clear.[2] After much slow and patient work it emerged that the various forms and colours of these parts represented different people. Her compulsion to measure and count proved to be derived from the impulse which had become obsessive, to find out for certain about the inside of her mother's body and the number of children there, the difference between the sexes, and so forth. In this case, too, the inhibition of her whole personality and intellectual growth had arisen from a very early repression of her powerful instinct for knowledge, which had changed into a defiant rejection of all knowledge. With the help of this drawing, measuring and counting we made considerable progress and Ilse's anxiety became less acute. Six months after the beginning of her treatment, therefore, I suggested that she should try again to carry on her analysis lying down, and she did so. Her anxiety grew more acute at once; but I was soon able to reduce it, and from that time on her analysis went faster. Owing to the poverty and monotony of her associations, this part of her analysis in no way came up to the normal course of analytic work at this age, it is true; but as it proceeded it approximated more and more closely to that standard. She now began to want very much to satisfy her teacher and get good reports from her, but her severe inhibition in learning rendered the fulfilment of this wish impossible. It was only now that

[1] An interpretation of this kind is not given in order to detect something (such as masturbation) which the child is consciously concealing and so to gain a hold over her. The object is to trace back the sense of guilt attaching to the masturbation (or whatever it may be) to its deeper sources and in that way to diminish it.

[2] Ilse had, in fact, no real interests that she could have talked about. She was, it is true, a passionate reader; but she did not care what the book was about, for reading was for her chiefly a means of escaping from reality.

she began to be fully conscious of the disappointment and suffering which her deficiencies caused her. She would cry for hours at home before beginning to write her essay for school, and would in fact fail to get it done. She would also be in despair if, before going to school, she found that she had not mended her stockings and they were in holes. Again and again her associations to her failure in learning led us to questions of a deficiency in her clothes or her body. For months on end her analytic hour was filled, along with stories about her school, with monotonous remarks about her cuffs, the collar of her blouse, her ties and every single item of her clothing—how they were too long or too short or dirty or not the right colour.[1]

My material for analysis was at this time mainly taken from the details of her failure in her homework.[2] To her unceasing complaints that she had nothing to write about the subject set I encouraged her to associate to that subject, and these forced phantasies[3] were very instructive. Doing her essay meant an acknowledgement of the fact of 'not-knowing', that is to say that she was ignorant of what went on when her parents copulated, or of what was inside her mother, etc.; and all the anxiety and defiance connected with this fundamental 'not-knowing' were stimulated anew in her by each school task. As in many other children, having to write an essay signified for her having to make a confession, and this touched her anxiety and feelings of guilt very closely. For instance, one of the subjects set, 'A Description of the Kurfürstendamm',[3a] led to associations about shop windows and their contents and about things she would like to possess, as, for instance, a very large decorated match-box which she had seen in a shop window when she was out walking with her mother. They had actually gone into the shop and her mother had struck one of the large matches to try it. Ilse would have liked to do the same but refrained out of fear of her mother and the shop assistant, who represented a father-imago. The match-box and its contents, like the contents of the shop windows, represented her mother's body, and the striking of the match meant coitus between her parents. Her envy of her mother, who possessed her father in copulation, and her aggressive impulses against her were the cause of her deepest feelings of guilt. Another subject for a composition was 'St. Bernard Dogs'. When Ilse had mentioned their cleverness in rescuing people from

[1] Cf. J. C. Flugel, 'The Psychology of Clothes' (1930).
[2] In a paper, 'History as Phantasy' (1929), Ella Sharpe has given an account of a case of an adult psychotic, in which for a long time she got her material for analysis almost entirely from the patient's interest in historical events and was able on that basis to penetrate to the deepest mental levels.
[3] Cf. Ferenczi, 'On Forced Phantasies' (1924).
[3a] One of the main shopping centres of Berlin.

89

freezing to death she began to have a great resistance. Her further associations showed that children buried in the snow were in her phantasy children who had been abandoned. It proved that the difficulties she felt about this subject were based on her death-wishes against her younger sisters, both before and after their birth, and her fear lest she should herself be abandoned by her mother as a punishment. Moreover, every school task she had to do, whether oral or written, stood to her for a confession about a whole number of things. And to these difficulties were added special inhibitions about mathematics, geometry, geography and so on.[1]

As Ilse's difficulties in learning continued to diminish, a very great change took place in her whole nature. She became capable of social adaptation, made friends with other girls and got on much better with her parents and her brothers and sisters. One could now call her a normal girl and her interests now approximated to what was adequate to her age; and as she was now good at school, a favourite with her mistresses and had become an almost too-obedient daughter, her family were completely satisfied with the success of her analysis and saw no reason for its continuance. But I did not share their opinion. It was obvious that at this point, when she was thirteen and physical puberty had already begun, Ilse had psychically only just accomplished a really successful transition to the latency period. By means of resolving anxiety quantities and reducing her sense of guilt, the analysis had enabled her to adapt herself socially, and to progress psychically to the latency period. However gratifying these changes might be, the person I saw before me was still a rather dependent child who was still excessively fixated to her mother. Though her circle of interests was greatly widening she was still hardly capable of having any ideas of her own. She usually prefaced her expressions with such words as 'Mother thinks'. Her wish to please, the great care that she now took of her appearance in contrast to her former total indifference to it, her need for love and recognition—all these sprang predominantly from her desire to please her mother and her mistresses; the same purpose served her desire to do better than her schoolmates. Her homosexual attitude was predominant and there were as yet scarcely any heterosexual impulses visible in her.

The continuation of the analysis, which now proceeded in a normal fashion, led to far-reaching changes not only in this respect, but in the whole development of Ilse's personality. In this she was very much helped by the fact that we were able to analyse the anxiety which menstruation aroused in her. Her excessive positive ties to her mother

[1] In my paper, 'The Role of the School in the Libidinal Development of the Child' (1923, *Writings*, 1) I have discussed the general significance of inhibitions associated with specific areas of learning.

were caused by anxiety and a sense of guilt. From time to time Ilse still had outbursts of rage against her mother though these had become less frequent. Further analysis completely uncovered her original attitude of rivalry with her mother and the intense hatred and envy she felt towards her, on account of her possession of the father, respectively of his penis, and of his love for her. In this way, her heterosexual trends had become stronger and her homosexual ones much weaker. It was only now that her psychological puberty really set in. Before this, she had not been in a position to criticize her mother and form her own opinions, because this would have signified making a violent sadistic attack upon her mother. The analysis of this sadism enabled Ilse—in keeping with her age—to achieve a greater self-reliance which became visible in her way of thinking and acting. At the same time, her opposition to her mother appeared more plainly, but it did not lead to special difficulties, since these were outweighed by her all-round improvement. Somewhat later, after an analysis extending over 425 hours, Ilse was able to achieve a stable and affectionate relationship with her mother and at the same time to establish a satisfactory heterosexual position.[1]

In this case, we see how the girl's failure to work over her overstrong sense of guilt was able to disturb not only her transition to the latency period but the whole course of her development. Her affects, which found an outlet in outbursts of rage, had been displaced; the modification of her anxiety went wrong. Ilse, who had the appearance of an unhappy and discontented individual, was not aware of her own anxiety nor of her dissatisfaction with herself. It was a great advance in her analysis when I was able to make her understand that she was unhappy and to show her that she felt inferior and unloved and that she was in despair about it and, in her hopelessness, would make no attempt to gain the love of others. In place of her former apparent indifference to affection and praise from the world around her, there then appeared an exaggerated longing for them, which led to that attitude of extreme obedience to her mother which is characteristic of the latency period. The later part of her analysis, which uncovered the deeper reasons for her severe feelings of guilt and for her failure, was far easier once she had become fully aware of her illness.

I mentioned earlier the sexual acts committed between Ilse and her brother, who was a year-and-a-half older than herself. Not long after I had begun her analysis I undertook the treatment of her brother as well. Both analyses showed that the sexual connection between them went back to early childhood and had been continued throughout

[1] Two and a half years after the completion of her analysis I heard that she was developing well in spite of great external difficulties.

the latency period, although at rare intervals and in a mitigated form. The remarkable thing was that Ilse had no conscious sense of guilt about it but detested her brother. The analysis of her brother had the effect of making him put a complete stop to these sexual relations, and this at first aroused a still more intense hatred of him in her. But later on in her analysis, along with the other changes brought about in her, she began to have strong feelings of guilt and anxiety[1] about these episodes.

Ilse's way of dealing with her feelings of guilt, which consisted of her refusing all responsibility for her actions and of a very hostile and defiant attitude to her environment, is, I have found, characteristic of a certain type of asocial individual. In Kenneth, for instance, who displayed such complete indifference to the opinions of others and such an extraordinary want of shame, there were similar mechanisms at work. And they are to be found even in the more normal, merely 'naughty' child though to a lesser extent. Analyses of children of every age go to show that the lessening of their latent feelings of guilt and anxiety leads to a better social adaptation and to a strengthening of their sense of personal responsibility—the more so the deeper the analysis goes.

This case also gives us certain indications for deciding which factors in the development of a girl are decisive for a successful transition to the latency period, and which for the further transition to puberty. As has already been said, we often find that at the age of puberty the girl is still in a protracted latency period. By analysing the early anxiety and feelings of guilt derived from her aggressiveness against her mother, we can enable her to make not only a satisfactory transition to the stage of puberty but a subsequent transition to adult life, and can thus ensure the complete development of her feminine sex-life and personality.

Finally I would like to draw attention to the technique employed in the treatment of this case. In the first part of it I used the technique belonging to the latency period, and in the second that belonging to puberty. I have repeatedly referred to the connecting links between the various forms of psycho-analytic technique appropriate to different stages. Let me emphasize that I regard the technique of early analysis as the basis of the technique applicable to children of every age. In the last chapter I have said that my method of analysing children of the latency period was based on the play technique I had worked out for small children. But as the cases discussed in the present chapter show, the technique of early analysis is indispensable for many patients at the age of puberty as well; for we shall fail with

[1] In Chapter VII we shall return to a fuller discussion of this relationship in another connection.

many of these often very difficult cases if we do not sufficiently take into account the adolescent's need for action and for expression of phantasy and are not careful to regulate the amount of anxiety liberated and, in general, do not adopt an exceedingly elastic technique.

In analysing the deepest strata of the mind we have to observe certain definite conditions. In comparison with the modified anxiety of the higher strata, the anxiety belonging to the deep levels is far greater both in amount and intensity, and it is therefore imperative that its liberation should be duly regulated. We do this by continually referring the anxiety back to its sources and resolving it, and by systematically analysing the transference-situation.

In the first chapters of this book I have described how, in cases where the child was timid or unfriendly towards me at first, I immediately began to analyse its negative transference. This method[1] aims at recognizing and interpreting the hidden signs of latent anxiety in good time, before they become manifest and lead to an anxiety-attack. In order to be able to do this, a thorough knowledge is indispensable, both of the anxiety-reactions of the earliest phases of the child's development, and of the defensive mechanisms employed by its ego against them. In fact, the analyst must have a theoretic knowledge of the structure of the deepest layers of the mind. His interpretative work must be directed to that part of the material which is associated with the greatest amount of latent anxiety and must uncover the anxiety-situations which have been activated. He must also establish the connection between that latent anxiety and (a) the particular sadistic phantasies underlying it, and (b) the defensive mechanisms employed by the ego to master it. That is to say, in resolving a given piece of anxiety by interpretation, he should follow up a little way the threats of the super-ego, the impulses of the id and the attempts of the ego to reconcile the two. In this way, step by step, the interpretation will be able to bring into consciousness the whole content of the particular piece of anxiety which is being stirred up at the time. To do this it is absolutely necessary that he should keep to strictly analytic methods in regard to his patient, since it is only by abstaining from exerting any educational or moral influence whatever on the child that he can ever analyse the deepest levels of its mind. For if he prevents the child from bringing out certain instinctual impulses he will inevitably keep down other id-impulses as well; and even in the small child it requires hard analytical work to make one's way down to the child's most primitive oral-sadistic and anal-sadistic phantasies.

Moreover, by having the quantity of its anxiety systematically

[1] Cf. Chapter II.

93

regulated, the child will not accumulate too much anxiety during intervals in its analysis, or if the treatment is prematurely broken off. In the case of such interruptions, it is true, the anxiety often does become more acute for the time being, but the child's ego is soon able to bind it and modify it, and even more so than before analysis. In some instances the child may escape even a passing phase of more acute anxiety of this kind.[1]

After having stressed the similarities between the age of puberty and the early period of the child's life, I will once more shortly review their differences. More so than in the latency period, the fuller development of the ego at the age of puberty and its more mature interests demand a technique approximating to that of adult analysis. In certain children or in certain phases of an analysis we may have to take recourse to other methods of representation, but, in general, in analyses at the age of puberty we must rely chiefly on verbal associations, as it is the language alone which enables the youngster to establish a complete relation with reality and with his normal field of interest.

For these reasons, the analysis of children at puberty demands a thorough knowledge of the technique of adult analysis. I consider a regular training in the analysis of adults as a necessary foundation for special training as a child analyst. No one who has not gained adequate experience and done a fair amount of work on adults should enter upon the technically more difficult field of child analysis. In order to be able to preserve the fundamental principles of analytic treatment in the modified form necessitated by the child's mechanisms at the various stages of its development, he must, besides being fully versed in the technique of early analysis, possess complete mastery of the technique employed in analysing adults.

[1] In a number of instances, ranging from children of three to twelve years of age, in which I had to break off analysis for external reasons after treatment of from three to nine months, I found that the child presented a considerably less disquieting picture than when it first came to me. Besides the cases of Rita, Trude and Ruth, which the reader will recall (Chapter II), I may mention the case of a boy of twelve who came to me with manifest ideas of being poisoned. After six months' analysis he had to go abroad. By that time not only had his fears been lessened, but he showed favourable changes in his general condition, which were observable, among other things in a greater ease of manner. (When last I heard of him, two and a half years after the end of his treatment, this improvement had been maintained.) In every instance, moreover, the child itself has felt better. And although an unfinished analysis of this sort cannot do more than lessen the child's neurosis, it does much, in my judgment, to obviate the danger of a psychosis or severe obsessional neurosis setting in later on. I have come to the conviction that every step, however slight, in the direction of resolving anxiety in the deepest levels of the mind effects, if not a cure, at least an improvement of the child's condition.

Chapter VI

NEUROSIS IN CHILDREN

So far, I have discussed the technique by which children can be as deeply analysed as grown-up persons. I shall now consider the problem of indications for treatment.

The first question that arises is: what difficulties are to be regarded as normal and what as neurotic in children—when are they simply being naughty and when are they really ill? In general, one expects to meet with certain typical difficulties, varying considerably in quantity and effect, which, so long as they do not exceed certain bounds, are regarded as part of the development of the child. As, however, a certain amount of difficulties is inevitable in the child's development, we are, I think, inclined to appreciate too little how far these everyday difficulties are to be regarded as a basis for, and indicative of, serious developmental disturbances.

More marked disturbances in eating habits and, above all, manifestations of anxiety, whether in the form of night-terrors or phobias, are generally recognized as definitely neurotic manifestations. But observations of small children show that their anxiety takes on very various and disguised forms, and that even at the early age of two or three years they exhibit modifications of anxiety which indicate a very complicated process of repression. After they have got over their night-terrors, for instance, they are still for some time subject to disturbances of sleep, such as getting off to sleep late, waking up early, having a restless or easily disturbed sleep, being unable to sleep in the afternoon—all of which I found in analysis to be modified forms of the original *pavor nocturnus*. To this group also belong the many fads and ceremonies, often of so disquieting a nature, which children indulge in at bedtime. In the same way, their original undisguised disturbances in eating* will often turn into a habit of eating slowly or not masticating properly or into a general lack of appetite or even merely into bad table manners.

It is easy to see that the anxiety children feel with regard to particular people often gives place to general timidity. Still later it appears often as no more than an inhibition in social intercourse or as shyness. All these degrees of fear are only modifications of their

* In Chapter IX I shall discuss the nature of the anxiety underlying infantile disturbances in eating.

original anxiety which, as in the case of fear of people, may determine their whole social behaviour later on. An outspoken phobia of certain animals will turn into a dislike of them or of animals in general. Fear of inanimate things, which to small children are always endowed with life, will come out later on, when they are grown-up, as an inhibition of activities connected with them. Thus in one instance a child's phobia of the telephone became, in later years, an aversion to telephoning; and in other cases, a fear of engines gave rise to a dislike of travelling or a tendency to get very tired on journeys. In others again, a fear of streets grew into an aversion to going out for walks; and so on. Into this class come inhibitions in sport and active games, which I have described in detail in my paper 'Early Analysis'.[1] These inhibitions can show themselves in all degrees, such as distaste for special forms of sport or general dislike of them, or liability to fatigue or clumsiness, etc. To this class, too, belong the peculiarities, habits and inhibitions of the normal adult.

The normal adult can rationalize his dislikes—which are never wanting—in all sorts of ways by calling the object of them 'boring', 'in bad taste' or 'unhygienic' and many other things, whereas in a child dislikes and habits of this kind which, it must be admitted, are more intense and less adapted socially than in the adult, are attributed to 'naughtiness'. Yet they are invariably an expression of anxiety and feelings of guilt. They are intimately related to phobias and usually to obsessional ceremonials as well and are determined by the child's complexes in every detail; and for this reason they are often very resistant to educative measures, though they can frequently be resolved by analysis like any neurotic symptom.

I can only mention here one or two instances from this interesting field of observation. In one boy, staring with wide open eyes and making a face; in another, blinking served to refute the fear of going blind. In yet a third, keeping his mouth open signified a confession of having performed *fellatio*, followed by whistling meaning the withdrawal of that confession. The unruly behaviour of children while being bathed or having their hair washed is, as I have repeatedly found, nothing but a hidden fear of being castrated or having their whole body destroyed. Nose-picking, in both children and adults, has turned out to represent, among other things, an anal attack on the bodies of their parents. The difficulties parents and nurses have in persuading children to perform the simplest services or acts of consideration—difficulties which often make things so unpleasant for the person in charge—invariably turn out to be determined by anxiety. A child's dislike, for instance, of taking an object out of a box in several cases proved to be due to the fact that doing so signified an

[1] (1923) [*Writings*, x].

aggressive attack on its mother's body and the materialization of this forbidden attack.

In children there is a kind of over-liveliness which often goes along with an overbearing and defiant manner and which people, from their own personal point of view, frequently mistake either for a special sign of 'temperament' or for disobedience mixed with defiance and contempt. Such behaviour is, too, an over-compensation for anxiety, and this method of working over anxiety greatly influences the child's character-formation and its later attitude to society.[1] The 'fidgetiness' which often accompanies this over-liveliness is, in my judgment, an important symptom. The motor discharges which the small child achieves through fidgetting often become condensed at the beginning of the latency period into definite stereotyped movements which are usually lost to view in the general picture of over-activity which the child presents. At the age of puberty, or sometimes even earlier, they reappear or become more obvious and form the basis of a tic.[2]

I have repeatedly pointed to the great importance of inhibitions in play which can be concealed under the most diverse forms. In analysis we can observe them in every degree of strength. Dislike of certain definite games and a lack of perseverance in any one game are examples of partial inhibition in play. Again, some children need someone who will take a large part in the play; they leave the initiative to him and do not fetch the toys themselves, etc. Others only like games that they can play exactly according to set rules, or only like certain kinds of games (in which case they usually play them with great assiduity). These children suffer from a powerful repression of phantasy, accompanied, as a rule, by compulsive traits; and their games have the character of an obsessional symptom rather than a sublimation.

There is a kind of play behind which—especially during the transition into the latency period—stereotyped or rigid movements are concealed. For instance, an eight-year-old boy used to play at being a policeman on point duty and used to carry out certain movements and repeated them for hours together, remaining motionless in certain attitudes for long periods at a time. In other cases, a peculiar overactivity closely related to tic is concealed in a particular game.

A dislike of active games in general and a lack of agility is a fore-runner of later inhibitions in sport and is always an important sign that something is wrong.

[1] Cf. Reich, 'Character Formation and the Phobias of Childhood' (1930).
[2] In my paper, 'A Contribution to the Psychogenesis of Tics' (1925), I have shown that a tic should often be regarded as a sign of deep-seated and concealed disturbances.

In many cases inhibitions in playing are the basis of inhibitions in learning. In several cases where children who were inhibited in play did become good at school it turned out that their impulse to learn was mainly compulsive, and some of them later on—especially at puberty—developed severe limitations in their capacity to learn. Inhibitions in learning, like inhibitions in play, can possess every degree of strength and every variety of form, such as indolence, lack of interest, strong dislike of particular subjects or the peculiar habit of refusing to do homework except at the last moment and then only in response to pressure. Such inhibitions in learning are often the basis of later vocational inhibitions whose earliest signs, therefore, are often already to be seen in the small child's inhibitions in play.

In my paper 'The Development of a Child' (1921),[1] I have said that the resistance children show to sexual enlightenment is a very important indication of something being wrong. If they abstain from asking any questions on the subject—and such an abstention often succeeds to, or alternates with, obsessive asking—this is to be regarded as a symptom founded upon often very serious disturbances of the instinct for knowledge. As is well known, the wearisome questionings of the child are often prolonged into the brooding mania of the adult with which neurotic disorders are always associated.

A trend to plaintiveness in children and a habit of falling down and knocking or hurting themselves are to be regarded as expressions of various fears and feelings of guilt. Analysis of children has convinced me that such recurrent minor accidents—and sometimes more serious ones—are substitutes for self-inflicted injuries of a graver kind and represent attempts at suicide with insufficient means. With many children, especially boys, excessive sensibility to pain is often replaced very early on by an exaggerated indifference to it, but this indifference is only an elaborate defence against, and modification of, anxiety.

The child's attitude towards presents is also very characteristic. Many children are quite insatiable in this respect, as no present can give them real and lasting satisfaction or lead to anything but disappointment. Others have too little desire for them and are equally indifferent to every gift. In adults we can observe the same two attitudes in many situations. Among women there are those who are always longing for new clothes but who never really enjoy them and apparently never have 'anything to put on'. These are generally women who are always hunting after amusement and who more often than not change their love-object very easily and cannot find true sexual satisfaction. Then there are those who are bored and desire nothing very much. In the analysis of children it becomes ultimately clear that presents signify all the love-gifts which were

[1] *Writings*, I.

denied to the child—its mother's milk and breast, its father's penis, urine, stool and babies. But presents are also evidence to the child that all those things which it had wanted to appropriate in a sadistic manner are now given to it voluntarily and in this way alleviate its sense of guilt. In its unconscious it regards not getting presents, like all other frustrations, as a punishment for the aggressive impulses that are bound up with its libidinal desires. In other cases, where the child's excessive sense of guilt is still more unfavourably placed or has not been successfully worked through, this together with its fear of fresh disappointments may lead it to suppress its libidinal desires altogether. Those children cannot enjoy presents at all.

The child's incapacity to tolerate frustration will make it unmanageable and badly adapted to reality, as this inability induces the child's unconscious to regard every frustration, inevitable as it is in the course of its upbringing, as a punishment. In bigger children—and in some cases in little children too—this incapacity to tolerate frustrations is often covered over by a seeming adaptation, on account of their need to please the people about them. An apparent adaptation of this kind is liable, especially in the latency period, to conceal more deeply seated difficulties.

The attitude many children have towards festivities and holidays is also very characteristic. They look forward to Chrstmas Day, Easter and so on with great impatience, only to be left completely unsatisfied by them when they are over. Days like these, and sometimes even Sundays, hold out the hope to a greater or lesser degree of a renewal, a 'fresh start' as it were, and in connection with the presents that are expected, of a making good of all the bad things that they have suffered and done. Family festivities touch very deeply the complexes connected with the child's situation in home-life. A birthday, for instance, always represents re-birth, and other children's birthdays stimulate the conflicts connected with the birth of real or expected brothers and sisters. The way in which children react to occasions of this kind may therefore be one of the signs of a neurosis in the child.

Dislike of the theatre, cinema and shows of all kinds is intimately connected with disturbances of the child's instinct for knowledge. The basis of this disturbance is, I have found, a repressed interest in the sexual life of its parents and also a defence against its own sexual life. This attitude, which brings about an inhibition of many sublimations, is ultimately due to anxiety and feelings of guilt belonging to a very early stage of development and arising from aggressive phantasies directed against sexual intercourse between the parents.

I should also like to emphasize the psychogenic element in the various physical illnesses to which children are liable. I have ascertained that many children found an expression for their anxiety and sense of guilt to a large measure in falling ill (in which case getting well has a reassuring effect) and that in general their frequent illnesses at a certain age are partly determined by neurosis. This psychogenic element has the effect of increasing not only the child's sensitivity to infection, but the severity and length of the illness itself.[1] In general, I have found that after a completed analysis the child is much less liable to colds in particular. In some cases its susceptibility to them has been almost entirely removed.

We know that neurosis and character-formation are intimately connected and that in many analyses of adults extensive changes of character take place as well. Now whereas the analysis of older children nearly always effects favourable changes in character, early analysis, in removing a neurosis, brings about a far-reaching removal of educational difficulties. There thus seems to be a certain analogy between the small child's educational difficulties and what in the older child and the adult are known as characterological difficulties. Following this analogy, it is a noteworthy fact that in talking of 'character' we think primarily of the individual himself even when his character has a disburbing influence on his environment, but that in talking of 'educational difficulties' we think first and foremost of the difficulties which the people in charge of the child have to contend with. In doing so we often overlook the fact that these educational difficulties are the expression of significant processes of development which reach completion with the decline of the Oedipus complex. They are therefore the after-effects of the developing or already formed character and the basis of the later neurosis or of any defect of development. They show themselves among other things, in excessive educational difficulties and it would be more correct to call them neurotic symptoms or characterological difficulties [rather than educational ones].

From what has been said so far, I conclude that the difficulties which are never lacking in the development of a child are neurotic in character. In other words, every child passes through a neurosis differing only in degree from one individual to another.[2] Since

[1] In some cases of whooping-cough, for instance, in which analytic treatment was resumed after only a short interruption, I have found that the coughing fits increased in violence during the first week of analysis but rapidly decreased after that and that the illness ended much sooner than usual. In these cases every coughing fit, owing to its unconscious meaning, released severe anxiety, and this anxiety, again, considerably reinforced the stimulus to cough.

[2] This view, which I have maintained for a number of years now, has lately received valuable support. In his book, *The Question of Lay Analysis* (1926), Freud writes: 'Since we have learnt how to look more sharply, we are tempted to say that neurosis in children is not the exception but the rule, as

psycho-analysis has been found to be the most efficacious means of removing the neuroses of adults, it seems logical to make use of psycho-analysis in combating the neuroses of children, and, moreover, seeing that every child goes through a neurosis, to apply it to all children. At present, owing to practical considerations, it is only possible to submit the neurotic difficulties of normal children to analytic treatment in rare instances. In describing indications for treatment, therefore, it is important to clarify what signs suggest the presence of a severe neurosis, a neurosis, that is, that places it beyond doubt that the child will suffer considerable difficulties in later years as well.

I shall not stop to discuss those infantile neuroses whose severity is unmistakable owing to the extent and character of the symptoms, but shall consider one or two cases which have not been recognized because insufficient attention has been paid to the specific indications of infantile neuroses. The reason why the neuroses of children have attracted so much less attention than the neuroses of adults is, I think, because in many respects their symptomatology differs essentially from that of adults. Analysts have known, it is true, that beneath the neurosis of the adult there always lay an infantile neurosis, but for a long time they have failed to draw the practical conclusion that neuroses must be, to say the least, extremely common among children—and this although the child itself puts before them evidence enough for such a view.

Comparison with the neuroses of adults cannot serve as a yardstick, since the child who most approximates to a non-neurotic adult is by no means the child who is least neurotic. Thus, for instance, a small child which fulfils all the requirements of its upbringing and does not let itself be dominated by its life of phantasy and instinct, which is in fact, to all appearances completely adapted to reality and, moreover, shows little sign of anxiety—such a child would assuredly not only be precocious and quite devoid of charm, but would be abnormal in the fullest sense of the word. If this picture is completed by the extensive repression of phantasy which is a necessary pre-condition of such a development, we should certainly have cause to regard that child's future with concern. A child whose development has been of this kind suffers, not from a quantitatively minor neurosis but from a symptomless neurosis; and as we know from the analysis of adults, such a neurosis is usually a serious one.

Normally, we should expect to see clear traces of the severe struggles and crises through which the child passes in the first years

though it could scarcely be avoided on the path from the innate disposition of infancy to civilized society' (*S.E.* **20,** p. 215).

of its life. These signs, however, differ in many ways from the symptoms of the neurotic adult. Up to a certain point, the normal child openly shows its ambivalence and affects; its subjection to instinctual urges and phantasies acts recognizably and so do the influences of its super-ego. It puts certain difficulties in the way of its adaptation to reality and therefore in the way of its upbringing and is by no means always an 'easy' child. But if the obstacles it presents to its adaptation to reality go beyond a certain limit, and its anxiety and ambivalence is too strong, in short, if the difficulties under which it suffers and which it makes its environment suffer are too great, then it ought to be called a decidedly neurotic child. Nevertheless, a neurosis of this type may often be less severe than the neuroses of those children in whom the repression of affect has been so crushing and has set in so early that there is hardly any sign left of emotion or anxiety. What actually differentiates the less neurotic from the more neurotic child is, besides the question of quantitative differences, above all the manner in which it masters its difficulties.

The signs and symptoms, which I described above, constitute a valuable point of departure for the study of the methods, often very obscure, by which the child has worked over its anxiety and of the basic attitude it has taken up. For example, it may be assumed that if a child does not like going to shows of any sort, such as the theatre or cinema, takes no pleasure in asking questions and is inhibited in its play or can only play certain games with no phantasy content, it is suffering from severe disturbances of its instinct for knowledge and from an extensive repression of its phantasy life, although it may be otherwise well-adapted and seem to have no very marked troubles. In cases of this kind the desire for knowledge will be satisfied at a later age mostly in a very obsessional way and in connection with this other neurotic disturbances may occur.

In many children the original inability to tolerate frustration becomes obscured by an extensive adaptation to the requirements of their upbringing. They very early become 'good' and 'co-operative' children. But it is precisely these children who most commonly have that attitude of indifference to presents and treats that has been mentioned above. If in addition to this attitude they show an extensive inhibition in playing and an excessive fixation to their objects, the probability of their developing a neurosis in later years is very great. Children like these have adopted a pessimistic outlook and an attitude of renunciation. Their chief aim is to fight off their anxiety and feelings of guilt at all costs, even if it means renouncing all happiness and all satisfaction of their instincts. At the same time they are more than ordinarily dependent upon their objects because they rely on their external environment for protection and support against their own anxiety and sense of guilt.[1] More obvious, though their true significance is not appreciated either, are the difficulties presented by those children whose insatiable craving for presents goes along with an incapacity to tolerate the frustrations imposed on them by their upbringing.

It is fairly certain that in the typical cases here described the prospects of the child's achieving real stability of mind in the future are not favourable. As a rule, too, the general impression the child makes—its way of walking, its facial expression, its movements and speech—betrays an unsuccessful internal adaptation. In any case, analysis alone can show how severe the disturbances are. I have again and again emphasized the fact that the presence of a psychosis or of psychotic traits can often only be recognized in a child after it has been analysed for a considerable length of time. This is because the psychoses of children, like their neuroses, differ in many ways from the psychoses of adults. In some children I have treated, whose neurosis at an early age already had the same character as a severe obsessional neurosis in an adult, analysis showed that strong paranoid features were present.[2]

The question now to be considered is: how does a child show that it is fairly well adapted internally? It is a favourable sign if it enjoys playing and gives free rein to its phantasy in doing so, being at the same time, as can be recognized from certain definite indications, sufficiently adapted to reality, and if it has really good—not over-affectionate—relations to its objects. Another good sign is if, together with this, it shows a relatively undisturbed development of its instinct for knowledge, which freely turns in a number of different directions, yet without having that character of compulsion and intensity which is typical of an obsessional neurosis. The emergence of a certain amount of affect and anxiety is also, I think, a pre-condition of a favourable development. These and other indications of a favourable prognosis have in my experience, however, only a relative value and are no absolute guarantee of the future; for it often depends on the unforeseeable external realities, favourable or unfavourable, which the child encounters as it grows up whether the neurosis of the child will reappear in the life of the adult or not.

Furthermore it seems to me that we do not know much about the mental structure and the unconscious difficulties of the normal individual, since he has been so much less the object of psycho-analytic investigation than the neurotic. Analytic experience of mentally healthy children of various ages has convinced me that even though their ego reacts in a normal way they too have to face great

[1] Cf. N. M. Searl, 'The Flight to Reality' (1929).
[2] Cf. the analyses of Erna (Chapter III) and Egon (Chapter IV).

quantities of anxiety, severe unconscious guilt and deep depression and that in some cases the only thing that distinguishes their difficulties from those of the neurotic child is that they are able to deal with them in a more hopeful and active manner. The result obtained by analytic treatment in these cases also seems to me to prove its value even for children who are only very slightly neurotic.[1] The assumption seems to be well-founded that by diminishing their anxiety and sense of guilt, and effecting fundamental changes in their sexual life, a great influence can be exerted not only on neurotic children but on the future of normal ones as well.[2]

The next question to be considered is at what point the analysis of a child is to be regarded as completed. In adults we can tell this from various signs, such as that the patient has become capable of working and loving, of looking after himself in the circumstances in which he is placed and of making whatever decisions are necessary in the conduct of his life. If we consider the factors which lead to failure in grown-up people and if we are alive to the presence of similar factors in children, we possess a reliable guide for the termination of an analysis.

The adult individual may succumb to a neurosis, to characterological defects, to disturbances of his capacity for sublimation or to disorders of his sexual life. An infantile neurosis can be detected at an early age, as I have endeavoured to show, by various slight but characteristic signs; the cure of the infantile neurosis is the best prophylaxis against the neurosis of the adult. Later characterological defects and difficulties are best prevented by being eliminated in childhood. The play of children, which enables us to penetrate so deeply into their minds, gives us a clear indication when their analysis can be considered as being completed in respect of their future capacity for sublimation. Before we can consider the analysis of a small child as completed, its inhibitions in playing must have been largely reduced.[3] This has been accomplished when its interest in play appropriate to its age has become not only deeper and more stable but has also been extended in various directions.

When, as a result of the analytic work, a child who starts with a single obsessive interest in play gains an ever-widening interest in games, this process is equivalent to the expansion of interests and the

[1] Cf. the analyses of Ludwig (Chapter V) and Inge (Chapter IV).

[2] This assumption is also supported by the fact that in a number of cases I have had, the child has successfully accomplished the transition to the next stage of development, even including in some instances the critical transition to puberty and the transition from that period into adult life.

[3] In older children inhibitions in learning and in active games must be similarly much reduced.

increase of capacity for sublimation which is the aim of the analysis of an adult. In this way, by understanding the play of children we can estimate their capacity for sublimation in future years; and we can also tell when an analysis has sufficiently guarded against future inhibitions of their capacity to learn and to work.

Finally, the development of the child's interest in play, and the variations in quantity and kind which they show, also permit reliable conclusions about its future sexual development. This may be illustrated by the analysis of two small children—a boy and a girl. Kurt, aged five, occupied himself at first, like most boys, with the toy motors and trains on my play-table. He picked them out from among the other toys and played some games with them. He compared their size and power, made them travel to a definite goal and expressed in this symbolic and, according to my experience, typical way, a comparison in respect of his penis, his potency and his personality as a whole with his father and brothers. It might have been assumed that these actions pointed to a normal and active heterosexual attitude in him. But this conflicted with his markedly apprehensive and unboyish nature;[1] and, as the analysis proceeded, the truth of this impression was confirmed. His games representing his rivalry with his father for the possession of his mother were very soon interrupted by the onset of severe anxiety. It appeared that he had developed a predominantly passive homosexual attitude, but, owing to anxiety, could not maintain this attitude either, and had therefore turned away from reality and found refuge in megalomanic phantasies. On this unrealistic basis he could thrust into the foreground and exaggerate both to himself and others, a portion of the active and masculine trends which still remained alive in him.

I have again and again observed that children's play, like dreams, has a façade and that we can only discover its latent content by means of a thorough analysis, in the same way as we discover the latent content of dreams. But play, owing to its closer relation to reality and its paramount role as the expression of the infantile mind, often undergoes a stronger secondary elaboration than the dream. For this reason it is only gradually, through the changes which the child's games undergo, that we can get to know the various currents of its mental life.

We have seen that in Kurt the active masculine attitude, which he exhibited in his first games in analysis, was for the most part only

[1] Kurt's passive attitude had been strengthened by the fact that he was the youngest by many years of a number of brothers. He was therefore in many ways in the situation of an only child, and he suffered much from comparisons with his active elder brothers whose superiority was all the more oppressive from their habit of bringing it home to him.

a pretence and that it was soon broken off by the appearance of severe anxiety. This marked the beginning of the analysis of his passive homosexual attitude, but it was only after a considerable period of treatment (which occupied in all about 450 sessions) that the anxiety which counteracted the homosexual position was to some degree reduced. Then the toy animals, which had originally represented imaginary allies in the fight against the father, emerged as children, and his passive feminine attitude and desire for children found a clearer expression.[1] The excessive fear of both parents had weakened both the feminine and the heterosexual position.[2]

Analysis of Kurt's fear of the 'mother with a penis' and of his excessive terror of his father had the effect of increasing and once more bringing to the fore his active heterosexual position. He was able to give a more sustained expression in his play to his feelings of rivalry with his father. He once more took up the games he had played at the beginning of his analysis but this time he played them more steadily and imaginatively. He would, for instance, take great pains to build up the garages in which the motors were housed and was indefatigable in adding fresh items towards their perfection; or he would construct different kinds of villages and towns for the cars to make expeditions to—expeditions which symbolized his rivalry with his father for the possession of his mother. In the pleasure and care he took in making these villages, towns and garages he gave expression to his desire to restore his mother whom he had attacked in phantasy. At the same time his attitude to his mother underwent a complete change in real life. As his anxiety and sense of guilt lessened, he became more capable of entertaining reactive tendencies and to have a much more affectionate attitude towards her.

The gradual strengthening of his heterosexual trends was registered in numerous alterations in his play. At first the details of his play showed that his pregenital fixations still predominated in his heterosexual relations or rather repeatedly replaced his genital fixations. For instance, the load which the train brought to the town or the van delivered at the house often symbolized excrements; and in that

[1] In my paper, 'Early Stages of the Oedipus Conflict' (1928), I have discussed the earliest foundation of the feminine position in the male child and have tried to show that his femininity complex undergoes a very early modification and becomes buried beneath the castration complex, to which it makes certain contributions. It is for this reason that the boy often very speedily relinquishes such games as playing with dolls, which correspond to his feminine components, and goes over to games which lay exaggerated emphasis on his masculinity.

[2] In this case also the aggressive feelings he had in regard to coitus between his parents proved to be the deepest motive force of his anxiety; and the 'woman with a penis' meant the mother who had incorporated his father's penis.

case it would be delivered at the back door. The fact that these games represented a violent kind of anal coitus with his mother appeared, among other things, from the fact that in unloading, say, coal from a van, the garden or house would often be damaged, the people in the house got angry and his game would soon be stopped by his own anxiety.

The conveying of loads of different kinds occupied, with its wealth of detail, the whole of one part of Kurt's analysis.[1] Sometimes it would be vans fetching goods from the market or taking them there, sometimes people going on a long journey with all their possessions. Here the further course of his play-associations showed that what was being represented was a flight and that the articles were things that had been seized or stolen from his mother's body. The variations in minor points were most instructive. The supremacy of his anal-sadistic phantasies was expressed by the use of the back entrance for the delivery of the goods. A little later on Kurt did the the same thing, but this time for the specific reason that he had to avoid the front entrance.[2] From his associations to the front garden (the female genitals) it appeared that his fixation on the anus was reinforced by his dislike of the female genitals, a dislike that was based on a fear of them which had many determinants, one important one being a phantasy of meeting his father's penis while he was copulating with his mother.

This fear, which often has an inhibiting effect, however, can also act as a stimulus to the development of certain sexual phantasies. The boy's attempt to retain his heterosexual impulses, in spite of his fear of his father's penis and his flight from it, can also lead to peculiarities in the sexual life of the adult. A typical boy's phantasy of this kind—and one which Kurt brought out, too—is of copulating with his mother jointly with his father or in turns with him. In this, combined genital and pre-genital phantasies or predominantly genital ones alone may be engaged. In Kurt's games, for instance two toy men or two carts would drive through one entrance or a building which represented his mother's body (another entrance being her anus). These two toy men would often agree to enter together or in turns; or else one of them would overpower or outwit the other. In this struggle the smaller man—Kurt himself—by

[1] This is, incidentally, a typical game among children.

[2] In this description I have only selected one or two of the play phantasies involved in order to illustrate by their development the development of play phantasies in general. The material quoted was supported by a number of representations of various kinds. Thus, for example, the carts that carried goods to the town took a road which was shown by various details to have the significance of the anus.

turning himself into a giant would gain the victory and would remove the bigger one—his father. But soon after, a reaction of anxiety would set in and he would use the other entrance, the back one, and give up the front one to the father figure. This example shows how the child's fear of castration impedes the establishment of his genital stage and strengthens his fixation, or rather regression, to pregenital stages. But the immediate result is not always a regression to the pregenital stage. If the child's anxiety is not too strong, he can have recourse to many kinds of phantasies belonging to the genital level besides the ones that have been mentioned here.

What the individual as a child shows us in these play phantasies will emerge in him in manhood as a necessary condition of his love life. Kurt's phantasies of the two toy men entering a building from different sides or using the same side, either together or alternately, either after a fight or by agreement, display the various ways in which an individual will actually behave in a 'triangular' situation in which he is the third party. In such a situation he may, for instance, take the line of the 'injured third party' or of the family friend who outwits the husband or fights him, and so on. Another effect of anxiety, on the other hand, may be to diminish the frequency of games of this sort representing coitus, and this effect will come out in later life in the diminished or disturbed potency of the individual in question. To what extent he will be able to live out the sexual phantasies of his childhood in later life will depend on other factors in his development as well, especially his experiences in reality. But fundamentally, the conditions under which he can love are foreshadowed in every particular in the play phantasies of his early years.

From the development of these phantasies, one can see that as the child's sexual impulses advance to the genital level his capacity for sublimation develops too. Kurt, for instance, made a house that was to be all his own. The house was his mother of whom he wanted to have sole possession. At the same time he could never do enough in the way of building his house well and making it beautiful.

Play phantasies of this kind already outline the detachment from his love-objects that the child will effect later on. Another small patient of mine used to represent his mother's body by means of maps. At first he wanted to have larger and larger sheets of paper so as to make the maps as large as possible; then, after his game had been interrupted by an anxiety-reaction, he began to do the opposite and make very small maps. By the smallness of the things, he attempted to depict a dissimilarity and detachment from his original large object—his mother—but this attempt failed, and his maps got bigger and bigger again until at last they reached their original size and he was once more interrupted in his drawing by anxiety. He brought out the same idea in the paper dolls which he cut out. The small doll, which he always ended by discarding in favour of a larger one, turned out to be a small girl friend of his whom he was trying to make his love-object instead of his mother. Thus we see that the individual's capacity for libidinal detachment from his objects at puberty has its roots in early years and that analysis of the small child is of great assistance in facilitating this process.

As his analysis goes forward the boy becomes increasingly able to carry out in games and sublimations the heterosexual phantasies in which he dares to fight his father for the possession of his mother. His pregenital fixations diminish and the struggle itself changes greatly in character. His sadism decreases, which facilitates the fight since it arouses less anxiety and guilt in him. Thus his increased ability to carry out his phantasies in games calmly and uninterruptedly and to introduce the element of reality into them more satisfactorily, is an indication that he possesses the foundations of sexual potency in later life. These changes in the character of his phantasies and games are always accompanied by other important changes in his whole behaviour, such as being more active and freer. This is seen from the removal of numerous inhibitions in him and from his changed attitude both to his immediate and his more distant environment.

I shall now describe the development of play phantasies in the course of an analysis of a little girl. Rita, aged two and three-quarters, was severely inhibited in play. The only thing she would do—and that only very unwillingly and with obvious inhibitions— was to play with her dolls and toy animals. Even this occupation had a clearly obsessional character. It consisted almost entirely of washing her dolls and continually changing their clothes in a compulsive way. As soon as she introduced any phantasy-element into these activities—that is, as soon as she began to play in the proper sense of the word, she had an immediate outbreak of anxiety and stopped the game.[1] Analysis showed that her feminine and maternal attitude was very poorly developed. In her play with her doll she played the part of mother only to a very slight degree; mainly she was identified with the doll. Her own acute fear of being dirty or destroyed inside or wicked urged her to keep on cleaning her doll—who represented her own person—and changing its clothes. Only after her castration complex had been analysed in part did it transpire that her obsessional play with her doll at the very beginning of the analysis had already given expression to her deepest anxiety, namely, her fear that her mother would take her children away from her.

[1] In Chapters I and II I have referred in another connection to the deeper causes of Rita's anxiety and the repression of her phantasies.

At the time when her castration complex was in the foreground, Rita made a toy bear represent the penis which she had stolen from her father[1] and with the help of which she wanted to supplant her father in the possession of her mother's love. The anxiety she experienced in this part of her analysis set in in connection with masculine phantasies of this kind. It was not until her deeper-lying anxiety belonging to the feminine and maternal position had been analysed that a genuinely maternal attitude towards her bear and her doll became apparent. While she was kissing the bear and hugging it and calling it pet names, Rita once said: 'Now I'm not a bit unhappy[2] any more because I've got such a dear little child after all.' The primacy she had now attained of the genital stage of a heterosexual and a maternal attitude found expression in many ways, among which was her changed attitude to her objects. Her aversion to her father, which before had been so marked, gave place to affection for him.[3]

The reason why we can foretell from the character and development of play phantasies in children what their sexual life will be in later years, is because the whole of their play and sublimations is based on masturbation phantasies. If, as I think, their games are a means of expressing their masturbation phantasies and finding an outlet for them, it becomes understandable that the character of their play phantasies will[4] indicate the nature of their later sexual life; and it also follows that child analysis is able not only to bring about a greater stability and capacity for sublimation in the child, but to ensure mental well-being and prospects of happiness in the adult.

---

[1] Rita used to pretend that she had got rid of the guard of the train and that she was now travelling with the bear to the house of a 'good' woman where she would be well looked after. But the guard came back and threatened her. This showed that her fear of her father, whose penis (the bear) she had stolen, prevented her from maintaining her identification with him.

[2] Rita suffered from periods of pronounced depression during which she sometimes brought to light quite extraordinarily strong feelings of guilt, and at others sat by herself and cried. When asked why she was crying she would answer: 'Because I'm so unhappy'; and when asked why she was unhappy she would answer: 'Because I'm crying.'

[3] Cf. Chapter II.

[4] In his course of lectures, 'On the Technique of Psycho-Analysis', delivered in Berlin in 1923, Hanns Sachs mentioned the evolution of masturbation phantasies from the anal-sadistic to the genital stage as one of the criteria which, in the analysis of an obsessional case, indicate that the treatment has been completed.

Chapter VII

THE SEXUAL ACTIVITIES
OF CHILDREN

ONE of the important achievements of psycho-analysis is the discovery that children possess a sexual life which finds utterance both in direct sexual activities and in sexual phantasies.

We know that masturbation in babies is a general occurrence and that masturbatory activities very commonly extend, in a greater or lesser degree, right up to the latency period, though, of course, we scarcely expect to find children, even small ones, masturbating openly. In the period immediately preceding puberty and particularly during puberty itself, masturbation becomes very frequent again. The period in which the child's sexual activities are least pronounced is the latency period. This is because the dissolution of the Oedipus complex is accompanied by a diminution of instinctual demands. On the other hand, it is still unexplained why, particularly in the latency period, the child's struggle against masturbation is at its height. Freud writes[1] 'The chief task during the latency period seems to be the fending-off of the temptation to masturbate.' His statement seems to support the view that during the latency period the pressure of the id has yet not diminished to the extent commonly accepted, or else that the force of the child's sense of guilt against the demands of the id has increased.

In my opinion, the strong sense of guilt which accompanies masturbatory activities in children is really aimed at the destructive trends which find expression in the masturbation-phantasies.[2] It is this sense of guilt which urges children to stop masturbating altogether and which, if it has been successful in doing so, often leads them on to a phobia of touching. That a fear of this kind is as important an indication of a disturbance in development as obsessive masturbation is perfectly evident from analyses of adults, where we see how the patient's excessive fear of masturbation often leads to grave disorders of his sexual life. Disturbances of this kind cannot, of course, actually be seen in the child, since they only emerge in later life in the form of impotence or frigidity according to

[1] Freud, *Inhibitions, Symptoms and Anxiety. S.E.* **20,** p. 116.
[2] Cf. Chapter VIII.

the sex of the individual; but their existence can be inferred from the presence of certain other difficulties which are invariable concomitants of a faulty sexual development.

Analyses of touching-phobias show that a too complete suppression of masturbation not only leads to all kinds of symptoms, particularly to tic,[1] but, by causing an excessive repression of masturbation phantasies, puts a grave obstacle in the way of the formation of sublimations—a task of the latency period which is of paramount importance from the cultural point of view.[2] For masturbation phantasies are not only the basis of all the child's play activities but a constituent of all its later sublimations. When these repressed phantasies are set free in analysis, the small child can be seen to play and the older one to learn and to develop sublimations and interests of every kind; while at the same time, if it has been suffering from a phobia of touching, it will start masturbating again. Also in cases of compulsive masturbation,[3] a much greater capacity for sublimation will be achieved, along with other changes according to the extent to which we succeed in dissolving that compulsion. In this case, however,[4] the child will continue to masturbate, though to a more moderate degree and not obsessively. Thus, as regards capacity for sublimation and masturbatory activity, analysis of obsessive masturbation and analysis of phobias of touching lead to the same result.

It would seem, then, that the decline of the Oedipus conflict normally ushers in a period in which the child's sexual desires are diminished though by no means entirely lost; and that a moderate amount of masturbation of a non-obsessive kind is a normal occurrence in children of all ages.

The factors underlying compulsive masturbation are operative in yet another form of infantile sexual activity. As I have repeatedly said, in my experience it is the regular thing for quite young children to enter into sexual relations with one another. Moreover, analyses

---

[1] Cf. Ferenczi, 'Psycho-Analytical Observations on Tic' (1919).

[2] In my paper, 'A Contribution to the Psychogenesis of Tics' (1925, *Writings*, 1), I have described a cause of tic during the analysis of which the patient gradually got rid of his symptom together with his fear of touching, at the same time as he resumed his long-forbidden practice of masturbation and along with it built up a number of sublimations.

[3] It nearly always happens that analysis of touching-phobias leads the patient through a temporary phase of obsessive masturbation, and vice versa. Another factor in obsessive masturbation is the patient's desire, based on his sense of guilt, to display his habit to the people about him. This also holds good for children of all ages who masturbate openly and to all appearance in an uninhibited manner.

[4] Cf. Chapter III.

of children in the latency and puberty periods have shown in a number of cases that mutual activities of this kind have not stopped with the onset of the latency period, or in other cases have been suddenly resumed for a time. The same factors were found to be operative in the main in every instance. I shall illustrate this by two cases, namely the relationship between two brothers of six and five years and that of a boy of fourteen and his sister of twelve years of age. As I analysed both partners in each case I was in a position to have a full view of the interaction of all factors.

The two brothers, Günther and Franz, had been brought up in poor but not unfavourable circumstances. Their parents got on well together; and although the mother had to do all the housework herself, she took an active and enlightened interest in her sons. She sent Günther to be analysed on account of his unusually inhibited and timid character and his obvious want of contact with reality. He was a secretive and extremely distrustful child, apparently incapable of any genuine feelings of affection. Franz, on the other hand, was aggressive, over-excitable and difficult to manage. The brothers got on very badly together, but on the whole Günther seemed to give way to his younger brother.[1] In their analysis, I was able to trace back their mutual sexual acts as far as the ages of about three and a half and two and a half years respectively,[2] but it is quite probable that they had begun even earlier. The analysis revealed that whereas neither had any conscious sense of guilt whatever about these acts (though they were careful to conceal them), both suffered from a very heavy one in the unconscious. To the elder brother, who had seduced the younger and sometimes forced him to perform them, the acts—which comprised mutual *fellatio*, masturbation and touching the anus with the fingers—were equivalent to castrating his brother (*fellatio* meant biting off his penis) and totally destroying his whole body by cutting and tearing him to pieces, poisoning or burning him, and so on. An analysis of the phantasies accompanying the acts showed that they not only represented destructive onslaughts upon his younger brother but that the latter stood for Günther's father and mother joined in sexual intercourse. Thus his behaviour was in a sense an actual enactment, though in a mitigated form, of his sadistic masturbatory phantasies against his parents.[3] Moreover, in doing these things, sometimes by force, to his [younger] brother, Günther was trying to assure himself that he would also come out best

---

[1] Analysis revealed the presence of strong psychotic traits in both boys. But we are solely concerned here with the analysis of their sexual relations.

[2] At that time their mother had noticed one or two occurrences of this kind.

[3] In his book *Der Schrecken* (1929), Reik has pointed out that anxiety increases feelings of hatred.

in his dangerous fight with his parents. His overwhelming fear of his parents increased his impulse to destroy them, and the subsequent attacks carried out in phantasy against them made his parents even more terrifying. Furthermore, his fear that his brother might betray him intensified his hatred of him and his desire to kill him by means of his practices with him.

Günther, who possessed an enormous amount of sadism, had a sexual life almost entirely lacking in positive elements. In his phantasy,[1] the various sexual procedures he undertook were nothing but a series of cruel and subtle tortures, designed in the end to put his object to death. His relations with his brother were continually arousing his anxiety along these lines, and served to increase those difficulties which had led to a completely abnormal psycho-sexual development in him.

As to the younger brother, Franz, his unconscious had a clear conception of the unconscious meaning of the acts and accordingly his terror of being castrated and killed by his elder brother had been heightened to an exaggerated degree. Yet he had never complained to anyone nor in any way allowed their relations to be discovered. He, the younger one, reacted to these activities which terrified him so much with a severe masochistic fixation and with a sense of guilt although he was the one who had been seduced. The following are some of the reasons for this attitude.

In his sadistic phantasies Franz identified himself with the brother who was doing him violence, and in this way obtained satisfaction of his sadistic trends, which, as we know, are one of the sources of masochism. But in thus identifying himself with the object of his fear he was also attempting to master his anxiety. In phantasy he was now the assailant and the enemy he was overpowering was his id[2] and also his brother's penis, internalized within himself, which represented his father's penis—his dangerous superego—and which he viewed as a persecutor. This persecutor would

---

[1] Cf. my paper, 'Early Stages of the Oedipus Conflict' (1928). In their total lack of any reaction-formations as well as in many other respects, these phantasies resembled the actions of criminals of a sadistic type. Günther felt no remorse or sorrow, but only fear of retaliation. But this fear was a constant incentive to him to repeat his sexual activities. Owing to his extremely abnormal character, in which the destructive instincts so greatly predominated over the libidinal ones that his sexual behaviour was equated with criminal actions (and we must not forget that among adult criminals perverse sexual acts often go along with criminal ones), his fear of retaliation, as we have seen, urged him to put his object out of the way. Every time Günther did violence to his brother he received assurance that he himself was not the victim.

[2] Cf. my paper, 'Personification in the Play of Children' (1929), in which these mechanisms are discussed at greater length.

be destroyed within by the attacks that were being made on his own body.[1, 2]

But since the boy could not maintain this alliance with a cruel external super-ego against his id and his internalized objects, because it constituted too great a menace to his ego, his hatred was continually being diverted to his external objects—which represented his own feeble and hated ego as well—so that he would, for instance, sometimes be brutal to children younger and weaker than himself. These displacements accounted for the hatred and rage which he showed at times during his analytic interview. He would, for instance, threaten me with a wooden spoon, wanting to push it into my mouth and calling me small, stupid and weak. The spoon symbolized his brother's penis being forcibly thrust into his own mouth. He had identified himself with his brother and thus turned his hatred of him against his own self. He passed on his rage against himself for being small and weak to other children less strong than him, and, incidentally, to me in the transference-situation. Alternately with the employment of this mechanism, he used in phantasy to reverse his relations with his elder brother so that he would view Günther's attacks on him as something that he, Franz, was doing to Günther. Since in his sadistic phantasies—this applies to Franz as well as to Günther—his brother was at the same time a substitute for his parents, he was put in the position of being his brother's accomplice in a joint attack on them, and consequently shared Günther's unconscious sense of guilt and fear of being found out by them. He had thus, like his brother, a strong unconscious motive for keeping the whole relationship secret.

A number of observations of this kind led me to the conclusion that it is the excessive pressure by the super-ego which determines a compulsive instigation of sexual activities, just as it determines a complete suppression of them, that is to say, that anxiety and a sense of guilt reinforces libidinal fixations and heightens libidinal desires.[3]

[1] In Chapter XI. I shall go more fully into this particular mechanism, which seems to me a fundamental one in the formation of feminine masochism.

[2] In her paper, 'Psychotic Mechanisms in Cultural Development' (1930), Melitta Schmideberg has pointed out that among primitive people the practice of expulsion of disease by violence aims at overcoming the patient's fear of the demon within him (his father's introjected penis).

[3] On this point, which is dealt with in greater detail in Chapter VIII, I find myself in agreement with Reik, who, in his 'Libido und Schuldgefühl' (1929), has pointed out that in certain instances activation of the sense of guilt can bring about a strengthening of the libido and an enlargement of instinctual satisfaction, and that in these cases an increase of anxiety coming from a bad conscience can actually enforce instinctual satisfaction.

An excessive sense of guilt and too great anxiety appear to *prevent* a lessening of the child's instinctual needs when the latency period sets in. And we have to add to this that in that period even a lessened sexual activity calls forth excessive reactions of guilt. The structure and dimensions of the child's neurosis will determine the outcome of the struggle in the latency period. A phobia of touching on the one hand and obsessive masturbation on the other are the two extremes of a complemental series that presents an almost infinite number of possible gradations and variations of the final result.

In the case of Günther and Franz it became clear that their compulsion to have sexual intercourse with one another was determined by a factor which would seem to be of general significance for the repetition-compulsion. When his anxiety concerns an unreal danger directed towards the inside of his body, the individual is impelled to turn that danger into a real and external one. (In the present instance, Franz's fear of his brother's internalized penis as a persecutor and his fear of his 'bad' internalized parents urged him to let himself be assaulted by his brother.) He will continually be bringing about an external danger-situation of this kind in a compulsive way since the fear of the real danger-situation[1] is nevertheless not so great as the anxiety he feels about the inside of his body and can also be better dealt with.

It would have been impossible to put a stop to the brother's sexual relations by external measures, since their home was not big enough for each to have a bedroom of his own. And even if such a measure had been practicable, in my experience it would have failed in a case like this, since the compulsion on both sides was so strong. As it turned out, when they were left alone together for only a few minutes in the day, they would use the time for some kind of mutual sexual touching which had the same significance for their unconscious as the complete performance of their various acts, imagined as being sadistic. It was only after a long analysis of both boys, during which I never once tried to influence them to give up their practices[2] but confined myself to the analysis by bringing to light the determin-

---

[1] M. N. Searl has pointed out the mechanism of flight into reality in her paper, 'The Flight to Reality' (1929).

[2] I may remark that in this particular case, where the evil consequences of the boys' relations were so striking I did not find it at all easy to keep to my absolute rule of abstaining from any interference of that kind. And yet it was precisely this case which brought me most convincing proof of the uselessness of any educational measures on the part of the analyst. Even if I had been able to stop their practices—which I was not—I should have done nothing towards the essential business of removing the underlying determinants of the situation and thus giving a new direction to the whole course of their hitherto faulty development.

ing cause of their sexual relations to each other, that their sexual activities gradually began to change, becoming at first less compulsive in character and finally ceasing altogether. It now became evident that the two had not grown indifferent about them, but that their sense of guilt as it became less acute urged them to renounce the practices. Whereas overwhelming anxiety and a sense of guilt originating in an early stage of development had led to a compulsion, that is to say, to a reinforcement of the fixation, a lessened sense of guilt showed itself in a different way, enabling them to give up their mutual sexual relations. Hand in hand with the gradual alteration and final cessation of their sexual practices, their personal attitude towards each other, which previously had been hostile and angry, gave way to a normal and friendly brotherly relation.

Coming to the second case, it will be sufficient for me to mention the facts and to state that, however different in detail, the same factors were operative as in the previous case. Ilse, aged twelve, and Gert, aged thirteen and a half, used to indulge from time to time in coitus-like acts which happened quite suddenly, and often after long intervals. The girl showed no conscious sense of guilt about them but the boy, who was much more normal, felt very guilty. The analysis of both children showed that they had had sexual relations with each other in earliest childhood which were only temporarily broken off at the beginning of the latency period; an overpowering sense of guilt generated an obsessive impulse in both of them, which from time to time, made them repeat their acts. During the latency period[1] the acts, as performed in early childhood, became not only less frequent but more limited in their scope. The children had given up *fellatio* and *cunnilingus* and for some time had not gone beyond touching and inspecting each other. During pre-puberty, however, they began having coitus-like contact once more. It was the brother who initiated these acts and they were compulsive in character. He used to do them on a sudden impulse and never thought about them before or after. He even used to 'forget' the event altogether between whiles. He had a partial amnesia of this kind for a number of things associatively connected with these

[1] In other instances, too, in which intercourse of this kind has been prolonged into the latency period, it has been my experience that only a portion of the original acts is continued (*fellatio* and *cunnilingus* being most often given up) and that even that remnant is performed more seldom—usually only quite occasionally. Nevertheless, in the child's unconscious they repeated the original relationship and all the acts performed at that time. For instance, after an attempt to have coitus with her brother, Ilse developed a rash round her mouth. This rash was an expression of her sense of guilt about *fellatio*, which she used to practice as a small child together with other sexual acts, but which she had given up since early childhood.

sexual relations, especially in regard to his early childhood. As far as the girl was concerned, she had often been the active partner in early childhood but later on she had only played a passive role.

As, under analysis, the profounder causes of this compulsion began to emerge in the two children, it was gradually resolved in both, until in the end the sexual relation between them stopped entirely. As in the previous case, their personal relations, which had originally been very bad, showed a remarkable improvement.

In these two cases and others like them the lifting of the compulsion is effected simultaneously with a number of important and interconnected changes. The analytically induced gradual decrease of [the child's] sense of guilt is accompanied by a lessening of sadism and a stronger emergence of the genital phase. These changes become evident in corresponding changes in [the child's] masturbation phantasies and, in the younger child, also in the play phantasies.

During analyses of children at the age of puberty a further alteration takes place in their masturbation phantasies. For instance, Gert had no conscious masturbation phantasies at all; but in the course of his analysis he began to have one about a girl whose naked body, but not her head, was visible. At a later stage the head began to appear and grew more and more distinct till at last it became recognizable as that of his sister. By that time, however, his compulsion was already done and his sexual relations with his sister had completely stopped. This shows the connection there was between the excessive repression of his desires and phantasies in regard to his sister and his obsessive impulse to have sexual relations with her. Later on still his phantasies underwent a further change and he saw other, unknown girls in his phantasy. Finally he had phantasies about one in particular, a friend of his sister's. This gradual alteration registered the process of libidinal detachment from his sister that was going on—a process which could not take place until his compulsive fixation on her, maintained by his excessive sense of guilt, had been removed in the course of analysis.[1]

In general, as regards the existence of sexual relations between children, especially between brothers and sisters, I may say on the basis of my observations that they are the rule in early childhood but are only prolonged into the latency period and puberty if the child's sense of guilt is excessive and has not been successfully worked over.[2] As far as we can judge, the effect of the sense of guilt

[1] Gert came to me on account of certain neurotic difficulties of a not very severe kind. His analysis lasted one year. Three years later I heard that he was doing well.

[2] In any case I think that such relations are much more frequent even during latency and puberty than is usually supposed.

THE SEXUAL ACTIVITIES OF CHILDREN

during the latency period is to allow the child to continue to masturbate, though in a lesser degree than before, but at the same time to make it give up its sexual activities with other children, whether its own brothers and sisters or not, as being too realistic an enactment of its incestuous and sadistic desires. During puberty the movement away from such relations is continued, in conformity with the aims of that period which involve a detachment from incestuous objects. But at a later stage of puberty the individual will normally enter into relations with new objects—a relationship based on his progressive detachment from the old objects and on different trends that act against incest.

The question that arises now is how far relations of this kind can be prevented from occurring in the first instance. It seems highly doubtful whether it is possible to do this without causing a good deal of harm in other ways, since, for instance, the children would have to be kept under regular surveillance and would suffer a serious curtailment of liberty; and whether in any case, however strictly they were watched, it could be done at all. Furthermore, although early experiences like these can do a lot of harm in some cases, in others they may influence the child's general development favourably. For besides satisfying the child's libido and his desire for sexual knowledge, relations of this kind serve the important function of reducing his excessive sense of guilt. The phantasies connected with these relations are based upon sadistic masturbation phantasies which generate the most intense feelings of guilt; for this reason, the fact that his proscribed phantasies against his parents are shared by a partner gives him the feeling of having an ally and this greatly lightens the burden of his anxiety.[1] On the other hand a relation of this kind gives rise to anxiety and a sense of guilt on its own account. Whether its effect will ultimately be good or bad—whether it will protect the child from anxiety or increase it—seems to depend upon the extent of his own sadism and more especially upon the attitude of his partner. From my knowledge of a number of cases, I should say that where the positive and libidinal factors predominate, such a relationship has a favourable influence upon the child's object relations and capacity for love;[2] but where destructive impulses and even acts of coercion on one side dominate, it can impair the whole development of the child in the gravest way.

In the matter of the sexual activities of children—as in some other matters—psycho-analytic knowledge has shown us the full import

[1] In his book, *Gemeinsame Tagträume* (1924), Hanns Sachs remarks upon the fact that when incestuous phantasies or day-dreams are shared the sense of guilt is lessened.
[2] Cf. Chapters XI and XII for a fuller consideration of these factors.

of certain developmental factors, but without offering us the possibility of suggesting any really reliable measures of a prophylactic kind. Freud says in the *Introductory Lectures*[1]: 'These facts have a certain interest from the point of view of education, which plans the prevention of neuroses by intervening at an early stage in children's sexual development. So long as one focuses attention principally on infantile sexual experiences, one must suppose that one has done everything for the prophylaxis of nervous illnesses by taking care that the child's development is delayed and that it is spared experiences of the sort. We already know, however, that the preconditions for the causation of neuroses are complex and cannot be influenced in general if we take account of only a single factor. Strict protection of the young loses value because it is powerless against the consitutional factor. Besides, it is more difficult to carry out than educationists imagine and it brings with it two fresh dangers which must not be underestimated: the fact that it may achieve too much—that it may encourage an excess of sexual repression, with damaging results, and the fact that it may send the child out into life without any defence against the onrush of sexual demands that is to be looked for at puberty. Thus it remains extremely doubtful how far prophylaxis in childhood can be carried with advantage and whether an altered attitude to the immediate situation may not offer a better angle of approach for the prevention of neuroses.'

[1] *Introductory Lectures on Psycho-Analysis* (1918), *S.E.* **16**, p. 364.

Part II

EARLY ANXIETY-SITUATIONS AND THEIR EFFECT ON THE DEVELOPMENT OF THE CHILD

Chapter VIII

EARLY STAGES OF THE OEDIPUS CONFLICT AND OF SUPER-EGO FORMATION

In the following chapters I intend to make a contribution to our knowledge of the origin and structure of the super-ego. The theoretical conclusions I am going to put forward are based on actual analyses of small children which enabled me to have a direct view of the earliest processes of mental development. These analyses have shown that oral frustrations release the Oedipus impulses and that the super-ego begins to be formed at the same time.[1] The genital impulses remain out of sight at first, since they do not as a rule assert themselves fully against the pre-genital impulses until the third year of life. This is the beginning of that developmental period which is characterized by the distinct demarcation of genital trends and which is known as the early flowering of sexuality and the phase of the Oedipus conflict.

In the following pages I shall outline the developmental processes which precede this early expansion of sexuality and try to show that the early stages of the Oedipus conflict and of the formation of the super-ego extend, roughly, from the middle of the first year to the third year of the child's life.

Normally the infant's pleasure in sucking is replaced by pleasure in biting. Lack of satisfaction at the oral sucking stage increases its need for satisfaction at the oral-biting stage.[2] Abraham's opinion that the child's inability to get sufficient pleasure in its sucking period is determined by the feeding situation, is borne out beyond doubt by general analytic observation. We also know that this

---

[1] Cf. my paper, 'Early Stages on the Oedipus Conflict' (1928, *Writings*, 1).

[2] In his 'The Influence of Oral Erotism on Character Formation' (1924), Abraham has pointed out (p. 397) that excess of satisfaction as well as want of it in the sucking period can lead to a specially strong fixation on pleasure in biting. In his 'Notes on Oral Character-Formation' (1925) Edward Glover lays special stress on the importance of oral frustration for a fixation of this kind, since he believes that whenever an excess of oral satisfaction leads to traumatic consequences other factors are at work as well. In my view, too, the results are essentially different in the two cases.

situation is one of the fundamental factors in the illnesses and development deficiencies of children. Nevertheless, unfavourable feeding conditions which we may regard as external frustrations, do not seem to be the only cause for the child's lack of pleasure at the sucking stage. This is seen from the fact that some children have no desire to suck—are 'lazy feeders'—although they receive sufficient nourishment. Their inability to obtain satisfaction from sucking is, I think, the consequence of an internal frustration and is derived, in my experience, from an abnormally increased oral sadism.[1] To all appearances these phenomena of early development are already the expression of the polarity between the life-instincts and the death-instincts. We may regard the force of the child's fixation at the oral-sucking level as an expression of the force of its libido, and, similarly, the early and powerful emergence of its oral sadism is a sign that its destructive instinctual components tip the balance.

As Abraham[2] and Ophuijsen have pointed out, a reinforcement from constitutional sources of the zones which are involved in biting, such as the muscles of the jaw, is a fundamental factor in the infant's fixation at the oral-sadistic level. The most serious deficiencies of development and psychic illnesses result where external frustrations—i.e. unfavourable feeding conditions—coincide with a constitutionally strengthened oral sadism which impairs the infant's enjoyment in sucking. Conversely, an oral sadism which sets in neither too soon nor too violently (and this presupposes that the sucking stage has run its course satisfactorily) seems to be a necessary condition for the normal development [of the child].[3]

If this is the case, time factors will take on a new importance side by side with quantitative ones. If the increase in the child's oral-

---

[1] Erna (cf. Chapter III) was a case in point. She had repeatedly injured her mother's breast by biting when she was still quite small and long before she had grown her teeth. She had also been a lazy feeder in infancy. I have come across other instances, too, of abnormally strong oral sadism in which the sucking period had brought with it no outward disturbance or difficulty but had been completely unsatisfactory for the child. Again, we get cases in which serious external disturbances in that period have led, not to an abnormally intense oral sadism, but to a strong fixation at the oral-sucking stage. Thus Ruth (Chapter II), who had a strong oral-sucking fixation of this kind, had gone hungry for months as an infant because her mother had too little milk. Another patient, who had never had the breast at all but had been bottle-fed, showed a strong oral sadism, it is true, but he also had a strong fixation at the oral-sucking stage.

[2] Abraham, 'A Short Study of the Development of the Libido' (1924), p. 451.

[3] Another developmental factor of basic importance is, I have found, the greater or lesser capacity of the immature ego to tolerate anxiety. This factor will be discussed later on.

sadistic trends sets in too violently, its object-relations and character formation will be dominated by its sadism and ambivalence,[1] and if it sets in too early, its ego will develop too soon. As we know, one factor in the genesis of obsessional neurosis is the development of its ego in advance of its libido.[2] A fundamental cause for a precocious development of the ego can be seen in a premature and excessive increase of its oral sadism which will exert great pressure on its as yet immature ego.

Concerning the origin of anxiety, Freud has broadened his original conception and now only gives a very limited validity to the hypothesis that anxiety arises from a direct transformation of libido. He shows that when the sucking infant is hungry it feels anxiety as a result of an increase of tension caused by its need, but that this early anxiety-situation has an earlier prototype. He says: 'The situation of non-satisfaction in which the amounts of stimulation rise to an unpleasurable height . . . must for the infant be analogous to the experience of being born—must be a repetition of the situation of danger. What both situations have in common is the economic disturbance raised by an accumulation of amounts of stimulation which require to be disposed of. It is this factor, then, which is the real essence of the "danger". In both cases, the reaction of anxiety sets in.'[3] On the other hand, he has difficulty in reconciling the fact 'that the anxiety felt in phobias is an ego anxiety and arises in the ego, and that it does not proceed out of repression but, on the contrary, sets repression in motion'[4] with his first statement that in certain cases anxiety arises from a tension of libido. The supposition[5] that 'when coitus is disturbed or sexual excitation interrupted or abstinence enforced, the ego scents certain dangers to which it reacts with anxiety' does not to his mind offer a satisfactory solution of the contradiction. In a later passage he once more returns to the problems from the discussion of other points. He relates the emergence of anxiety to 'a situation analogous to birth . . . in which the ego is helpless in the face of a constantly increasing instinctual demand— the earliest and original determinant of anxiety.[6] He defines as the nucleus of the danger-situation the 'admission of helplessness in the face of it [the danger]—physical helplessness if the danger is real and psychical helplessness if it is instinctual'[7].

The clearest instance of transformation of unsatisfied libido into

---

[1] Cf. Abraham, 'The Influence of Oral Erotism on Character-Formation' (1924) (p. 398); also Edward Glover, 'The Significance of the Mouth in Psycho-Analysis' (1924).

[2] Cf. Freud, 'The Predisposition to Obsessional Neurosis' (1913).

[3] *Inhibitions, Symptoms and Anxiety* (1926), *S.E.* **20**, p. 137.

[4] *ibid.*, p. 110.   [5] *ibid.*, p. 110.   [6] *ibid.*, p. 144.   [7] *ibid.*, p. 166.

anxiety is, I think, the reaction of the suckling to tensions caused by physical needs. Such a reaction, however, is without doubt not only one of anxiety but of rage as well.[1] It is difficult to say at what time the fusion of the destructive and libidinal instincts occurs. There is a good deal of evidence for the view that it has existed from birth and that the tension caused by need merely serves to strengthen the sadistic instincts of the infant. We know, however, that the destructive instinct is directed against the organism itself and must therefore be regarded by the ego as a danger. I believe it is this danger which is felt by the individual as anxiety.[2] Therefore anxiety would originate from aggression.[3] But since, as we know, libidinal frustration heightens the sadistic instincts, unsatisfied libido would, according to this view, indirectly liberate anxiety or increase it. On this theory Freud's suggestion that the ego scents a danger in abstinence would be a solution of the problem after all. My only contention is that the danger which he calls 'psychical helplessness—if it [the danger] is instinctual' arises from the destructive instincts.

Freud tells us that the narcissistic libido of the organism thrusts the death-instinct outwards towards its objects in order to prevent it from destroying the organism itself. He considers this process fundamental to the individual's relations to his objects and to the mechanism of projection. He goes on to say: 'Another portion [of the death-instinct] does not share this transposition outwards; it remains inside the organism and, with the help of the accompanying sexual excitation described above, becomes libidinally bound there. It is

---

[1] Cf. Ferenczi, 'The Problem of the Acceptance of Unpleasant Ideas' (1926). In his paper, 'The Problem of Melancholia' (1928), Radó has pointed out the importance of rage in the reaction of the infant to hunger, but the inferences he has drawn from it are different from those I shall put forward in the following pages.

[2] In *Inhibitions, Symptoms and Anxiety* (1926), Freud considers that in some cases a certain amount of instinctual anxiety which has become released from the destructive instinct may enter into reality anxiety. His actual words are: 'It may quite often happen that although a danger situation is correctly estimated in itself, a certain amount of instinctual anxiety is added to the realistic anxiety. In that case the instinctual demand before whose satisfaction the ego recoils is a masochistic one: the instinct of destruction directed against the subject himself. Perhaps an addition of this kind explains cases in which reactions of anxiety are exaggerated, inexpedient or paralysing.' (*S.E.* **20**, p. 168 n.)

[3] Since writing this book I find that Therese Benedek, starting from a different line of approach, has also come to the conclusion that anxiety originates in the destructive instinct. She says: 'Anxiety, therefore, is not a fear of death but the perception of the death-instinct that has been liberated in the organism—the perception of primary masochism' ('Todestrieb und Angst', 1931).

in this portion that we have to recognize the original erotogenic masochism.'[1]

It seems to me that the ego has yet another means of mastering those destructive impulses which still remain in the organism. It can mobilize one part of them as a defence against the other part. In this way the id will undergo a split which is, I think, the first step in the formation of instinctual inhibitions and of the super-ego and which may be the same thing as primal repression.[2] We may suppose that a split of this sort is rendered possible by the fact that, as soon as the process of incorporation has begun, the incorporated object becomes the vehicle of defence against the destructive impulses within the organism.[3]

The anxiety evoked in the child by his destructive instinctual impulses makes itself felt in the ego, I think, in two directions. In the first place it implies the annihilation of his own body by his destructive impulses, which is a fear of an internal instinctual danger;[4] but in the second place it focuses his fears on his *external* object, against whom his sadistic feelings are directed, as a source of danger. The onset of the development of its ego which is accom-

---

[1] 'The Economic Problem in Masochism' (1924), *S.E.* **19**, p. 163/4.

[2] In *'Inhibitions, Symptoms and Anxiety'* (1926) (*S.E.* **20**, p. 94), Freud writes: 'We cannot at present say whether it is perhaps the emergence of the super-ego which provides the time of demarcation between primal repression and after-pressure. At any rate the earliest outbreaks of anxiety, which are of a very intense kind, occur before the super-ego has become differentiated. It is highly probable that the immediate precipitating causes of primal repressions are quantitative factors, such as an excessive degree of excitation and the breaking through of the protective shield against stimuli.'

[3] The process by which the object is internalized will be discussed later on. At present it is enough to say that, in my opinion, the incorporated object at once assumes the role of a super-ego.

[4] In early analysis we come across numerous representations of this anxiety. Here is an example: A five-year-old boy used to pretend that he had all sorts of wild animals, such as elephants, leopards, hyenas and wolves, to help him against his enemies. Each animal had a special function. The elephants were to stamp the foe to a pulp, the leopards to tear him to bits and the hyenas and wolves to eat him up. He sometimes imagined that these wild animals who were in his service would turn against him, and this idea used to arouse very great anxiety in him. It turned out that the animals stood in his unconscious for the various sources of his sadism—the elephant being his muscular sadism; the animals that tore, his teeth and nails; and the wolves, his excrements. His fear that those dangerous animals which he had tamed would themselves exterminate him was referable to his fear of his own sadism as a dangerous internal enemy. Let me also remind the reader of the common expression 'to burst with rage'. In my analyses of small children I have repeatedly come across representations of the idea underlying this figure of speech.

panied by the growing ability to test reality leads the child to experience his mother as someone who can give or withhold satisfaction and in this way it acquires the knowledge of the power of his object in relation to the satisfaction of his needs—a knowledge which seems to be the earliest basis in external reality for his fear of the object. In this connection it would appear that he reacts to his intolerable fear of instinctual dangers by shifting the full impact of the instinctual dangers on to his object, thus transforming internal dangers into external ones. Against these external dangers his immature ego then seeks to defend itself by destroying his object.

We must now go on to consider in what way a deflection of the death-instinct outwards influences the relations of the child to his objects and leads to the full development of his sadism. His growing oral sadism reaches its climax during and after weaning and leads to the fullest activation and development of sadistic tendencies flowing from every source. His oral-sadistic phantasies, which seem to form a link[1] between the oral-sucking and oral-biting stages, have a quite definite character and contain ideas that he gets possession of the contents of his mother's breast by sucking and scooping it out. This desire to suck and scoop out, first directed to her breast, soon extends to the inside of her body.[2] In my article, 'Early Stages of the Oedipus Conflict',[3] I have described an early stage of development which is governed by the child's aggressive trends against its mother's body and in which its predominant wish is to rob her body of its contents and destroy it.

As far as can be seen, the sadistic tendency most closely allied to oral sadism is urethral sadism. Observations have confirmed that children's phantasies of flooding and destroying by means of enormous quantities of urine in terms of soaking, drowning, burning and poisoning are a sadistic reaction to their having been deprived

---

[1] Abraham has drawn attention to the vampire-like behaviour of some people and has explained it as being the effect of a regression from the oral-sadistic to the oral-sucking stage. ('The Influence of Oral Erotism on Character Formation', 1924, p. 401.)

[2] In discussing this subject with me, Edward Glover suggested that the feeling of emptiness in its body which the small child experiences as a result of lack of oral satisfaction might be a point of departure for phantasies of assault on its mother's body, since it might give rise to phantasies of the mother's body being full of all the desired nourishment. Going over my data once more, I find that his supposition is completely borne out. It seems to me to throw fresh light upon the steps by which the transition is effected from sucking out and devouring the mother's breast to attacking the inside of her body. In this connection Dr Glover also mentioned Radó's theory of an 'alimentary orgasm' ('The Psychic Effects of Intoxicants', 1926), in virtue of which satisfaction passes over from the mouth to the stomach and intestines.

[3] (1928, *Writings*, 1).

of fluid by their mother and are ultimately directed against her breast. I should like in this connection to point out the great importance, hitherto little recognized, of urethral sadism in the development of the child.[1] Phantasies, familiar to analysts, of flooding and destroying things by means of great quantities of urine,[2] and the more generally known connection between playing with fire and bed-wetting,[3] are merely the more visible and less repressed signs of the sadistic impulses which are attached to the function of urinating. In analysing both children and adults I have constantly come across phantasies in which urine was imagined as a burning, corroding and poisoning liquid and as a secret and insidious poison. These urethral-sadistic phantasies have a fundamental share in giving the penis the unconscious significance of an instrument of cruelty and in bringing about disturbances of sexual potency in the male. In a number of instances I have found that bed-wetting was caused by phantasies of this kind.

Every other vehicle of sadistic attack that the child employs, such as anal sadism and muscular sadism, is in the first instance levelled against its mother's frustrating breast; but it is soon directed to the inside of her body, which thus becomes at once the target of every highly intensified and effective instrument of sadism. In early analysis these anal-sadistic destructive desires of the small child constantly alternate with desires to destroy its mother's body by devouring and wetting it; but their original aim of eating up and destroying her breast is always discernible in them.[4]

[1] In his 'The Narcissistic Evaluation of Excretory Processes in Dreams and Neurosis' (1920) in connection with a case of strongly developed urethral sadism, Abraham states that in neurotic persons 'we find the functions and products of the bowel and bladder used as vehicles of hostile impulses' (p. 319).

[2] Cf. in especial Freud, The Interpretation of Dreams (1900), and Three Essays on the Theory of Sexuality (1905); also Sadger, 'Über Urethralerotik' (1910); Abraham, 'Ejaculatio Praecox' (1917) and 'The Narcissistic Evaluation of Excretory Processes in Dreams and Neurosis' (1920), and Rank, Psychoanalytische Beiträge zur Mythenforschung (1919).

[3] Cf. Freud's remarks on this connection in his 'Fragment of an Analysis of a Case of Hysteria' (1905), S.E. 7, p. 71–72.

[4] In his 'Short Study of the Development of the Libido' (1924) (p. 474) Abraham has pointed out that criminal phantasies of manic patients are for the most part directed against their mother, and he gives a striking example of this in a patient who identified himself in his imagination with the Emperor Nero, who killed his mother and wanted to burn down Rome (a mother symbol). But according to Abraham these destructive impulses of the son against his mother are secondary in character, being originally aimed at his father. In my view these attacks on her body have their origin in oral-sadistic attacks upon her breast and are therefore primary; but in so far as they are reinforced by his original hatred of his father's penis as he imagines it to exist

The phase of life in which the child's phantasies of sadistically attacking the inside of its mother's body are predominant, is initiated by the oral-sadistic stage of development and comes to an end with the decline of the earlier anal-sadistic stage and embraces the period when sadism is at its height in every area.

Abraham's work has shown that the pleasure the infant gets from biting is not only due to libidinal satsfaction of its erotogenic zones but is connected with clearly marked destructive cravings which aim at the annihilation of its object. This is still more so in the phase when the sadism is at the height of its development. The idea of an infant of from six to twelve months trying to destroy its mother by every method at the disposal of its sadistic trends—with its teeth, nails and excreta and with the whole of its body, transformed in phantasy into all kinds of dangerous weapons—presents a horrifying, not to say an unbelievable picture to our minds. And it is difficult, as I know from my own experience, to bring oneself to recognize that such an abhorrent idea answers to the truth. But the abundance, force and multiplicity of the cruel phantasies which accompany these cravings are displayed before our eyes in early analyses so clearly and forcibly that they leave no room for doubt. We are already familiar with those sadistic phantasies of the child which find their culmination in cannibalism, and this makes it easier for us to accept the further fact that as its methods of sadistic attack become enlarged so do its sadistic phantasies gain in fullness and vigour. This element of escalation of impulse seems to me to be the key to the whole matter. If what intensifies sadism is libidinal frustration, we can readily understand that the destructive cravings which are fused with the libidinal ones and cannot be gratified—in the first instance, that is, oral-sadistic cravings—should lead to a further intensification of sadism and to an activation of all its methods.

In early analyses we find, furthermore, that oral frustration arouses in the child an unconscious knowledge that its parents enjoy mutual sexual pleasures and a belief at first that these are of an oral sort. Under the pressure of its own frustration it reacts to this phantasy with envy of its parents, and this in turn reinforces its hatred of them. Its cravings to scoop and suck out now lead it to want to suck out and devour all the fluids and other substances which its parents (or rather their organs) contain, including what they have

---

inside her body and are centred upon that object and culminate in its destruction, they are directed against his father to an extent sufficient to influence the whole course of his Oedipus conflict. Thus it is true to say that the son's primary hatred of his father is in part displaced on to his mother. In Chapter XII, we shall discuss in detail the significance of this displacement in the sexual development of the male child.

received from one another in oral copulation.[1] Freud has shown that the sexual theories of children are a phylogenetic heritage, and from what has been said above it appears to me that an unconscious knowledge of this kind about sexual intercourse between the parents, together with phantasies concerning it, already emerges at this very early stage of development. Oral envy is one of the motive forces which make children of both sexes want to push their way into their mother's body and which arouse the desire for knowledge allied to it.[2] Their destructive impulses, however, soon cease to be directed against the mother alone and become extended to the father. For they imagine that his penis is incorporated by her during oral copulation and remains inside her (the father being equipped with a great many), so that their attacks on her body are also levelled at his penis inside it.

I think that the reason why the boy has in the deepest layers of his mind such a tremendous fear of his mother as the castrator, and why he harbours the idea so closely associated with that fear, of the 'woman with a penis', is that he is afraid of her as a person whose body contains his father's penis; so that ultimately what he is afraid of is his father's penis incorporated in his mother.[3] The displacement of feelings of hatred and anxiety from the father's penis to the mother's body which harbours it is very important, I think, in the origin of mental disorders and is an underlying factor in disturbances of sexual development and in the adoption of a homosexual attitude.[4] This displacement, I think, occurs in this way: the fear of his

[1] In a short communication, 'A Paranoiac Mechanism as seen in the Analysis of a Child' (1928), M. N. Searl has reported a case of intensely oral-sadistic phantasies of this kind, in which the child's craving to suck out of its father what he had taken from its mother's breast was bound up with paranoic mechanisms. The great power exerted by phantasies of this sort, which are connected with an intense oral sadism and which consequently pave the way for particularly aggressive impulses against the inside of the mother's body, is, I have since found, characteristic of psychotic disorders.

[2] Cf. Abraham, 'Psycho-Analytical Studies on Character-Formation' (1925).

[3] In his 'Homosexualität und Ödipuskomplex' (1926) Felix Boehm draws attention to the significance of phantasies frequently found in men that their father's penis has been retained by their mother after copulation and is hidden inside her vagina. He also points out that 'the various notions of a concealed female penis exert a pathological influence in virtue of the fact that they are brought into unconscious relation with the idea of a large and dreaded penis belonging to the father, which is hidden inside the mother'. In psycho-analytical literature frequent mention is made of phantasies of meeting the father's penis in the mother's womb and of witnessing copulation between the parents, or of being damaged by it, during intra–uterine life.

[4] Cf. Chapter XII.

father's penis incorporated by his mother is worked over by the well-known mechanism of displacement on to the less disturbing fear of the maternal penis. The fear of the paternal penis incorporated by the mother is so overwhelming, because at this early stage of development the principle of *pars pro toto* holds good and the penis also represents the father in person. Thus the penis inside the mother represents a combination of father and mother in one person,[1] this combination being regarded as a particularly terrifying and threatening one. As I pointed out earlier, at its period of maximal strength the child's sadism is centred round coitus between his parents. The death-wishes he feels against them during the primal scene or in his primal phantasies are associated with sadistic phantasies which are extraordinarily rich in content and which involve the sadistic destruction of his parents both singly and together.

The child also has phantasies in which his parents destroy each other by means of their genitals and excrements which are felt to be dangerous weapons. These phantasies have important effects and are very numerous, containing such ideas as that the penis, incorporated in the mother, turns into a dangerous animal or into weapons loaded with explosive substances; or that her vagina, too, is transformed into a dangerous animal or some instrument of death, as, for instance, a poisoned mouse-trap. Since such phantasies are wish-phantasies and since his sexual theories are largely fed by sadistic desires, the child has a sense of guilt about the injuries which, in his phantasy, his parents inflict on each other.

In addition to the quantitative increase which the child's sadism undergoes at every point of origin, qualitative changes take place in it and serve to heighten it still further. In the later part of the sadistic phase, the child's imaginary attacks on his object, which are of a very violent nature and made by every method at the disposal of his sadism, become extended to include secret and surreptitious attacks by particularly subtle methods, which make them all the more dangerous. In the first part of this phase, for instance, where open violence reigns, excrements are regarded as instruments of direct assault; but later they acquire significance as substances of an explosive or poisonous kind. All these elements taken together give rise to sadistic phantasies whose number, variety and richness are all but inexhaustible. Moreover, these sadistic impulses against his

---

[1] I have noticed in boys' analyses time and again that attempts to attack me were directed more especially against my head or feet or nose. The analysis of these attacks showed that they were directed against these parts of the body not only as such, but that my head, feet and nose symbolized the penis. I have found that it was not the female penis which they were thus attacking but the father's penis which had been incorporated in me or affixed to my person.

father and mother copulating together lead the child to expect punishment jointly from both parents. In this early stage, however, his anxiety serves to intensify his sadism and to increase his impulse to destroy the dangerous object, so that he brings a still greater amount of sadistic and destructive wishes to bear upon his combined parents and is correspondingly more afraid of them as a hostile entity.

According to my view, the Oedipus conflict sets in in the boy as soon as he begins to have feelings of hatred against his father's penis and to want to achieve genital union with his mother and destroy his father's penis which he supposes to be inside her body. I consider that early genital impulses and phantasies, which set in during the phase dominated by sadism, constitute in children of both sexes the early stages of the Oedipus conflict, because they satisfy the accepted criteria for it. Although the child's pre-genital impulses are still predominant, it is already beginning to feel, in addition to oral, urethral and anal desires, genital desires for the parent of the opposite sex and jealousy and hatred of the parent of the same sex and to experience a conflict between its love and its hatred of the latter even at this early stage. We may even go so far as to say that the Oedipus conflict owes its very acuteness to this early situation. The small girl, for instance, while turning from her mother with feelings of hatred and disappointment and directing her oral and genital desires towards her father, is yet bound to her mother by the powerful ties of her oral fixations and of her helplessness in general; and the small boy is drawn to his father by his positive oral attachment, and away from him by feelings of hatred that arise from the early Oedipus situation. But the conflict is not so clearly visible in this stage of the child's development as it is later on. This, I think, is partly due to the fact that the small child has less means of giving expression to its feelings and that its relations to its objects at this early stage of development are as yet confused and vague. A part of its reactions to its objects are passed on to its phantasy-objects;[1] and it often directs the bulk of its anxiety and hatred towards the latter—especially towards internalized objects—so that its attitude towards its parents only reflects a portion of the difficulties it experiences in its attitude to its object.[2] But these difficulties find expression in a

---

[1] It attaches to its phantasy-objects not only feelings of hatred and anxiety but positive feelings as well. In doing this it withdraws them from its real objects, and if its relations to its phantasy-objects are too powerful, both in a negative and a positive sense, it cannot adequately attach either its sadistic phantasies or its restitutive ones to its real objects, with the result that it undergoes disturbances of its adaptation to reality and of its object-relationships.

[2] I shall discuss these object-relations later on.

number of other ways. It has been my experience, for instance, that the night-terrors and phobias of small children are already due to an Oedipus conflict.

I do not think that a sharp distinction can be made between the early stages of the Oedipus conflict and the later ones. Since, as far as my observations show, the genital impulses set in at the same time as the pre-genital ones and influence and modify them, and since as a result of this early association, they themselves bear traces of certain pre-genital impulses even in later stages of development,[1] the attainment of the genital stage merely means a strengthening of the genital impulses. That the pre-genital and genital impulses are thus merged together is seen from the well-known fact that when children witness the primal scene or have primal phantasies—both events of a genital character—they experience very powerful pre-genital impulses, such as bed-wetting and defaecating, accompanied by sadistic phantasies directed towards their copulating parents.

According to my observation, the child's masturbation phantasies have as their nucleus early sadistic phantasies centred upon its parents' copulation. It is those destructive impulses, fused with libidinal ones, which cause the super-ego to put up defences against masturbation phantasies and, incidentally, against masturbation itself. The child's sense of guilt about its early genital masturbation is thus derived from its sadistic phantasies directed against its parents. And since, furthermore, those masturbation phantasies contain the essence of its Oedipus conflict and can therefore be regarded as the focal point of its whole sexual life, the sense of guilt it has on account of its libidinal impulses is really a reaction to the destructive impulses that are fused with them.[2] If this is so, then not only would it be the incestuous trends which give rise in the first instance to a sense of guilt, but horror of incest itself would ultimately be derived from the destructive impulses which are bound up permanently with the child's earliest incestuous desires.

If we are right in supposing that the child's Oedipus trends set in

[1] I do not, for instance, think that Fenichel is justified in differentiating 'pre-genital precursors of the Oedipus complex' from the Oedipus complex itself, as he does in his 'Pregenital Antecedents of the Oedipus Complex' (1930).

[2] In a paper, 'The Importance of Symbol-Formation in the Development of the Ego', which I read at the Psycho-Analytical Congress held in Oxford in 1929, I stated the view as follows: 'It is only in the later stages of the Oedipus conflict that the defence against the libidinal impulses makes its appearance; in the earlier stages it is against the accompanying destructive impulses that the defence is directed.' *Writings*, 1.

At the same Congress Ernest Jones, in his paper, 'Fear, Guilt and Hate' (1929), laid stress upon the importance of the aggressive tendencies in giving rise to the sense of guilt.

when the sadism is at its height, we are led to the conclusion that it is chiefly impulses of hate which initiate the Oedipus conflict and the formation of the super-ego and which govern the earliest and most decisive stages of both. Such a view, though it may at first sight seem alien to the accepted theory of psycho-analysis, nevertheless fits in with our knowledge of the fact that the development of the libido proceeds from the pre-genital to the genital stage. Freud has repeatedly pointed out that hatred precedes the development of love. He writes:[1] 'Hate as a relation to objects, is older than love. It derives from the narcissistic ego's primordial repudiation of the external world with its outpouring of the stream of stimuli', and again:[2] 'The ego hates, abhors and pursues with intent to destroy all objects which are a source of unpleasurable feelings for it, without taking into account whether they mean a frustration of sexual satisfaction or of the satisfaction of self-preservative needs.'[3]

Originally it was believed that the formation of the super-ego begins in the phallic phase. In his 'Dissolution of the Oedipus Complex' (1924) Freud states that the Oedipus complex is succeeded by the erection of the super-ego—that it falls to pieces and the super-ego takes its place.[4, 4a] Again, in his *Inhibitions, Symptoms and Anxiety* (1926),[5] we read: 'The anxiety felt in animal phobias is, therefore, an affective reaction on the part of the ego to danger; and the danger which is being signalled in this way is the danger of castration. This anxiety differs in no respect from the realistic anxiety which the ego normally feels in situations of danger, except that its content remains unconscious and only becomes conscious in the form of a distortion.' If this were so, however, then the anxiety

---

[1] 'Instincts and their Vicissitudes' (1915), p. 139.

[2] *ibid.*, p. 138.

[3] In his *Civilization and its Discontents* (1930), he goes still further and says: 'It [aggressiveness] forms the basis of every relation of affection and love among people (with the single exception, perhaps, of the mother's relation to her male child)' (*S.E.* **21**, p. 113). My own view that the Oedipus conflict starts under the primacy of sadism seems to me to supplement what Freud says, since it gives another reason why hatred should be the basis of object-relationships in the fact that the child forms its relation with its parents—a relation that is so fundamental and so decisive for all its future object-relationships — during the time when its sadistic trends are at their height. The ambivalence it feels towards its mother's breast as its first object becomes strengthened by the increasing oral frustration it undergoes and by the onset of its Oedipus conflict, until it grows into fully-developed sadism.

[4] *S.E.* **19,** p. 177.

[4a] The author apparently quoted from memory as the exact wording quoted could not be found at the place mentioned; but in substance the quotation remains correct. See *S.E.* **19,** p. 177.

[5] *S.E.* **20,** p. 126.

ects children until the beginning of the latency period
related solely to fear of castration in the case of the boy and
osing love in the case of the girl, and the super-ego would
form until the pre-genital stages had been left behind and
.... be effected by a regression to the oral stage. Freud[1] writes:
'At the very beginning, in the individual's primitive oral phase,
object cathexis and identification are no doubt indistinguishable
from each other'; and[2] 'it' (the super-ego) 'is in fact a precipitate
of the first object cathexes of the id, and is the heir to the Oedipus
complex after its demise'.

According to my observations, the formation of the super-ego is a
simpler and more direct process. The Oedipus conflict and the
super-ego set in under the supremacy of the pre-genital impulses,
and the objects which have been introjected in the oral-sadistic
phase—the first object cathexes and identifications—form the
beginnings of the early super-ego.[3] Moreover, what initiates the
formation of the super-ego and governs its earliest stages are the
destructive impulses and the anxiety they arouse. Also in my view,
the significance of the objects for the formation of the super-ego
remains fully valid; but it appears in a different light if we regard
the impulses of the individual as the fundamental factor in the
formation of the super-ego. I found that the earliest identifications
of the child give an unreal and distorted image of the objects on
which they are based. As we know from Abraham,[4] in an early
stage of development both real and introjected objects are mainly
represented by their organs. We also know that the father's penis is an
anxiety object *par excellence* and is equated with dangerous weapons
of various kinds and with animals which poison and devour, while
in the unconscious the vagina represents a dangerous opening.[5]
These equations as I learnt to recognize them, are a universal
mechanism of fundamental importance in the formation of the
super-ego. As far as I can judge, the nucleus of the super-ego is to be
found in the partial incorporation that takes place during the

[1] *The Ego and the Id, S.E.* **19**, p. 29.
[2] *The Question of Lay Analysis* (1927), *S.E.* **20**, p. 223.
[3] In her paper, 'Privation and Guilt' (1929), Susan Isaacs points out that
Freud's 'primary identification' probably plays a greater part in the formation
of the super-ego than was originally supposed.
[4] Abraham writes: 'Another point to be noted in regard to the part of the
body that has been introjected, is that the penis is regularly equated with the
female breast . . .' ('A Short Study of the Development of the Libido, viewed
in the Light of Mental Disorders.' (1924), *Selected Papers*, p. 490.
[5] Cf. the phantasy, so often mentioned in psycho-analytic literature, of the
vagina dentata.

cannibalistic phase of development;[1] and the child's early imagos take the imprint of those pre-genital impulses.[2]

It would follow logically that the ego would regard the internalized object as so cruel an enemy of the id from the fact that the destructive instinct which the ego has turned outward has become directed against that object, and consequently nothing but hostility against the id can be expected. But as far as can be seen, a phylogenetic factor is also involved in the origin of the very early and intense anxiety which, in my experience, the child feels in respect of his internalized object. The father of the primal horde was the external power which enforced an inhibition of instinct.[3] The fear of his father which man had acquired in the course of history would, when he began to internalize his object, serve in part as a defence against the anxiety to which his destructive instinct gave rise.[4]

[1] In the next chapter, and more especially in Chapter XI, I shall try to show that the child introjects [unrealistic] imagos, both phantasized good imagos and phantasized bad ones, and that gradually, as his adaptation to reality and the formation of his super-ego go forward, those imagos approximate more and more closely to the real objects they represent. In this chapter I only intend to give a picture of the development of the child's sadistic trends and their connection with his early super-ego formation and anxiety-situations.

[2] In my 'Early Stages of the Oedipus Conflict' (1928) I wrote: 'It does not seem clear why a child of, say, four years old should set up in his mind an unreal, phantastic image of parents who devour, cut and bite. But it is clear why in a child of about one year old the anxiety caused by the beginning of the Oedipus conflict takes the form of a dread of being devoured and destroyed. The child himself desires to destroy the libidinal object by biting, devouring and cutting it, which leads to anxiety, since the awakening of the Oedipus tendencies is followed by introjection of the object, which then becomes one from which punishment is to be expected. The child then dreads a punishment corresponding to the offence: the super-ego becomes something which bites, devours and cuts.'

[3] Cf. Freud, *Totem and Taboo* (1913).

[4] The ego would, as it were, play off its two enemies, the object and the destructive instinct, against one another, although in so doing it would find itself in a very perilous position between the two opposed forces. That the dreaded father should in part be a protection against the destructive instinct may also be due to the admiration for his power which the individual would have acquired in the same phylogenetic way. This possibility receives support from the fact that in early analysis we find that quite small children of both sexes are not only afraid of their father but have a feeling of boundless admiration for his power — a feeling which is very deep-lying and primary in character. And we must remember that as children grow older, the part their super-ego plays, though that of a severe father, is not that of an unkind one. Freud concludes his paper on 'Humour' (1928) with these words: 'And, finally, if the super-ego tries, by means of humour, to console the ego and protect it from suffering, this does not contradict its origin in the parental agency.' *S.E.* **21**, p. 166.

Concerning the formation of the super-ego, Freud seems to follow two lines of thought, which are to some extent mutually complementary. According to one, the severity of the super-ego is derived from the severity of the real father whose prohibitions and commands it repeats.[1] According to the other, as indicated in one or two passages in his writings, its severity is an outcome of the destructive impulses of the subject.[2]

Psycho-analysis has not followed up the second line of thought. As its literature shows, it has adopted the theory that the super-ego is derived from parental authority and has made this theory the basis of all further enquiry into the subject. Nevertheless, Freud has recently, in part, confirmed my own view,[3] which lays emphasis on

[1] In his 'The Dissolution of the Oedipus Complex' (1924) Freud says that the ego of the child turns away from the Oedipus complex in consequence of the threat of castration. 'The authority of the father or the parents is introjected into the ego and there it forms the nucleus of the super-ego, which takes over the severity of the father and perpetuates his prohibition against incest, and so insures the ego against a recurrence of the libidinal object-cathexis' (S.E. **19,** pp. 176–7). In The Ego and the Id (1923) we are told: 'Its (the super-ego's) 'relation to the ego is not exhausted by the precept: "You *ought to be* like this (like your father) — that is, you may not do all that he does; some things are his prerogative." This double aspect of the ego-ideal derives from the fact that the ego-ideal had the task of repressing the Oedipus complex; indeed, it is to that revolutionary event that it owes its existence. Clearly the repression of the Oedipus complex was no easy task. The child's parents, and especially his father, were perceived as the obstacle to a realization of his Oedipus wishes; so his infantile ego fortified itself for the carrying out of the repression by erecting this same obstacle within itself. It borrowed strength to do this, so to speak, from the father, and his loan was an extraordinarily momentous act. The super-ego retains the character of the father, while the more powerful the Oedipus complex was and the more rapidly it succumbed to repression (under the influence of authority, religious teaching, schooling and reading), the stricter will be the domination of the super-ego over the ego later on — in the form of conscience or perhaps of an unconscious sense of guilt. I shall presently bring forward a suggestion about the source of its power to dominate in this way — the source, that is, of its compulsive character which manifests itself in the form of a categorical imperative' (S.E. **19,** pp. 34–5).

[2] In The Ego and the Id (1923) he says: 'Every such identification is in the nature of a desexualization or even of a sublimation. It now seems as though when a transformation of this kind takes place, an instinctual defusion occurs at the same time. After sublimation the erotic component no longer has the power to bind the whole of the destructiveness that was combined with it, and this is released in the form of an inclination to aggression and destruction. This defusion would be the source of the general character of harshness and cruelty exhibited by the ideal — its dictatorial "Thou shalt".' (S.E. **19,** pp. 54–5.)

[3] My views are in agreement with those of Ernest Jones, Edward Glover, Joan Riviere and M. N. Searl, who, approaching the subject from different standpoints, have come to the conclusion that the child's early phantasy life and libidinal development play a large part in the evolution of the super-ego.

the importance of the impulses of the individual as a factor in the origin of his super-ego and on the fact that his super-ego is not identical with his real objects.[1]

It appears to me to be justified to call the early identifications made by the child 'early stages of super-ego formation' in the same way as I have used the term 'early stages of the Oedipus conflict'. Already in the earliest stages of the child's development the effects of these object cathexes exert an influence of a kind which characterizes them as a super-ego, although they differ in quality and influence from the identifications belonging to later stages. And cruel as this super-ego formed under the supremacy of sadism may be, it nevertheless even becomes at this early stage, the agency from which instinctual inhibitions proceed, as it takes over the ego's defence against the destructive instinct.

Fenichel has applied certain criteria[2] which differentiate the 'precursors of the super-ego' (as he calls those early identifications in accordance with a suggestion made by Reich)[3] from the super-ego itself. These precursors exist, he thinks, in a scattered state and independently of one another, and lack the unity, the severity, the opposition to the ego, the quality of being unconscious and the great power which characterize the actual super-ego as inheritor of the Oedipus complex. In my opinion such a differentiation is incorrect in several respects. As far as I have been able to observe, it is precisely the early super-ego which is especially severe; and under normal conditions, in no period of life is the opposition between ego and super-ego so strong as in early childhood. Indeed, this latter fact explains why in the first stages of life the tension between the two is chiefly felt as anxiety. Furthermore, I have found that the commands and prohibitions of the super-ego are no less unconscious in the small child than in the adult, and that they are by no means identical with

---

Cf. 'Symposium on Child Analysis' (1926); also a paper by Ernest Jones on 'The Origin and Structure of the Super-ego' (1926), in which he points out that 'there is every reason to think that the concept of the super-ego is a nodal point where we may expect all the obscure problems of Oedipus complex and narcissism on the one hand, and hate and sadism on the other, to meet' (p. 304).

[1] In his *Civilization and its Discontents* (1930) we read: 'Experience shows, however, that the severity of the super-ego which a child develops in no way corresponds to the severity of treatment which he has himself met with' and that 'the original severity of the ego does not—or does not so much—represent the severity which one has experienced from it (the object), or which one attributes to it; it represents rather one's own aggressiveness towards it.' (*S.E.* **21**, pp. 129–30.)

[2] Fenichel, 'Identification' (1926).

[3] Cf. Reich, *Der Triebhafte Charakter* (1925).

the commands that come from its real objects. Fenichel is right, I think, in saying that the super-ego of the child is not yet as organized as that of the adult. But this point of difference, apart from not being universally true, since many small children exhibit a well-organized super-ego and many adults a weakly-organized one, seems to me merely to be in keeping with the lesser degree of organization of the small child's mind as compared to the adult's. We also know that small children have a less highly-organized ego than children in the latency period, yet this does not mean that they have no ego, but only precursors of an ego.

I have already said that in the phase when the sadism is at its height a further increase of sadistic trends leads to an increase of anxiety. The threats of the early super-ego against the id contain in detail the whole range of sadistic phantasies that were directed to the object, which are now turned back against the ego item by item. Thus the pressure of anxiety exerted in this early stage will correspond in quantity to the extent of sadism originally present, and in quality to the variety and wealth of the accompanying sadistic phantasies.[1]

The gradual overcoming of sadism and anxiety[2] is a result of the progressive development of the libido. But the very excess of his anxiety is also an incentive for the individual to overcome it. Anxiety assists the several erotogenic zones to grow in strength and gain the upper hand one after another. The supremacy of the oral- and urethral-sadistic impulses is replaced by the supremacy of the anal-sadistic impulses; and since the mechanisms belonging to the early anal-sadistic stage, however powerful they may be, are already acting in the service of the defences against anxiety arising from the earlier periods of this phase, it follows that that very anxiety which is pre-eminently an inhibiting agency in the development of the individual is at the same time a factor of fundamental importance in promoting the growth of his ego[3] and of his sexual life.

In this stage, his methods of defence are violent in the extreme, since they are proportionate to the excessive pressure of anxiety. We know that in the early anal-sadistic stage what he is ejecting is his object, which he perceives as something hostile to him and which he equates with excrement. But as I see it, what is already being ejected in the early anal-sadistic stage is the terrifying super-ego which he has introjected in the oral-sadistic phase. Thus his act of ejection is a

my paper, 'Infantile Anxiety Situations Reflected in a Work of Art' *Writings*, **1**).
he next chapter for a fuller discussion of this point.
hapter X, about the significance of anxiety in the development of the

means of defence employed by his fear-ridden ego against his super-ego; it expels his internalized objects and at the same time projects them into the outerworld. The mechanisms of projection and expulsion in the individual are closely bound up with the process of super-ego formation. Just as his ego tries to defend itself against his super-ego by violently ejecting it and thus destroying it, so it also tries to rid itself of his destructive trends by forcible expulsion. Freud[1] considers the idea of defence as well-fitted for 'a general designation for all the techniques which the ego makes use of in conflicts which may lead to a neurosis, while we retain the word "repression" for the special method of defence which the line of approach taken by our investigations made us better acquainted with in the first instance'. He furthermore emphasizes the possibility 'that repression is a process which has a special relation to the *genital* organization of the libido and that the ego resorts to other methods of defence when it has to secure itself against the libido on other levels of organization'[2]. My view is also supported by Abraham in a passage in which he says that 'the tendency to spare the object and to preserve it has grown out of the more primitive destructive tendency by a process of repression'.[3]

Concerning the dividing line between the two anal-sadistic stages the same author writes as follows:[4] 'In regarding this dividing line as extremely important we find ourselves in agreement with the ordinary medical view. For the division that we psycho-analysts have made on the strength of empirical data coincides in fact with the classification into neurosis and psychosis made by clinical medicine. But analysts, of course, would not attempt to make a rigid separation between neurotic and psychotic affections. They are, on the contrary, aware that the libido of any individual may regress beyond this dividing line between the two anal-sadistic phases, given a sufficiently exciting cause of illness, and given certain points of fixation in his libidinal development which facilitate a regression of this nature.'

As we know, the normal man does not differ from the neurotic in structural, but in quantitative factors. The above quotations from Abraham show that he, too, sees the difference between the psychotic and the neurotic as one of degree only. My own psycho-analytical work with children has not only confirmed me in the opinion that the points of fixation for psychoses lie in the stages of development preceding the second anal level, but has also convinced me that these

---

[1] '*Inhibitions, Symptoms and Anxiety*', S.E. **20**, p. 163.
[2] *ibid.*, p. 125.
[3] 'A Short Study of the Development of the Libido' (1924), p. 428.
[4] *ibid.*, p. 433.

points of fixation apply in the same way to neurotic and normal children, though in a minor degree.

We know that the psychotic has a far greater quantity of anxiety than the neurotic; yet there is so far no explanation of the fact that such an overwhelming anxiety can come into being in those very early stages of development in which, according to the findings of Freud and Abraham, the fixations for the psychoses are situated. Freud's latest theories, brought forward in his *Inhibitions, Symptoms and Anxiety*, rule out the possibility that this immense quantity of anxiety might arise from the transformation of unsatisfied libido into anxiety. Nor can we assume that the child's fear of being devoured, cut up and killed by its parents is a realistic fear. But if we suppose that this excessive anxiety can only be an effect of intra-psychic processes we shall not be so far from the theory which I put forward that early anxiety is caused by destructive trends and the pressure of the early super-ego. The pressure which in an early stage of the child's development the super-ego exerts in defence against his destructive trends and which corresponds both in degree and kind to his sadistic phantasies, is reflected, as I see it, in the earliest anxiety-situations. These anxiety-situations are closely related to the sadistic phase. Furthermore they trigger off special mechanisms of defence on the part of his ego and determine the specific character of his psychotic disorder, as well as his development in general.[1]

Before attempting to study the relationship between early anxiety-situations and the specific character of psychotic disorders, however, let me first turn to the way in which the formation of the super-ego and the development of object-relations affect each other. If it is true that the super-ego is formed at such an early stage of ego development, which is still so far removed from reality, we must review the growth of object-relations in a new light. The fact that the image of his objects is distorted by the individual's own sadistic impulses has the following consequences: it not only puts a different complexion on the influence exerted by real objects and by his relations to them, on the formation of his super-ego, but, in contrast to the theory hitherto accepted, it also increases the importance of his super-ego formation in regard to his object-relations. When, as a small child, he first begins to introject his objects—and these, it must be remembered, are yet only very vaguely demarcated by his various organs—his fear of those introjected objects sets in motion the mechanisms of ejection and projection, as I have tried to show; and there now follows a reciprocal action between projection and

---

[1] In *Inhibitions, Symptoms and Anxiety* (1926), Freud writes: 'It is possible, however, that there is a fairly close relationship between the danger-situation operative and the form taken by the ensuing neurosis.' (*S.E.* **20**, p. 142.)

introjection, which seems to be of fundamental importance not only for the formation of his super-ego but for the development of his object-relations and his adaptation to reality. The steady and continual urge he is under to project his terrifying identifications on to his objects results, it would seem, in an increased impulse to repeat the process of introjection again and again, and is thus itself a decisive factor in the evolution of his relationship to objects.[1]

The interaction between object-relation and super-ego also finds expression, I think, in the fact that at every stage of development the methods which the ego uses in its dealings with its object correspond exactly to those used by the super-ego towards the ego, and by the ego towards the super-ego and the id. In the sadistic phase the individual protects himself from his fear of his violent object, both introjected and external, by redoubling his own destructive attacks upon it in his imagination. Getting rid of his object would partly serve the purpose of silencing the intolerable threats of his super-ego. A reaction of this kind presupposes that the mechanism of projection is initiated along two lines—one by which the ego is putting the object in the place of the super-ego from which it wants to free itself, and another by which it is making the object stand for the id of which it also wants to be freed. In this way the amount of hatred which was primarily directed against the object is augmented by the amount meant for the id and the super-ego.[2] Thus it would seem that in people in whom the early anxiety-situations are too powerful and who have retained the defensive mechanisms belonging to that early stage, fear of the super-ego, if for external or intra-psychic reasons it oversteps certain bounds, will compel them to destroy their object and will form the basis for the development of a criminal type of behaviour.[3]

These too-powerful early anxiety-situations are also, I think, of fundamental importance in schizophrenia. But I can only support this view here by putting forward one or two suggestions. As has already been pointed out, by projecting his terrifying super-ego on to his objects, the individual increases his hatred of those objects and thus also his fear of them, with the result that, if his aggression and

[1] In his 'Instincts and their Vicissitudes' (1915), Freud writes: 'In so far as the objects which are presented to it are sources of pleasure, it [the ego] takes them into itself, "introjects" them (to use Ferenczi's term [1909]; and, on the other hand, it expels whatever within itself becomes the cause of unpleasure (see below, the mechanism of projection).' (*S.E.* **14**, p. 136.)

[2] Theodor Reik says in his paper 'Angst und Hass' (1929) that anxiety increases hatred.

[3] If crime does indeed spring from early anxiety in this way, our only hope of understanding the criminal and perhaps reforming him would seem to be to analyse the deepest levels of his mental life.

anxiety are excessive, his external world is changed into a place of terror and his objects into enemies and he is threatened with persecution both from the external world and from his introjected enemies. If his anxiety is too immense or if his ego cannot tolerate it, he will try to evade his fear of external enemies by putting his mechanisms of projection out of action; this would at the same time prevent any further introjection of objects from taking place and put an end to the growth of his relation to reality,[1, 2] and he would be all the more exposed to fear of his already introjected objects. This fear would take various forms of being attacked and injured by an enemy within him from whom there was no escape. A fear of this kind is probably one of the deepest sources of hypochondria, and the excess of it, insusceptible as it is to any modification or displacement, would obviously call out particularly violent methods of defence. A disturbance of the mechanism of projection seems, moreover, to go along with a negation of intra-psychic reality.[3] The person thus affected denies,[4] and, so to speak, eliminates,[5] not only the *source* of his anxiety, but its affect as well. A whole number of phenomena belonging to the syndrome of schizophrenia can be explained as an attempt to ward off, master or contend with an internal enemy. Catatonia, for instance, could be regarded as an attempt to paralyse the introjected object and keep it immovable and so render it innocuous.[6]

The earliest period of the sadistic phase is characterized by the great violence of the attack made on the object. In a later period of

[1] Cf. my paper, 'The Importance of Symbol-Formation in the Development of the Ego' (1930, *Writings*, 1).

[2] Melitta Schmideberg has pointed out that the schizophrenic cuts himself off from the external world by taking refuge in his 'good' internal object — which he accomplishes by ceasing to project and by over-compensating his love of his internal object in a narcissistic way and thus evading his fear of his 'bad' introjected and external objects. ('The Role of Psychotic Mechanisms in Cultural Development', 1930, and 'A Contribution to the Psychology of Persecutory Ideas and Delusions', 1931.)

[3] In his paper, 'Stages in the Development of a Sense of Reality' (1913), Ferenczi has remarked that the complete denial of reality is a very early form of mental reaction and that the points of fixation for psychoses should be situated in a correspondingly early stage of development.

[4] According to Melitta Schmideberg, denial of the affect of anxiety is in part utilized to deny the existence of the introjected object with which the affects are equated ('A Contribution to the Psychology of Persecutory Ideas and Delusions', 1931).

[5] In his 'Scotomisation in Schizophrenia' (1926), Laforgue has suggested the name 'scotomization' for this defensive mechanism and has drawn attention to its importance in schizophrenia.

[6] According to Melitta Schmideberg, catatonia represents death and is a means of escaping from the various forms of attack which the patient dreads (cf. op. cit.).

this phase, coinciding with the early anal stage in which the anal-sadistic impulses take the lead, more secret methods of attack prevail, such as the use of poisonous and explosive weapons. Excrements now represent poisons,[1] and in its phantasies the child uses faeces as persecuting agencies[2] against its objects and secretly and surreptitiously inserts them by a kind of magic (which I consider to be the basis of black magic) into the anus and other bodily apertures of those objects and leaves them there.[3] In consequence it begins to be afraid of its own excrement, as a substance which is dangerous and harmful to its own body, and of the incorporated excrements of its objects from whom it expects similar secret attacks through the same dangerous medium. Thus its phantasies lead to a fear of having a multitude of persecutors inside its body and of being poisoned, and are the basis of hypochondriacal fears. They also serve to increase the fear aroused by the equation of the introjected object with faeces,[4] for that object is made still more dangerous by being linked to the poisonous and destructive scybalum. And the fact that, in consequence of its urethral-sadistic impulses, the child also thinks of urine as something dangerous, as something that burns, cuts and poisons, prepares it unconsciously to regard the penis as a sadistic organ and to dread its father's (the persecutor's)[5] dangerous penis within itself. In this way the sadistic transformation of its excrements into

[1] Cf. my paper, 'The Importance of Symbol-Formation in the Development of the Ego' (1930), also 'A Contribution to the Theory of Intellectual Inhibition' (1931) [both in *Writings*, 1]. More recently, in a paper entitled Respiratory Introjection' (1931), Fenichel has described a class of sadistic phantasies in which the excreta are instruments of killing, the faeces by poisoning and exploding, and the urine by poisoning. According to him these phantasies bring on a fear of being poisoned by excreta. His paper seems to me to corroborate the views already put forward by me in the above-mentioned articles.

[2] Cf. Ophuijsen, 'On the Origin of the Feeling of Persecution' (1920), and Stärcke, 'The Reversal of the Libido-Sign in Delusions of Persecution' (1920). According to them the paranoic's idea of the persecutor is derived from the unconscious idea that persecutor and scybalum are simply treated as equivalent things and that the scybalum represents his persecutor's penis. I have found that the fear of pieces of stool as persecutors was ultimately derived from sadistic phantasies in which urine and faeces were employed as poisonous and destructive weapons against the mother's body.

[3] Róheim, in his 'Nach dem Tode des Urvaters' (1923), has shown that in primitive tribes the black magician kills a man or makes him ill by magically inserting excrements or their equivalents into his body.

[4] Abraham ('A Short Study of the Development of the Libido', 1924) has shown that the hated object is equated with faeces. Cf. also Róheim, 'Nach dem Tode des Urvaters' (1923), and Simmel, 'The Doctor-Game Illness, and the Profession of Medicine' (1926).

[5] Cf. my paper, 'A Contribution to the Theory of Intellectual Inhibition' (1931, *Writings*, 1).

poisonous matter, which the child feels to have been achieved in its phantasy, increases its anxiety of the internalized persecutor.

In the period in which attacks by means of poisonous excreta predominate, the child's fears of analogous attacks upon itself on the part of its introjected and external objects become more manifold, in accordance with the greater variety and subtlety of its own sadistic procedures; and they push the effectiveness of its mechanisms of projection to their furthest limits. Its anxiety spreads out and is distributed over many objects and sources of danger in the outer world, so that it is now afraid of being attacked by a multitude of persecutors.[1] The quality of secrecy and cunning which it attributes to those attacks leads it to observe the world about it with a watchful and suspicious eye and increases its relations to reality, though in a one-sided way; while its fear of the introjected object is a constant incentive to keep the mechanisms of projection in operation.

The fixation point for paranoia is, I think, the period when sadism is at its height, in which the child's attacks upon the interior of its mother's body and the penis it presupposes to be there are carried out by means of poisonous and dangerous excreta;[2] and delusions of reference and persecution seem to me to spring from these anxiety-situations.[3]

[1] The fear of numerous persecutors has not only an anal-sadistic origin, as being a fear of many persecuting faeces, but an oral one as well. In my experience the child's sexual theory, according to which its mother incorporates a new penis every time she copulates and its father is provided with a quantity of penises, contributes to its fear of having a great number of persecutors. Melitta Schmideberg regards this multiplicity of persecutors as being a projection of the child's own oral-sadistic attacks on its father's penis, each separate bit of his penis becoming a new object of anxiety (cf. her paper, 'The Role of Psychotic Mechanisms in Cultural Development', 1930).

[2] Cf. also my paper, 'The Importance of Symbol-Formation in the Development of the Ego' (1930). I find myself in agreement with Abraham's view that in the paranoic the libido regresses to the earlier anal stage, as I assume that the phase of sadism at its height is introduced by the oral-sadistic trends and terminates with the decline of the earlier anal stage. The period of this phase which has been described above and which I consider to be fundamental for paranoia will be seen to be under the supremacy of the earlier anal stage. What has been said here supplements, I think, the findings of Abraham. It shows that in the above-mentioned phase the various means of sadism are employed in conjunction and to their fullest capacity, and that the fundamental importance of the urethral-sadistic trends is stressed side by side with the oral-sadistic ones. It has also furnished a certain amount of information about the structure of those phantasies in which the anal-sadistic trends belonging to the earlier anal stage find expression.

[3] Melitta Schmideberg has since brought forward two cases in which delusional ideas of persecution and reference were derived from anxiety-situations of this kind (cf. her paper, 'A Contribution to the Psychology of Persecutory Ideas and Delusions', 1931).

According to my view, the child's fear of its introjected objec. urges it to project that fear into the external world.[1] In doing this it equates its organs, faeces and all manner of things, as well as its internalized objects, with its external objects; and it also distributes its fear of its external object over a great number of objects by equating one with another.[2, 3]

A relation of this kind to many objects, based in part on anxiety, is, I think, a further advance [on the part of the individual] in the establishment of a relationship to objects and an adaptation to reality; for his original object-relation only included one object, i.e., his mother's breast as representing his mother. In the phantasy of the small child, however, these multiple objects are situated in the very place which is the chief objective of his destructive and libidinal trends and also of his awakening desire for knowledge—namely, inside his mother's body. As his sadistic trends increase and he takes possession in phantasy of the interior of his mother's body, that part of her becomes the representative of the object, and at the same time symbolizes the external world and reality. Originally [the child's] object which is represented by [his mother's] breast is identical with the external world. But now the inside of her body represents object and outer world in a more extended sense, because it has become the place which contains more manifold objects by reason of the wider distribution of his anxiety.

Thus the child's sadistic phantasies about the interior of his mother's body lay down for him a fundamental relation to the external world and to reality. But his aggression and the anxiety he has in consequence of it, is one of the fundamental factors of his object-relations. At the same time, his libido is also active and influences the object-relations. His libidinal relations to his objects and the influence exerted by reality counteract his fear of internal

---

[1] The child's destructive desires against its objects, as represented by bodily organs, arouse its fear of those organs and objects. Such a fear, together with its libidinal interests, leads it to equate those organs with other things, which thus in their turn become objects of anxiety, so that it is continually moving away from them and making fresh equations; and in this way stimulates the development of symbols. (Cf. my paper, 'The Importance of Symbol-Formation in the Development of the Ego', 1930 [*Writings*, **1**]).

[2] As Ferenczi has shown, the small child seeks to rediscover its own organs and their functions in every outside thing by means of identification—which is the precursor of symbolization.

[3] According to Ernest Jones ('The Theory of Symbolism', 1916) the pleasure-principle enables the individual to liken quite different things to each other if the interest they arouse is of a similar kind. This view lays stress on the importance of libidinal interest as a basic factor in processes of identification and symbolization.

and external enemies. His belief in the existence of kindly and helpful figures—a belief which is founded upon the efficacy of his libido[1]—enables his reality-objects to emerge ever more powerfully and his phantastic imagos to recede into the background.

The interaction between super-ego formation and object-relation, based on an interaction between projection and introjection, profoundly influences his development. In the early stages, the projection of his terrifying imagos into the external world turns that world into a place of danger and his objects into enemies; while the simultaneous introjections of real objects which are in fact well-disposed to him, works in the opposite direction and lessens the force of his fear of the terrifying imagos. Viewed in this light, super-ego formation, object-relations and adaptation to reality are the result of an interaction between the projection of the individual's sadistic impulses and the introjection of his objects.

[1] Cf. my paper, 'Personification in the Play of Children' (1929, *Writings*, **1**).

Chapter IX

THE RELATIONS BETWEEN
OBSESSIONAL NEUROSIS AND
THE EARLY STAGES OF
THE SUPER-EGO

IN the previous chapter we considered the content and effects of the early anxiety-situations of the individual. We shall now go on to examine the way in which his libido and his relations to real objects bring about a modification of those anxiety-situations.

Oral frustration leads to a search for new sources of gratification.[1] As a result the little girl turns away from her mother. The father's penis now becomes an early object of oral gratification, but at the same time genital tendencies make their appearance.[2]

So far as the boy is concerned he also develops a positive relationship to the father's penis out of the oral position of sucking, as breast and penis are equated.[3] The oral fixation to the father's penis belonging to the sucking stage appears to me to be a fundamental factor in the establishment of true homosexuality.[4] Normally the boy's fixation on the father's penis is counteracted by feelings of hatred and anxiety that stem from awakening Oedipus tendencies.[5]

---

[1] In his 'Notes on Oral Character-Formation' (1925), Edward Glover has pointed out that frustration is a stimulating factor in the development of the individual.

[2] Cf. my papers, 'The Psychological Principles of Early Analysis' (1926) and 'Early Stages of the Oedipus Conflict' (1928) [both in *Writings*, 1].

[3] In his paper, 'Nach dem Tode des Urvaters' (1923), Róheim argues that through having devoured the corpse of their primal father his sons came to look on him as the nourishing mother. In this way, he thinks, they transferred the love which they had hitherto felt for their mother alone, to their father as well; and their attitude to him, from having been a purely negative one, acquired a positive element.

[4] Cf. Freud, *Leonardo da Vinci and a Memory of his Childhood* (1910). We shall follow these developmental processes more closely in Chapter XII in discussing the sexual development of the boy.

[5] The following example, taken from direct observation, illustrates the course of such a change from like to dislike. In the months which followed his weaning, a small boy showed a preference for fish foods as well as a great interest in fish in general. At the age of one he used often to look on with

If all goes well his good attitude to the father's penis is the foundation of a good relationship to his own sex and at the same time enables the boy to complete his heterosexual development. Whilst, however, in the boy an oral-sucking relation to his father's penis may, under certain circumstances, lead to homosexuality, in the girl it is normally the precursor of heterosexual impulses and of the Oedipus conflict. As the girl turns towards the father her libidinal desires find a new aim; correspondingly the boy, by turning anew to the mother, regains her as a genital love object. The genital asserts itself.

In that early phase of development in which, as I have called it, sadism is at its height, I have found that all the pre-genital stages and the genital stage as well are cathected in rapid succession. What then happens is that the libido gradually consolidates its position by its struggle with the destructive instinctual drives.

Side by side with the polarity of the life-instinct and the death-instinct, we may, I think, place their interaction as a fundamental factor in the dynamic processes of the mind. There is an indissoluble bond between the libido and destructive tendencies which puts the former to a great extent in the power of the latter. But the vicious circle dominated by the death-instinct, in which aggression gives rise to anxiety and anxiety reinforces aggression can be broken by the libidinal forces when these have gained in strength; in the early stages of development, the life-instinct has to exert its power to the utmost in order to maintain itself against the death-instinct. But this very necessity stimulates sexual development.

Since genital impulses remain concealed for a long time, we are not able to discern clearly the fluctuations and interminglings of the various stages of development which result from the conflict between destructive and libidinal impulses. The emergence of the stages of organization with which we are acquainted corresponds, I would say, not only to the positions which the libido has won and established in its struggle with the destructive instinct, but, since these two components are for ever united as well as opposed, to a growing adjustment between them.

Analyses of the deepest mental levels uncover a flourishing sadism of which comparatively little is visible in the small child. My

---

intense and obviously pleasurable interest while his mother killed and prepared fish in the kitchen. Soon afterwards he developed a great dislike of fish foods, which spread to a dislike of seeing fish and then to a regular fish phobia. Experience of numerous early analyses in which attacks on fishes, snakes and lizards have been seen to represent attacks on the father's penis enable us, I think, to understand the child's behaviour. The killing of fish by his mother satisfied his sadistic impulses against his father's penis in a very high degree, and this made him afraid of his father, or, more correctly, of his father's penis.

contention, that in the earliest stages of development the child goes through a phase when its sadism is at its height in all its fields of origin, is only an amplification of the accepted and well established theory that a stage of oral sadism (cannibalism) is followed by one of anal sadism. We must also bear in mind that those cannibalistic tendencies themselves find no expression commensurate with their psychological import; for normally we only get comparatively faint indications of the small child's impulses to destroy its objects. What we see are only derivatives of its phantasies.

The assumption that the extravagant phantasies which arise in a very early stage of the child's development never become conscious could well help to explain the phenomenon that the child expresses its sadistic impulses towards real objects only in an attenuated form. It should, moreover, be remembered that the stage of development of the ego in which these phantasies originate is an early one and that the child's relations to reality are as yet undeveloped and dominated by its phantasy life. A further reason may be found in the relative proportions of the child's size and strength compared with those of the adult and its biological dependence on him; for we see how much more strongly it manifests its destructive instincts towards inanimate things, small animals and so on. The fact that genital impulses, although hidden from view, already exert a restraining influence on the sadism of the young child, may contribute to an early lessening of the sadism expressed towards external objects.

As far as can be seen, there exists in the quite small child, side by side with its relations to real objects, a relationship to unreal imagos which are experienced both as excessively good and as excessively bad, but on a different plane. Ordinarily, these two kinds of object-relations intermingle and colour each other to an ever increasing extent. (This is the process which I have described as an interaction between super-ego formation and object-relations.) But in the mind of the quite small child its real objects and its imaginary ones are still widely separated; and this may in part account for its not exhibiting as much sadism and anxiety towards its real objects as would be expected from the character of its phantasies.

As we know, and as Abraham especially has pointed out, the nature of the child's object-relations and character-formation is very strongly determined by whether its predominant fixations are situated in the oral-sucking stage or in the oral-sadistic one. In my opinion this factor is decisive for the formation of the super-ego as well. The introjection of a kindly mother influences the formation of a friendly father-imago, owing to the equation of breast with penis.[1]

[1] Abraham writes, in 'A Short Study of the Development of the Libido' (1924), p. 490: 'Another point to be noted in regard to the part of the body

In the construction of the super-ego, too, fixations in the oral-sucking stage will counteract the anxiety-provoking identifications which are made under the sway of oral-sadistic impulses.

As the sadistic tendencies of the child diminish, the threats made by his super-ego become somewhat reduced in violence and the reactions of his ego also undergo a change. The child's overwhelming fear of the super-ego and of objects which dominates the earliest stages of development precipitates violent reactions. It would seem that the ego tries to defend itself at first against the super-ego by scotomizing it—to use Laforgue's word—and then by ejecting it. As soon as it attempts to outwit the super-ego[1] and to evade the latter's opposition to the id-impulses, it is, I think, beginning to react in a way which takes cognizance of the power of the super-ego. As the later anal stage sets in, the ego recognizes that power ever more clearly and is led to make progressive attempts to come to terms with it. With the recognition of the power of the super-ego the ego also recognizes the necessity of submitting itself to the commands of the super-ego. At the same time a step has been made towards a recognition of intrapsychic reality, which also depends on the recognition of external reality; the former is the precondition for the latter.[2] The relations of ego to the id, which in a somewhat earlier stage has been one of ejection, becomes in the later anal stage one of suppression of instincts—or rather, of repression in the true sense of the word.[3]

Since the hatred relating to the super-ego and to the id is displaced onto the object, the quantity of hatred for the object is now also reduced.[3a] As the libidinal components increase and effect a diminution of the destructive elements the primary sadistic tendencies

---

that has been introjected is that the penis is regularly equated with the female breast, and that other parts of the body, such as the finger, the foot, hair, faeces and buttocks, can be made to stand for those two organs in a secondary way . . .'

[1] In his *Psychoanalysis of the Total Personality* (1927) Alexander has pointed out that the id in a sense bribes the super-ego and that this 'understanding' between them enables it to carry out its forbidden actions.

[2] In his 'Problem of the Acceptance of Unpleasant Ideas' (1926), Ferenczi remarks that knowledge of external reality goes along with knowledge of psychical reality.

[3] In his *Inhibitions, Symptoms and Anxiety* (1926), Freud says: 'Nevertheless, we shall bear in mind for future consideration the possibility that repression is a process which has a special relation to the *genital* organization of the libido, and that the ego resorts to other methods of defence when it has to secure itself against the libido on other levels of organization . . .' (*S.E.* **21**, p. 125.)

[3a] This sentence is obscure and should be understood in the light of the preceding sentence that the hatred of the object is reduced owing to the ejection and repression of the instincts.

directed against the object, too, decrease. When this happens the ego seems to become more conscious of its fear of retribution by its object. To submission to the severe super-ego and acknowledgement of the prohibitions imposed by the super-ego is thus added an acknowledgement of the power of the object. This is reinforced by the ego's tendencies to equate super-ego and object. This equation is a further step in the modification of anxiety which promotes the development of its relation to external reality by means of the mechanisms of projection and displacement. The ego now tries to master anxiety by attempting to satisfy the demands both of the external and internalized objects. This induces the ego to shield its objects—a reaction which Abraham has allocated to the later anal stage. This changed method of behaviour towards the object may show itself in two ways: the individual may turn away from it, on account of his fear of it as a source of danger and also in order to shield it from his own sadistic impulses; or he may turn towards it with greater positive feeling. This process of relating to objects is brought about by a splitting up of the mother-imago into a good and a bad one. The existence of this type of ambivalence towards the object indicates a further step in the development of object-relations, and also helps to modify the child's fear of the super-ego. This fear is displaced onto the external object and then spread over several objects by means of displacement. As a result certain persons take on the significance of the attacked and therefore threatening object, others—particularly the mother—take on the significance of the kindly and protecting object.

The individual becomes increasingly successful in overcoming anxiety thanks to the progressive development of the infant towards the genital stage during which it introjects more friendly imagos, resulting in a change in the character of the super-ego's methods.

When the hitherto overpowering threats of the super-ego become toned down into admonitions and reproaches the ego can find support against them in its positive relationships. It can now employ restitutive mechanisms and reaction-formations of pity towards its objects so as to placate the super-ego;[1] and the love and recognition it receives from those objects and the external world are regarded as both a demonstration and a measure of the approval of the super-ego. In this connection the mechanism of splitting the imagos is important; the ego turns away from the object that threatens danger, but it turns towards the friendly object in an attempt to repair the imaginary

---

[1] In his paper, 'The Psychology of Pity' (1930), Jekels shows that the person who feels compassion for his object treats it as he would like to be treated by his own super-ego.

injuries it has inflicted. The process of sublimation can now set in,[1,2] for the restitutive tendencies of the individual towards this object are a fundamental motive force in all his sublimations, even his very earliest ones, such as quite primitive manifestations of the impulse to play. A pre-condition for the development of restitutive tendencies and of sublimations is that the pressure exerted by the super-ego should be mitigated and felt by the ego as a sense of guilt. The qualitative changes of the super-ego which are initiated by the accentuation of genital impulses and object relations influence the relation of the super-ego to the ego and precipitate a sense of guilt. Should such feelings of guilt become too overpowering their effect will once more be felt by the ego as anxiety.[3] If this line of thought is correct, then it would be not a deficiency in the super-ego but a qualitative difference in it that gives rise to a lack of social feeling in certain individuals, including criminals and so-called 'asocial' persons.[4]

In my view, in the earlier anal stage the child is making a defence against the terrifying imagos which it has introjected in the oral-sadistic phase. Ejecting the super-ego would represent a step in overcoming anxiety. This step could not succeed at this stage because the anxiety to be overcome is still too powerful and because the method of violent ejection continually arouses fresh anxiety. The anxiety which cannot be allayed in this way urges the child to cathect the next highest level of the libido—the later anal stage—and thus acts as a promoting agency in its development.

We know that super-ego and object in the adult are by no means identical; nor are they so at any time in childhood, as I have tried to show. The discrepancy of super-ego and ego resulting in an endeavour of the ego to make real objects and their imagos interchangeable is in my view a fundamental factor in development.[5] This development shows itself in the following way: the discrepancy between object and super-ego becomes smaller and the imagos move closer to real objects, as a result of the increased predominance of the

[1] Cf. my paper 'Infantile Anxiety-Situations Reflected in a Work of Art' (1929).

[2] Ella Sharpe has shown that in sublimation the child projects its introjected parents on to an external object upon whom it satisfies its sadistic and restitutive trends and with whom it thus connects its feelings of magical omnipotence. (Cf. her paper 'Certain Aspects of Sublimations and Delusions', 1930.).

[3] Cf. also Ernest Jones's contribution to this subject, 'Fear, Guilt and Hate' (1929).

[4] In his paper, 'Identification' (1926), Fenichel also takes this view.

[5] The importance of this factor for the development of the ego and for its relationship to reality is examined at greater length in Chapter X.

genital level; further, the phantastic and anxiety-provoking imagos which belong to the earliest phase of development retreat into the background and at the same time the mental balance of the individual becomes more stable and the modification of early anxiety situations is more successful.[1a]

As the genital impulses gradually gain in strength, the suppression of the id by the ego loses much of its violence, too, making a better understanding between them possible.

Thus the more positive object-relationship which goes along with the advent of the genital stage may also be regarded as a sign of a satisfactory relation between super-ego and ego and between ego and id.

We have already been told that the fixation-points for the psychoses are to be found in the earliest stages of development and that the boundary between the earlier and later anal stage forms the line of demarcation between psychosis and neuroses. I am inclined to go a step further and regard those fixation-points as points of departure not only for subsequent illnesses but for disturbances which the child undergoes during the earliest stages of its life. In the last chapter[2] we have seen that the excessively powerful anxiety situations that arise when sadism is at its height are a fundamental aetiological factor in psychotic disorders. But I also found that in the earliest phases of development the child normally passes through anxiety-situations of a psychotic character. If, whether for external or internal reasons, those early situations are activated to a high degree, the child will exhibit psychotic traits. And if it is too hard pressed by its fear-arousing imagos and cannot sufficiently counteract them with the aid of its helpful imagos and its real objects, the child will suffer a psychotic disturbance[3] which resembles an adult psychosis and often extends into an actual psychosis in later life, or forms the basis of severe illnesses or other impairments of development.

Since these anxiety situations become active from time to time in every child and reach a certain strength, every child will periodically exhibit psychotic phenomena. The change between excessive high spirits and extreme sadness which is characteristic of melancholic

[1a] The verbal translation of this sentence is: The smaller this discrepancy becomes, the more the imagos under the predominance of the genital phase become closer to real objects; the more the phantastic anxiety-producing imagos which belong to the earliest stage of development retreat into the background, the more stable does the psychic balance of the individual become and the better does the modification of early anxiety-situations succeed.

[2] Cf. also my paper, 'Personification in the Play of Children' (1929, Writings, 1).

[3] The reader will recall the cases of Erna (Chapter III), Egon (Chapter IV) and Ilse (Chapter V).

disorders, is regularly found in small children. The depth and the character of the sadness children feel is usually not appreciated because it is of such frequent occurrence and undergoes such rapid changes. But analytic observation has taught me that their sadness and depression, though not so acute as the melancholic depression of the adult, have the same causes and can be accompanied by thoughts of suicide. The minor and major accidents that befall children and the hurts they do themselves are often, I have found, attempts at suicide, undertaken with as yet ineffective means. The withdrawal from reality which is a criterion of psychosis is considered in the child still largely as a normal phenomenon. Paranoid traits which are active in the small child are less easy to observe since they are linked with the tendency to secrecy and deception which are characteristic of this disorder. It is a known fact that small children feel themselves hemmed in and pursued by phantastic figures. In analysing some quite young children[1] I found that when they were alone, especially at night, they had the feeling of being surrounded by all sorts of persecutors like sorcerers, witches, devils, phantastic figures and animals and that their fears about them had the character of a paranoid anxiety.

Infantile neuroses present a composite picture made up of the various psychotic and neurotic traits and mechanisms which we find singly and in a more or less pure form in adults. In this complicated picture sometimes the features of this disorder, sometimes of that, are more strongly emphasized. But in many instances the picture of the infantile neuroses is completely obscured by the fact that the various disorders and the defences employed against them are all at work at the same time.

In his book, *Inhibitions Symptoms and Anxiety*,[2] Freud declares that 'the earliest phobias of infancy [have] so far not been explained' and '[that] it is not at all clear what their relation is to the undoubted neuroses that appear later on in childhood'. In my experience those early phobias contain anxieties arising in the early stages of the formation of the super-ego. The earliest anxiety-situations of the child appear about the middle of the first year of its life and are brought on by an increase of sadism. They consist of fears of violent (i.e. devouring, cutting, castrating) objects, both external and introjected; and such fears cannot be sufficiently modified at such an early stage.

The difficulties small children often have in eating are also closely connected, according to my experience, with their earliest anxiety-situations and invariably have paranoid origins. In the cannibalistic

[1] The child's belief in imaginary, helpful figures, such as fairies or Father Christmas, helps it to conceal and overcome its fear of its bad imagos.
[2] *S.E.* **20**, p. 136.

phase children equate every kind of food with their objects, as represented by their organs, so that it takes on the significance of their father's penis and their mother's breast and is loved, hated and feared like these. Liquid foods are likened to milk, faeces, urine and semen, and solid foods to faeces and other substances of the body. Thus food is able to give rise to all those fears of being poisoned and destroyed inside, which children feel in relation to their internalized objects and excrements if their early anxiety-situations are strongly operative.

Infantile animal phobias are an expression of early anxiety of this kind. They are based on the ejection of the terrifying super-ego which is characteristic of the earlier anal stage. The infantile animal phobias thus represent a process, made up of several moves, whereby the child modifies its fear of its terrifying super-ego and id. The first move is to eject the super-ego and the id and to project them into the outside world, whereby the super-ego is equated with the real object. The second move, familiar to us as a displacement onto an animal of the fear felt of the real father, is in many cases based on a modification of the equation in phantasy of the super-ego and of the id with wild and dangerous animals which is characteristic for the earliest stages of ego-development. In place of the wild animal a less ferocious one is chosen as an anxiety object in the outside world. The fact that the anxiety-animal not only attracts to itself the child's fear of its father but often also the child's admiration of him, is a sign that the formation of an ideal is taking place.[1] Animal phobias are already a far-reaching modification of the fear of the super-ego; and we see here what a close connection there is between super-ego, object-relationship and animal phobias.

Freud writes:[2] 'On a previous occasion I have stated that phobias have the character of a projection in that they replace an internal, instinctual danger by an external, perceptual one. The advantage of this is that the subject can protect himself against an external danger by fleeing from it and avoiding perception of it, whereas it is useless to

[1] Abraham told me the following story as a good example of how a small child's hatred of an animal could already contain a fear of being reproved by it. He had given a picture-book to a small relative of his, a boy of not yet one and a half years of age, and was showing him the pictures and reading the text aloud to him. On one page there was a picture of a pig who was telling a small child to be clean. The words, and the picture too, obviously displeased the boy, for he wanted to turn the page over at once, and when Abraham returned to the picture he would not look at it. Later on Abraham learnt that though the boy was very fond of the picture-book he could not bear the page with the pig on it. In telling me this story Abraham added: 'His super-ego must at that time have been a pig.'

[2] *Inhibitions, Symptoms and Anxiety* (1926). *S.E.* **20**, p. 126.

flee from dangers that arise from within. This statement of mine was not incorrect, but it did not go below the surface of things. For an instinctual demand is, after all, not dangerous in itself; it only becomes so inasmuch as it entails a real external danger, the danger of castration. Thus what happens in a phobia in the last resort is merely that one external danger is replaced by another.' But I venture to think that what lies at the root of a phobia is ultimately an internal danger. It is the person's fear of his own destructive instinct and of his introjected parents. In the same passage, in describing the advantages of substitutive formations, Freud says:[1] 'For the anxiety belonging to a phobia is conditional; it only emerges when the object of it is perceived—and rightly so, since it is only then that the danger situation is present. There is no need to be afraid of being castrated by a father who is not there. On the other hand one cannot get rid of a father; he can appear whenever he chooses. But if he is replaced by an animal, all one has to do is to avoid the sight of it—that is, its presence—in order to be free from danger and anxiety.'

Such an advantage would be even greater if by means of an animal phobia the ego could not only bring about a displacement from one external object to another but also a projection of a much feared object from which, because internalized, there was no escape, onto another, external one, and one less feared at that. Regarded in this light castration anxiety is not only a distortion of the sentence: 'bitten by the horse (devoured by the wolf) instead of being castrated by the father' but also an earlier anxiety of a devouring super-ego which is the basis of animal phobia.

As an illustration of what I mean let us take two well-known cases of an animal phobia—that of Little Hans and that of the Wolf Man. Freud has pointed out[2] that in spite of certain similarities these two phobias differ from one another in many respects. As regards the differences we observe that Little Hans's phobia contained many traits of positive feeling. His anxiety-animal was not a terrifying one in itself, and he felt a certain amount of friendliness towards it, as was shown by his playing at horses with his father just before his phobia came on. His relation to his parents and to his environment was on the whole very good; and his general development showed that he had successfully surmounted the anal-sadistic stage and attained the genital stage. His animal phobia exhibited only a few traces of that type of anxiety which belongs to the earliest stages, in which the super-ego is equated with a wild and terrifying animal and the child's fear of its object is correspondingly intense. In the main he seemed to have overcome and modified that early anxiety quite well. Freud says of him: ' "Hans" seems, in fact, to have been a normal boy with

[1] ibid., S.E. **20**, p. 125. [2] ibid., S.E. **20**, p. 107.

what is called a "positive" Oedipus complex.' So that his infantile neurosis may be regarded as a mild, even 'normal' one; his anxiety, as we know, was readily dissipated by a short piece of analysis.

The neurosis of the so-called Wolf Man, a four-year-old boy, presents quite a different picture. The development of this boy cannot be described as normal. Freud writes of him: '. . . His attitude to female objects had been disturbed by an early seduction and his passive, feminine side was strongly developed. The analysis of his wolf-dream revealed very little intentional aggressiveness towards his father, but it brought forward unmistakable proof that what repression overtook was his passive tender attitude to his father. In his case, too, the other factors may have been operative as well; but they were not in evidence.'[1] The analysis of the wolf-man 'shows that the idea of being devoured by the father gives expression, in a form that has undergone regressive degradation, to a passive, tender impulse to be loved by him in a genital-erotic sense'.[2]

Regarded in the light of our previous discussion, this idea is seen not only to express a passive tender yearning which has been degraded by regression, but, over and above this, to be a relic of a very early stage of development.[3] If we look upon the boy's fear of being devoured by a wolf not only as a substitute by distortion for the idea of being castrated by his father, but, as I would suggest, as a primary anxiety which has persisted in an unchanged form along with later, modified versions of it, then it would follow that there had been a fear of the father active in him which must have decisively influenced the course of his abnormal development. In the phase when sadism is at its height, ushered in by the oral-sadistic instincts, the child's desire to introject his father's penis, together with his intense oral-sadistic hostile impulses, give rise to fears of a dangerous, devouring animal which he equates with his father's penis. How far he can succeed in overcoming and modifying this fear of his father will in part depend on the magnitude of his destructive tendencies. The Wolf Man did not overcome this early anxiety. His fear of the wolf, which stood for his fear of his father, showed that he had retained the image of his father as a devouring wolf in subsequent years. For, as we

---

[1] *ibid.*   [2] *ibid.*, p. 105.

[3] It seems to me important not merely from a theoretical point of view, but from a therapeutic one as well, to decide whether at the outbreak of the child's neurosis his idea of being devoured was receiving a regressive cathexis only, or whether it had retained its original activity side by side with later modifications; for we are concerned not only with the content of an idea but, above all, with the anxiety attached to it. We cannot fully understand such an anxiety, either in its quantitative or its qualitative aspect, until we have recognized it as an anxiety which underlies neurosis and which is specific for psychosis.

know, he rediscovered this wolf in his later father-imagos, and his whole development was governed by that overwhelming fear.[1] In my view, this enormous fear of his father was an underlying factor in the production of his inverted Oedipus complex. In analysing several highly neurotic boys, of between four and five years of age, who exhibited paranoid traits[2] and in whom the inverted Oedipus complex was predominant, I became convinced that this course of development was greatly determined by an excessive fear of their father, which was still active in the deepest mental layers and which had been generated by extremely strong primary impulses of agression against him.

The struggle which would result from a direct Oedipus situation could not be waged in phantasy against a dangerous, devouring father of this sort and so the heterosexual position had to be abandoned. In the Wolf Man, too, these anxiety-situations appear to me fundamental for his passive attitude to his father, and his sister's seduction of him merely served to strengthen and confirm him in the attitude to which his fear of his father had led him. We are told that 'from the time of the decisive dream onward, the boy became naughty, tormenting and sadistic', and soon afterwards developed a genuine obsessional neurosis which turned out in analysis to be a very severe one. These facts seem to bear out my view that even at the time of his wolf phobia he was engaged in warding off his aggressive tendencies.[3] That in Hans's phobia his defence against the aggressive impulses should be so clearly visible whilst in that of the Wolf Man it should be so deeply concealed, seems to me to be explained by the fact that in the latter the much greater anxiety—or primary sadism —had been dealt with in a far more abnormal way. And the fact that Hans's neurosis showed no obsessional traits, whereas the Wolf Man quickly developed a regular obsessional neurosis, agrees with my idea that if obsessional features appear too strongly and too early in an infantile neurosis we must infer that very serious disturbances are going on.[4]

In those analyses of boys on which my present conclusions are based, I was able to trace their abnormal development back to an overstrong sadism, or rather to sadism which had not been successfully modified and which had led to excessive anxiety in a very early

[1] Cf. Ruth Mack-Brunswick, 'A Supplement to Freud's "History of an Obsessional Neurosis" ' (1928).

[2] My analyses of adults have corroborated these findings.

[3] In the last passage quoted above, Freud seems to leave open the possibility that a defence against sadistic impulses may also have played a part, though not a manifest one, in the structure of the Wolf Man's illness.

[4] Cf. Chapter VI on this point.

stage of life. The result of this had been a very extensive exclusion of reality and the production of severe obsessional and paranoid traits. The reinforcement of the libidinal impulses and homosexual components that took place in these boys served to ward off and modify the fear of their father which had been aroused so early in them. This mode of dealing with anxiety is, I think, a fundamental aetiological factor in the homosexuality of paranoics,[1,2] and the fact that the Wolf Man developed paranoia in later life tends to support my view.[3]

In his *The Ego and the Id*[4] (1923), in speaking about the love-relations of the paranoic, Freud seems to bear out my line of thought. He says: 'There is another possible mechanism, however, which we have come to know of by analytic investigation of the processes concerned in the change in paranoia. An ambivalent attitude is present from the outset and the transformation is effected by means of a reactive displacement of cathexis, energy being withdrawn from the erotic impulse and added to the hostile one.'

In the Wolf Man's phobia I believe I could clearly recognize the unmodified anxiety belonging to the earliest stages. His object-relations were also much less successful than those of Little Hans; and his insufficiently established genital stage and the effect of overpowering anal-sadistic impulses became evident in the severe obsessional neurosis that so soon made its appearance. It would appear that Little Hans had been better able to modify his threatening and terrible super-ego into a less dangerous imago and to overcome his sadism and anxiety. His greater success in this respect also found expression in his more positive object-relationship to both his parents and in the fact that his active and heterosexual attitude was predominant and that he had satisfactorily attained the genital stage of development.

Let us briefly summarize my findings about the evolution of phobias. The anxiety of the earliest anxiety-situations finds expression in the phobias babies have at the breast. Infantile animal phobias beginning in the earlier anal stage continue to involve intensely terrifying objects. In the later anal stage, and still more in the genital stage, these anxiety objects are greatly modified.

The process of modification of a phobia is, I believe, linked with

[1] In Chapter III, in discussing a case with paranoid traits, I have tried to establish a similar theory of the origin of female homosexuality. The reader may also remember what was said in connection with Egon's analysis (Chapter IV). I shall return to the subject in Chapter XII.

[2] Róheim comes to the same conclusion on the basis of his ethnological data (cf. his paper 'Das Völkerpsychologische in Freud's Massenpsychologie und Ich analyse' (1922).

[3] Cf. Ruth Mack-Brunswick, op. cit.

[4] *S.E.* **19,** p. 43–4.

those mechanisms starting in the later anal stage upon which the obsessional neuroses are based. It seems to me that obsessional neurosis is an attempt to cure the psychotic conditions of the earliest phases,[1] and that in infantile neuroses both obsessional mechanisms and those belonging to a previous stage of development are already operative.

At first glance it would seem that my idea of the important role which certain elements of obsessional neurosis play in the clinical picture of infantile neuroses is at variance with what Freud has said concerning the starting-point of obsessional neurosis. Nevertheless, I believe that the disagreement can be explained away in one fundamental point. It is true that according to my findings the origins of obsessional neurosis lie in the early period of childhood; but the synthesis of the isolated obsessional traits into an organized entity which we come to regard as an obsessional neurosis does not emerge until the later period of childhood, that is, until the beginning of the latency period. The accepted theory is that fixations at the anal-sadistic stage do not come into force as factors in obsessional neurosis until later on, as the result of a regression to them. My view is that the true starting point for obsessional neurosis — the point at which the child develops obsessional symptoms and obsessional mechanisms — falls in that period of life which is governed by the later anal stage. The fact that this early obsessional illness presents a somewhat different picture from the later full-blown obsessional neurosis is understandable if we recollect that it is not until later, in the latency period, that the more mature ego, with its altered relationship to reality, sets to work to elaborate and synthesize those obsessional features which have been active since early childhood.[2] Another reason why the obsessional traits of the small child are often not easily discernible is that they operate side by side with earlier disorders which have not yet been overcome together with various other defensive mechanisms.

Nevertheless, as I have tried to show,[2a] young children too frequently exhibit traits of a distinctly obsessional character, and there also exist infantile neuroses in which a true obsessional neurosis

---

[1] Obsessional neurosis is only one of the methods of cure attempted by the ego in order to overcome this early infantile psychotic anxiety. Another method will be discussed in Chapter XII.

[2] I shall consider these changes in greater detail in Chapter X, where I have tried to show that in the latency period the child is enabled by its obsessional neurosis to meet the requirements of its ego, super-ego and id, whereas at an earlier age, when its ego is still immature, it is not as yet able to master its anxiety in this way.

[2a] See Chapter VI.

already dominates the picture.[1] In my experience this happens when the early anxiety-situations are too powerful and have not been sufficiently modified, resulting in a very grave obsessional neurosis.

In thus distinguishing between the early origin of obsessional traits and, later, obsessional neuroses proper I have, I hope, been able to bring the view put forward here concerning the genesis of obsessional neurosis more into line with the accepted theory. In his *Inhibitions, Symptoms and Anxiety* Freud says: 'Obsessional neurosis originates . . . in . . . the necessity of fending off the libidinal demands of the Oedipus complex'. He continues: 'The genital organization of the libido turns out to be feeble and insufficiently resistant, so that when the ego begins its defensive efforts the first thing it succeeds in doing is to throw back the genital organization (of the phallic phase), in whole or in part, to the earlier sadistic-anal level. This fact of regression is decisive for all that follows.' If we regard as regression the fluctuation between the various libidinal positions—such fluctuation is, in my opinion, characteristic of the early stages of development as regression in which the already cathected genital position is repeatedly abandoned for a time until it has been properly strengthened and established and if my contention that the Oedipus situation begins very early is correct, then the view here maintained about the origin of the obsessional neurosis would not be in contradiction with Freud's view as quoted above. My thesis would go to bear out another suggestion of his which he has only put forward quite tentatively. He writes: 'Perhaps regression is the result not of a constitutional factor but of a time-factor. It may be that regression is rendered possible not because the genital organization of the libido is too feeble but because the opposition of the ego begins too early, while the sadistic phase is at its height.' In arguing against this idea he continues: 'I am not prepared to express a definite opinion on this point but I may say that analytic observation does not speak in favour of such an assumption. It shows rather that, by the time an obsessional neurosis is entered upon, the phallic stage has already been reached.

---

[1] Cf. also the case of Rita (Chapter III), who came to analysis when she was two and three-quarter years old and already had a number of marked obsessional symptoms, chief among which were a complicated bed-ceremonial and an exaggerated love of order and cleanliness. The latter found expression in a great many habits that betrayed the obsessional bent of her character and the way in which it pervaded her whole personality. Moreover, these habits were already of long standing. Her bed-ceremonial, for instance, had begun some time in her second year and had steadily grown ever since. Erna (Chapter III), who came to me at the age of six, had certain obsessional symptoms which also went back to the end of her second year. In this very severe case the neurosis very early on showed many similarities with an adult obsessional neurosis.

Moreover, the onset of this neurosis belongs to a later time of life than that of hysteria—to the second period of childhood, after the latency period has set in.'[1] These objections would be eliminated if, as I assert, obsessional neurosis has its origin in the first period of childhood but does not become manifest as obsessional neurosis proper till the beginning of the latency period.

The view that obsessional mechanisms begin to become active very early in childhood, in the second year, is part of my general thesis that the super-ego is formed in the earliest stages of the child's life, being first felt by the ego as anxiety and then, as the early anal-sadistic stage gradually comes to a close, as a sense of guilt as well. This thesis once more differs from the theory as we have known it hitherto. In the first part of this book I have given the empirical data upon which it is based; now I should like to give a theoretical reason to support it. To turn to Freud once more.[2] 'In the [obsessional neurosis], the mainspring of all later symptom-formation is clearly the ego's fear of its super-ego.' My contention that the obsessional neurosis is a means of modifying early anxiety-situations and that the severe super-ego in the obsessional neurosis is no other than the un-modified, terrifying super-ego belonging to early stages of the child's development, brings us, I think, nearer to a solution of the problem of why the super-ego should in fact be such a severe one in this neurosis.

The child's feelings of guilt which are bound up with its urethral- and anal-sadistic tendencies are derived, I have found, from the phantasied attacks it makes on its mother's body during the phase when sadism is at its height.[3] In early analysis we get to know the child's fear of its bad mother who demands back from it the faeces and the children it has stolen from her. Hence the real mother (or nurse) who makes demands of cleanliness upon it turns at once into a terrifying person, one who not only insists upon its giving up its faeces, but, as its terrified imagination tells it, who intends to tear

---

[1] *Inhibitions, Symptoms and Anxiety* (1926), *S.E.* **20**, pp. 113–14.
[2] *ibid.*, p. 128.
[3] The generally accepted view, that what happens is that the sense of guilt which is aroused in the genital stage is associated by regression with training in cleanliness, does not take into account the severity of the feelings of guilt in question nor the closeness of their union with the pre-genital trends. The permanent impression made on the adult by his early training and the way in which it influences the whole of his later development—as we see over and over again in analyses of adults—points to the existence of a deeper and more direct connection between that early training and severe feelings of guilt. In his 'Psycho-Analysis of Sexual Habits' (1925), Ferenczi suggests that there is a more direct connection between the two and that there may be a kind of physiological precursor of the super-ego which he calls 'sphincter morality'.

them by force out of its body. Another, yet more overwhelming, source of fear arises from its introjected imagos from whom, because of its own destructive phantasies directed against external objects, it anticipates attacks of an equally savage kind inside itself.

In this phase, in consequence of likening excrement with dangerous, poisonous, burning substances and with offensive weapons of every kind, the child becomes terrified of its own excreta as something which will destroy its body. This sadistic equation of excreta with destructive substances, together with its phantasies of attacks undertaken with their help, furthermore lead the child to fear that similar attacks may be made against it both by its external and its internal objects and to feel a terror of excreta and of dirt in general. These sources of anxiety, all the more overwhelming because they are so manifold, are, in my experience, the deepest causes of the child's feelings of anxiety and guilt in connection with its training in cleanliness.

The child's reaction-formations of disgust, order and cleanliness, arise, therefore, from the anxiety, fed from various sources, which originates in its earliest danger-situations. When, at the onset of the second anal stage, the child's relations to the object have developed, its reaction-formation of pity comes, as we know, more especially to the fore. Moreover, as I have stressed before, the contentment of its objects is also a guarantee of the child's own safety and a safeguard against destruction from without and from within, and the restoration of its objects is a necessary condition for its body to remain intact.[1]

The anxiety arising from the early danger-situations is, in my opinion, closely associated with the origins of obsessions and obsessional symptoms. It is concerned with manifold injuries and acts of destruction done inside the body, and therefore it is inside the body that restitution has to be made. But there is no certainty of knowledge about the inside of the body, whether its own or that of its objects. The child cannot ascertain how far its fear of internal injuries and attacks is well founded, nor how far it has succeeded in making them good by means of its obsessional acts. The child's

---

[1] The view that reaction-formations and feelings of guilt set in at a very early period of ego-development—as early as in the second year—is supported by Abraham in one or two passages. In his 'Short Study of the Development of the Libido' (1924), he says: 'In the stage of narcissism with a cannibalistic sexual aim the first evidence of an instinctual inhibition appears in the shape of morbid anxiety. The process of overcoming the cannibalistic impulses is intimately associated with a sense of guilt which comes into the foreground as a typical inhibitory phenomenon belonging to the third stage' (p. 496).

resulting state of uncertainty which becomes allied to, and increases, its intense anxiety, together with the impossibility of obtaining secure knowledge of the phantasied destruction, gives rise to an obsessive desire for knowledge. The child tries to overcome its anxiety, the imaginary nature of which defies critical inspection, by laying extra emphasis upon reality, by being over-precise, and so on. The doubt which results from this uncertainty[1] plays a part not only in creating an obsessional character, but in stimulating exactness and order and the observance of certain rules and rituals, and the like.

Another element which has an important bearing on the character of obsessions is the intensity and multiplicity of the anxiety arising from various sources, which is attached to the earliest danger situations. This intensity and multiplicity of the anxiety produces an equally strong impulsion to set the defensive mechanisms in motion. It induces the child to clean and put together in an obsessive manner whatever it has dirtied or broken or spoiled in any way. It has to beautify and restore the damaged thing in all manner of ways in accordance with the variety of its sadistic phantasies and the details contained in them.

The coercion which the obsessional neurotic often applies to other people as well, is, I would say, the result of a manifold projection. In the first place he is trying to throw off the intolerable compulsion under which he is suffering by treating his object as though it were his id or his super-ego and by displacing the coercion outside. In doing this he is, incidentally, satisfying his primary sadism by tormenting and subjugating his object. In the second place he is turning outward on to his external objects what is ultimately a fear of being destroyed or attacked by his introjected objects. This fear has aroused a compulsion in him to control and rule his imagos. This compulsion (which can in fact never be satisfied) is turned against external objects.

If I am correct in my view that the magnitude and intensity of obsessional activities, and the severity of the neurosis are equivalent to the extent and character of the anxiety arising from the earliest danger-situations, we shall be in a better position to understand the close connection which we know to exist between paranoia and the more severe forms of obsessional neurosis. According to Abraham, in paranoia the libido regresses to the earlier of the two anal-sadistic stages. From what I have been able to discover, I should be inclined to go further and say that in the early anal-sadistic stage, the

---

[1] In his 'Notes upon a Case of Obsessional Neurosis' (1909), Freud remarks: 'The *compulsion*, on the other hand, is an attempt at a compensation for the doubt and at a correction of the intolerable conditions of inhibition to which the doubt bears witness' (*S.E.* **10,** p. 243).

individual, if his early anxiety-situations are strongly operative, actually passes through rudimentary paranoid states which he normally overcomes in the next stage (the second anal-sadistic one), and that the severity of his obsessional illness depends on the severity of the paranoid disturbances that have immediately preceded it. If his obsessional mechanisms cannot adequately overcome those disturbances his underlying paranoid traits will often come to the surface, or he may succumb to a regular paranoia.

We know that the suppression of obsessive acts arouses anxiety and that therefore those acts serve the purpose of mastering anxiety. If we assume that the anxiety thus overcome belongs to the earliest anxiety-situations and culminates in the child's fear of having its own body and that of its object destroyed in a number of ways, we shall, I believe, be better able to understand the deeper meaning of many obsessive acts. The compulsive accumulation of things as well as the compulsive giving away of them becomes for instance more intelligible as soon as we are able to recognize more clearly the nature of the anxiety and sense of guilt which underlie an exchange of goods on the anal level.

In play analysis compulsive taking and giving back again finds very diverse expression. It occurs, together with anxiety and guilt, as a reaction to preceding representations of acts of robbery and destruction. Children, for instance, will transfer the whole or part of the contents of one box to another and carefully arrange them there and preserve them with every show of anxiety, and will—if they are old enough—count them over one by one. The contents are very varied and include burnt matches, whose ash the child will often go to the trouble of rubbing off, paper patterns, pencils, bricks for building, bits of string and so on. They represent all the things the child has taken out of his mother's body—his father's penis, children, pieces of stool, urine, milk, etc. He may behave in the same way with writing blocks, tearing out the leaves and preserving them carefully somewhere else.

We then often see that in consequence of his rising anxiety, the child not only puts back what he has symbolically taken out of his mother's body, but also that by doing so, his compulsion to give, or rather to return, is not being satisfied. He is incessantly compelled to supplement in all sorts of ways, what he gives back, and in doing so, his primary sadistic tendencies continually break through his reactive ones.

My little patient John, aged five, a very neurotic child, developed in this stage of his analysis a counting mania—a symptom which had not been much noticed, as it was such a usual occurrence at his age. In his analysis he used carefully to mark the position of his toy men and other playthings on a sheet of paper on which he had placed them, before transferring them on to another sheet. But he not only wanted to know exactly where they had been before, so as to be able to replace them in identically the same place; he would also count them over and over again in order to make sure of the number of things (i.e. the bits of faeces, his father's penis and the children) which he had taken (out of his mother's body) and which he had to give back. While he was doing this he would call me stupid and naughty and say: 'One *can't* take thirteen from ten or seven from two.' This fear of having to give back more than they possess is typical in children and can be explained amongst other things by the difference in size between them and grown-up people, and by the extent of their sense of guilt. They feel that they cannot give back out of their own small body all that they have taken out of their mother's body which is so huge in comparison; and the weight of this guilt, which reproaches them ceaselessly with robbing and destroying their mother or both parents, strengthens their feeling of never being able to give back enough. The feeling of 'not knowing' which they have at a very early age adds considerably to their anxiety. This is a subject I shall return to later on.

Very often children will be interrupted in their representations of 'giving back' by having to go to the lavatory to defaecate. Another small patient of mine, also a five-year-old boy, used sometimes to have to go to the lavatory four or five times during his hour at this stage of his analysis. When he came back he would count obsessively, and by getting up to high numbers convinced himself that he possessed enough to pay back what he had stolen. Viewed in this light, the anal-sadistic heaping up of possessions which seems to arise simply from the pleasure of amassing for its own sake takes on another aspect. Analyses of adults, too, have shown me that the wish to have a capital sum in hand for any contingency is really a desire for security, by being armed against an attack on the part of the mother they have robbed—a mother who was as often as not in point of fact, long since dead—and to be able to give back to her what they have stolen. On the other hand, the fear of being deprived of the contents of their own body compels them continually to accumulate more money so as to have 'reserves' to fall back on. For instance, after John and I had agreed that his fear of no longer being able to give his mother back all the stool and the children he had stolen from her, was driving him to go on cutting things up and stealing them, he gave me further reasons why he could not restore everything he had taken. He said that his stool had melted away in the meanwhile; that, after all, he had been passing it out all the time, and even if he were to go on and on making more, he could never make enough now. And, besides, he did not know if it would be 'good enough'. By 'good enough' he meant in the first instance equal in value to what he had stolen out of his mother's body. (Hence, his care in choosing the shapes and colours he used in the scenes which represented restitution.) But in a deeper sense it meant innocuous,[1a] free from poison.[2] On the other hand, his frequent constipation was due to his need to store up his faeces and keep them inside so that he should not himself be empty. These many conflicting tendencies, of which I have mentioned only a few, aroused very severe anxiety in him. Whenever there was an increase in his fear of not being able to produce the right kind of thing or to give enough, or of not being able to repair what he had damaged, his primary destructive trends once more broke out in full force. He would tear, cut to pieces and burn the things he had made when moved by reactive tendencies—the box which he had stuck together and filled up and which represented his mother, or the piece of paper on which he had drawn (perhaps a plan of a town)—and his thirst for destruction would then be insatiable. At the same time the primitive sadistic significance of urinating and defaecating became clearly visible. Tearing, cutting up and burning paper alternated with wetting things with water, smearing them with ashes or smudging with a pencil and so on—all these actions served the same destructive purposes. Wetting and smearing meant soaking, drowning or poisoning. Wet paper squashed into balls, for instance, represented especially poisonous missiles because of being a mixture of urine and stool. These details clearly showed that the sadistic significance of urinating and defaecating was the most deeply seated cause of his sense of guilt and that it was this sense of guilt that led to the impulse to make restitution which found expression in his obsessional mechanisms.

The fact that an increase of anxiety will lead to a regression to the defensive mechanisms of earlier stages shows how fateful is the influence exerted by the overwhelmingly powerful super-ego belonging to the earliest period of development. The pressure exerted by this early super-ego increases the sadistic fixations of the child, with the result that he has constantly to be repeating his original destructive acts in a compulsive way. His fear of not being able to put things right again arouses his still deeper fear of being exposed to the revenge of the objects which, in his phantasy, he has killed and which keep on coming back again, and sets in motion the defensive mechanisms that belong to earlier stages; for the object that cannot be

[1a] In German 'nicht beschädigend' ('not damaging'). Compare footnote (2).

[2] In his paper, 'Fear, Guilt and Hate' (1929), Ernest Jones has pointed out that the word 'innocent' denotes 'not hurting', so that to be innocent means to do no harm.

placated or satisfied must be put away. The weak ego of the child cannot come to terms with such an unreasonably menacing super-ego, and it is not until a rather more advanced stage has been reached that its anxiety is also felt as a sense of guilt and sets the obsessional mechanisms in motion. One is amazed to discover that at this period of its analysis the child not only obeys its sadistic phantasies, under an intense pressure of anxiety, but also that the mastering of anxiety has become its greatest pleasure.

Directly the child's anxiety increases, its desire for possession is overshadowed by its need to have the wherewithal to meet the threats of its super-ego and objects, and becomes a desire to be able to give back. But this desire cannot be fulfilled if its anxiety and conflict are too great, and so we see the very neurotic child labouring under a constant compulsion to take in order to be able to give. (This psychological factor, it may be remarked, enters into all the functional disturbances of the bowels that we meet with and into many bodily ailments as well.) Conversely, as the violence of its anxiety decreases, its reactive trends also lose their character of violence and compulsion and become steadier in their application and make their effect felt in a more gentle and continuous way with less liability to interruption from destructive trends. And now the child's idea that the restoration of its own person depends on the restoration of its objects comes out more and more strongly. Its destructive trends have not, indeed, become inoperative, but they have lost their character of violence and have become more adaptable to the demands of the super-ego. The second part of the two-stage action of obsessional neurosis — the reaction-formation — also contains destructive elements. These are now more clearly directed by the super-ego + ego and are free to pursue the aims sanctioned by them.

There is, as we know, a close connection between obsessive acts and the 'omnipotence of thoughts'. Freud has pointed out[1] that the primary obsessive actions of primitive peoples are essentially magical in character. He says: 'If they are not charms, they are at all events counter-charms, designed to ward off the expectations of disaster with which the neurosis usually starts'; and again:[2] 'The protective formulas of obsessional neurosis, too, have their counterpart in the formulas of magic. It is possible, however, to describe the course of development of obsessive acts; we can show how they begin by being as remote as possible from anything sexual — magical defences against evil wishes — and how they end by being substitutes for the forbidden sexual act and the closest possible imitations of it.' From this we see that obsessive acts are counter-magic, evil wishes (i.e.

---

[1] *Totem and Taboo* (1913) (*S.E.* **13**, p. 87). [2] *ibid.*, pp. 87–8.

death-wishes),[1] and at the same time a shield against sexual acts.

We should expect to find that these three elements which have united in a defensive action would also be present in those phantasies and deeds which have aroused a sense of guilt in the first place and thus called that defensive action into being. This mixture of magic, evil wishes and sexual activities is to be found, I think, in a situation which has been described in detail in the last chapter—in the masturbatory activities of the infant.

I pointed out there that the developmental stages in which the Oedipus conflict and its accompanying sadistic masturbation phantasies begin to arise centre around copulation between the parents and are concerned with sadistic attacks on them, and that they thus become one of the deepest sources of the child's sense of guilt. And I came to the conclusion that it is the sense of guilt arising from destructive impulses directed against its parents which makes masturbation and sexual behaviour in general something wicked and forbidden to the child, and that this guilt is therefore due to the child's destructive instincts and not to its libidinal and incestuous ones.[2]

The phase in which, according to my view, the onset of the Oedipus conflict and its accompanying sadistic masturbation phantasies arise is the phase of narcissism—a phase in which the subject has, to quote Freud.[3] '. . . . a high valuation [of his own psychic acts]—in our eyes [what amounts to] an *over-valuation*—to psychical acts.' This phase is characterized by a sense of omnipotence on the part of the child in regard to the functions of its bladder and bowels and a consequent belief in the omnipotence of its thoughts.[4] As the

[1] Concerning the obsessional neurotic, Freud says, in *Totem and Taboo* (1913): 'Nevertheless, his sense of guilt has a justification: it is founded on the intense and frequent death-wishes against his fellow which are unconsciously at work in him.' (*S.E.* **13**, p. 87.)

[2] In Chapter I, I have already pointed out the agreement between my own views on this subject and some conclusions that Freud has come to in his *Civilization and its Discontents* (1930). He says there: '. . . it is after all only the aggressiveness which is transformed into a sense of guilt, by being suppressed and made over to the super-ego. I am convinced that many processes will admit of a simpler and clearer exposition if the findings of psycho-analysis with regard to the derivation of the sense of guilt are restricted to the aggressive instincts.' (*S.E.* **21**, p. 138.) And again: 'It now seems plausible to formulate the following proposition. When an instinctual trend undergoes repression, its libidinal elements are turned into symptoms, and its aggressive components into a sense of guilt' (p. 139).

[3] *Totem and Taboo* (1913) (*S.E.* **13**, p. 89).

[4] Ferenczi has drawn attention, in his 'Stages in the Development of a Sense of Reality' (1913), to the connection between anal functions and the omnipotence of words and gestures. Cf. also Abraham, 'The Narcissistic Evaluation of Excretory Processes in Dreams and Neurosis' (1920).

result of this it feels guilty on account of the manifold assaults on its parents which it carries out in its phantasy. But this excess of guilt which results from a belief in the omnipotence of their excrements and thoughts is, I think, one factor which causes neurotics and primitive peoples to retain or regress to their original feeling of omnipotence. When their sense of guilt sets in motion obsessive actions as a defence, they will employ the feeling of omnipotence for the purpose of making restitution. But this feeling of omnipotence must now be sustained in a compulsive and exaggerated way, for the restitution, too, like the original destruction, is based upon 'omnipotence'.

Freud has said:[1] 'It is difficult to judge whether the obsessive or protective acts performed by obsessional neurotics follow the law of similarity (or, as the case may be, of contrast); they have been distorted by being displaced on to something very small, some action in itself of the greatest triviality.' Early analysis brings complete proof of the fact that the restitutive mechanisms are ultimately based on this law of similarity (or contrast) both in quantity, quality and in every detail. If a child has retained very strong primary feelings of omnipotence in association with its sadistic phantasies, it follows that it will have to have a very strong belief in the creative omnipotence that is to help it to make restitution. Analysis of children and adults shows very clearly how large a part this factor plays in promoting or inhibiting such constructive and reactive actions. The subject's sense of omnipotence with regard to his ability to make restitution is by no means equal to his sense of omnipotence in regard to his ability to destroy; for we must remember that his reaction-formations set in at a stage of ego-development and object-relationship which presupposes a much more advanced relationship to reality. Thus where an exaggerated sense of omnipotence is a necessary condition for making restitution, his belief in the possibility of being able to do so will be handicapped from the outset.[2]

In some analyses I have found that the inhibiting effect which resulted from this disparity between those feelings of omnipotence which were connected with destruction, and those connected with restitution, was reinforced by a particular factor. If the patient's primary sadism and sense of omnipotence had been exceedingly strong, his reactive trends were correspondingly powerful; his restitutive trends were based on megalomanic phantasies of excep-

---

[1] *Totem and Taboo* (1913) (*S.E.* **13**, p. 87).

[2] In a discussion on this subject Miss Searl pointed out that the child's impulse to restore things is also hindered by its early experience of the fact that it is easy to break things but exceedingly difficult to put them together again. Factual evidence of this kind must, I think, contribute to an increase in its doubts about its creative powers.

tional magnitude. In the child's phantasy, the havoc his destructive powers had wrought was something unique and gigantic, and therefore the effect of restitution had to be of an extraordinary and earth-shattering magnitude too. This in itself would be a sufficient impediment to the fulfilment of his constructive trends (although it may be mentioned that two of my patients did undoubtedly possess unusual artistic and creative gifts), but this impediment was yet further reinforced by the following factors. Side by side with these megalo-manic phantasies, the child had very strong doubts as to whether he possessed the omnipotence necessary for making restitution on this scale. In consequence he tried to deny his omnipotence in his acts of destruction as well. But, in addition, every indication that he was using his omnipotence in a positive sense would be proof of his having used it in a negative sense, and must therefore be avoided until he could bring forward absolute proof that his constructive omnipotence fully counterbalanced its opposite. In the two adult cases I have in mind, the 'all or nothing' attitude which resulted from these conflicting trends led to severe inhibitions in their capacity to work; whilst in one or two child-patients, it strongly helped to inhibit the formation of sublimations.

This mechanism, however, does not seem to be typical for obsessional neurosis. The patients in whom I have observed it presented a clinical picture of a mixed type, not a purely obsessional one. By virtue of the mechanism of 'displacement on to something very small', which plays so great a part in his neurosis, the obsessional patient can seek in very slight achievements a proof of his constructive omnipotence[1] and his capacity to make complete restitution. It thus appears that the doubt in his constructive omnipotence is an essential incentive to repeat his actions compulsively.

It is well known what close ties there are between the instinct for knowledge and sadism. Freud writes,[2] 'we often gain an impression that the instinct for knowledge can actually take the place of sadism in the mechanism of obsessional neurosis'. From what I have been able to observe, the connection between the two is formed in a very early stage of ego-development, during the phase at which sadism is at its height. At this time, the child's instinct for knowledge is activated by its awakening Oedipus conflict and, to begin with, is put into the service of its oral-sadistic trends.[3] My experience has shown

---

[1] In his 'Notes upon a Case of Obsessional Neurosis' (1909) (*S.E.* **10,** p. 241), Freud remarks that doubt is in reality a doubt of one's own love and that 'a man who doubts his own love may, or rather *must*, doubt every lesser thing'.

[2] 'The Predisposition to Obsessional Neurosis' (1913).

[3] Cf. Abraham, 'Psycho-Analytical Studies on Character-Formation' (1925).

me that the first object of this instinct for knowledge is the interior of the mother's body, which the child first of all regards as an object of oral gratification and then as the scene where intercourse between its parents takes place, and where in its phantasy the father's penis and the children are situated. At the same time as it wants to force its way into its mother's body in order to take possession of the contents and to destroy them, it wants to know what is going on and what things look like in there. In this way, its wish to know what there is in the interior of her body is equated in many ways with its wish to force a way inside her, and the one desire reinforces and stands for the other. Thus the instinct for knowledge becomes linked at its source with sadism when it is at its height, which makes it easier to understand why that bond should be so close, and why the instinct for knowledge should arouse feelings of guilt in the individual.

We see the small child overwhelmed by a crowd of questions and problems which its intellect is as yet utterly unfit to deal with. The typical reproach, which it makes against its mother principally, is that she does not answer these questions, and no more satisfies its desire to know than she has satisfied its oral desires. This reproach plays an important part both in the development of the child's character and in its instinct for knowledge. How far back such an accusation goes, can be seen from another reproach which the child habitually makes in close association with it, viz. that it could not understand what grown-up people were saying or the words they used: and this second complaint must refer to a time before it was able to speak. Moreover, the child attaches an extraordinary amount of affect to these two reproaches, whether they appear singly or in combination, and at these moments it is likely to talk in its analysis in such a way as not to be understood—this occurred in the case of my little patient Rita[1] at the age of only two years and nine months— and will at the same time reproduce reactions of rage. It cannot put the questions it wants to ask into words, and would not be able to understand any answer that was given in words. But, in part at least, these questions have never been conscious at all. The disappointment to which the first stirrings of the instinct for knowledge originating in the earlies stages of ego-development are doomed, is, I think, the deepest source of severe disturbance of that instinct in general.[2]

We have seen that sadistic impulses against its mother's body activate the child's instinct for knowledge in the first place, but the

[1] Cf. Chapter II.

[2] In addition the hatred felt for people who speak another language and the difficulty experienced in learning a foreign language seem to me to be derived from these earliest disturbances of the desire for knowledge.

anxiety which soon follows as a reaction to such impulses gives a further very important impetus to the increase and intensification of that instinct. The urge the child feels to find out what happens inside its mother's body and its own, is reinforced by its fear of the dangers which it supposes the former to contain, and also by its fear of the dangerous introjected objects and occurrences within itself. Knowledge is now a means of mastering anxiety; this leads to an impetus to acquire knowledge which becomes an important factor both in the development of its instinct for knowledge and in its inhibition. For, as in the case of the development of the libido, so, too, in that of the development of the instinct to know, anxiety acts both as a promoting and inhibiting factor. We have had occasion in earlier pages to discuss some examples of severe disturbances of the instinct for knowledge.[1] In these cases the child's terror of knowing anything about the fearful destruction it had done to its mother's body in phantasy and the consequent counter-attacks and perils it was exposed to, etc., was so tremendous that it set up a radical disturbance of its instinct for knowledge as a whole. The child's original excessively strong and unsatisfied desire to get information about the nature, size and number of its father's penises, excrements and children inside its mother had turned into a compulsion to measure, add up and count things, and so on.

As the libidinal impulses of children grow stronger and their destructive ones get weaker, so qualitative changes continually take place in their super-ego, whose effects are now felt by the ego as predominantly admonitory influences. And, as anxiety diminishes, the restitutive mechanisms become less obsessive in character and work more steadily, efficiently and with more satisfactory results; and then the reactions corresponding to the genital stage emerge more clearly.

The genital stage would thus be characterized by the fact that in the interactions which take place between projection and introjection and between super-ego formation and object-relations— interactions which govern the whole of the child's early development—the positive element has attained predominance.

[1] Cf. Erna (Chapter III), Kenneth (Chapter IV) and Ilse (Chapter V).

Chapter X

THE SIGNIFICANCE OF
EARLY ANXIETY-SITUATIONS IN
THE DEVELOPMENT OF THE EGO

ONE of the main problems presented by psycho-analysis is that of anxiety and its modification. The various psycho-neurotic illnesses to which the individual is liable can be looked upon as more or less unsuccessful attempts to master anxiety. But side by side with these methods of modifying anxiety, which may be considered as pathological, there are a number of normal methods, and they have an outstanding importance for the development of the ego. It is to some of these that we shall turn our attention in this chapter.

At the beginning of its development, the ego is subjected to the pressure of early anxiety-situations. Weak as it still is, the ego is exposed on the one hand to the violent demands of the id, and on the other, to the threats of a cruel super-ego, and it has to exert its powers to the utmost to satisfy both sides. Freud's description of the ego as a 'poor creature owing service to three masters and consequently menaced by three dangers'[1] is especially true of the feeble and immature ego of the small child, whose principal task it is to master the pressure of anxiety it is under.[2]

In its play, even the quite small child will attempt to overcome its unpleasurable experiences as Freud demonstrated in the play of a small boy of one and a half.[3] The child threw away a wooden reel tied to a piece of string so that it disappeared and then (by pulling it back into sight again) made it reappear. By doing this over and over again, he attempted to master an unpleasant event—the temporary absence of the mother—psychically. Freud has recognized in his

---

[1] *The Ego and the Id* (1923) (*S.E.* **19,** p. 56).

[2] In some extreme cases this pressure can be so forcible as to arrest completely the development of the ego. But even in less abnormal cases it can act not only as a promoting agency but as a retarding one in that development. In order for it to have a favourable effect, as in all developmental processes, a certain optimum relation between the co-operating factors is required. (Cf. my paper 'The Importance of Symbol-Formation in the Development of the Ego', 1930, *Writings*, **1**).

[3] *Beyond the Pleasure Principle* (1920) (*S.E.* **18,** p. 14).

behaviour a function of general importance in the play of children. Through play the child turns the experience it has passively endured into an active one and changes unpleasure into pleasure by giving its originally unpleasurable experience a happy ending.

Early analysis has shown that in play the child not only overcomes painful reality, but at the same time it also uses it to master its instinctual fears and internal dangers by projecting them into the outer world.[1]

The endeavour made by the ego to displace intra-psychic processes into the outer world and let them run their course there seems to be connected with another mental function, one which Freud has recognized in dreams of patients suffering from a traumatic neurosis.[2]

The displacement of dangers, instinctual and internal ones, on to the external world permits the child not only to master anxiety better but also to become more prepared for them.[3] The child's ever-renewed attempts to master anxiety in its play also seem to me to involve a 'control of stimuli by developing apprehension'.[4] The displacement of the child's anxiety arising from intra-psychic causes into the external world—a displacement which goes along with the deflection of its destructive instinct outwards—has the further effect of increasing the importance of its objects, for it is in relation to those objects—or their substitutes—that both its positive and reactive trends are being confirmed[4a]. The objects thus become a

[1] Freud regards the origins of projection as a 'particular way of dealing with any internal excitations which produce too great an increase of unpleasure. There is a tendency to treat them as though they were acting, not from the inside, but from the outside, so that it may be possible to bring the shield against stimuli into operation as a means of defence against them. This is the origin of *projection*, which is destined to play such a large part in the causation of pathological processes.' (*Beyond the Pleasure Principle*, 1920, *S.E.* **18**, p. 29.)

[2] Freud writes: 'These dreams are endeavouring to master the stimulus retrospectively, by developing the anxiety whose omission was the cause of the traumatic neurosis. They thus afford us a view of a function of the mental apparatus which, though it does not contradict the pleasure principle, is nevertheless independent of it and seems to be more primitive than the purpose of gaining pleasure and avoiding unpleasure.' (*Beyond the Pleasure Principle*, *S.E.* **18**, p. 32.)

[3] In the two previous chapters we have seen that in the earliest stage of the development of the individual, his ego is not sufficiently able to tolerate his instinctual anxiety and his fear of his internalized objects, and tries to protect itself in part by scotomizing and denying psychical reality.

[4] Concerning the close relations between dreams and play, cf. Chapter I of this book; and also my paper, 'Personification in the Play of Children' (1929).

[4a] German text has 'betätigt' (activated). Translator takes it to be a misprint for 'bestätigt'.

source of danger to the child, and yet, in so far as they appear kindly, they also represent a support against anxiety.

Freud interpreted the throwing away of the reel also as an expression of the child's sadistic and revengeful impulses against the mother who had abandoned it.[1] On the other hand, that the child made the reel to reappear, expressing the return of the mother, seems to represent a magic restoration[2] of the mother who was destroyed in the earlier part of the play, as throwing away being equated with killing.

Besides the relief which projection affords by enabling internal instinctual stimuli to be treated as external ones, the displacement of anxiety relating to internal dangers to the outer world gives additional advantages. The child's instinct for knowledge, which, together with its sadistic impulses, has been directed towards the interior of its mother's body, is intensified by its fear of the dangers and acts of destruction which are going on there and inside its own body and which the child has no means of controlling. Real [external] dangers can be more easily mastered because the child is able to find out more about their nature and to test whether the measures it has adopted against them have been successful. This need to test by reality is a strong incentive for the development of its instinct for knowledge as well as many other activities. All those activities which help the child to defend itself from danger, which refute its fears and which enable it to make restitution to its object, have, in the same way as the early manifestations of the impulse to play, the purpose of mastering anxiety in regard to dangers both from without and within, both real and imaginary.

In consequence of the interaction of introjection and projection— a process which corresponds to the interaction of super-ego formation and object-relationship[3]—the child finds a refutation of what it fears in the outer world, and at the same time allays its anxiety by introjecting its real, 'good' objects. Since the presence and love of its real objects also has the purpose of lessening the small child's fear of its introjected objects and its sense of guilt, its fear of internal dangers strengthens its fixation upon its mother and increases its need for love and help significantly. Freud has explained that those expressions of anxiety in small children which are intelligible to us can be reduced to a single source—'missing someone who is loved or longed-for'[4]—and he traces that anxiety back to a stage in

---

[1] *Beyond the Pleasure Principle*, *S.E.* **18,** pp. 14–16.

[2] I have pointed out in Chapter IX of this book that the sense of guilt acts as an impetus for earliest activities and sublimations.

[3] Cf. Chapter IX.

[4] *Inhibitions, Symptoms and Anxiety* (1926) (*S.E.* **20,** p. 136).

which the immature individual was entirely dependent on its mother. Missing the loved or longed-for person, experiencing a loss of love or a loss of object as a danger, being frightened of being alone in the dark, or with an unknown person—all these things are, I have found, modified forms of early anxiety-situations, that is, of the small child's fear of dangerous internalized and external objects. At a somewhat later stage of development there is added to this fear a concern for the object itself. The child now fears that its mother will die in consequence of its phantasied attacks upon her and, in addition, is afraid that it will be left all alone in its helpless state. Freud says,[1] concerning this: 'It [the infant] cannot as yet distinguish between temporary absence and permanent loss. As soon as it loses sight of its mother it behaves as if it were never going to see her again; and repeated consoling experiences to the contrary are necessary before it learns that her disappearance is usually followed by her reappearance'.[2]

According to my observation of children, the mother has to prove again and again by her presence that she is not the 'bad', attacking mother. The child requires a real object to combat its fear of its terrifying introjected objects and of its super-ego. Furthermore, the presence of the mother is used as evidence that she is not dead. As its relationship to reality advances the child makes increasing use of its relations to its objects and its various activities and sublimation as a help against its fear of its super-ego and its destructive impulses. My starting point was that anxiety stimulates the development of the

[1] *ibid.*, p. 169.

[2] But the small child will only allow itself to be convinced by comforting experiences of this kind provided that its earliest anxiety-situations do not predominate and that in the formation of its super-ego its relations to its real objects are sufficiently brought into play. I have over and over again found that in older children the absence of their mother reactivated the earliest anxiety-situations under whose pressure they had, as small children, felt her temporary absence as a permanent one. In my paper, 'Personification in the Play of Children' (1929), I have reported the case of a boy of six who made me play the part of a 'fairy mamma' who was to protect him against his 'bad' combined parents and kill them. I had, furthermore, to change over and over again from the 'fairy mamma' to the 'bad mamma' all at once. As the 'fairy mamma' I had to heal the fatal wounds he had received from a huge wild animal (the 'bad' combined parents); but the next moment I had to go away and come back as the 'bad mamma' and attack him. He said 'Whenever the fairy mamma goes out of the room you never know if she won't come back all of a sudden as the bad mamma'. This boy, who had an unusually strong fixation on his mother since his earliest years, lived in the perpetual belief that some harm had befallen his parents and his brothers and sisters. It came out that even if he had only just seen his mother the minute before he felt no security that she had not died in the meanwhile.

ego. What happens is that in its efforts to master anxiety, the child's ego summons to its assistance its relations to its objects and to reality. Those efforts are therefore of fundamental importance for the child's adaptation to reality and for the development of its ego.

The small child's super-ego and objects are not identical; but it is continually endeavouring to make them interchangeable, partly so as to lessen its fear of its super-ego, partly so as to be better able to comply with the requirements of its real objects, which do not coincide with the phantastic commands of its introjected objects. Thus the ego of the small child is burdened with the conflict between the super-ego and the id as well as with the conflicting demands of the super-ego itself which contains various imagos that have been formed in the course of development. In addition to all this the child has to cope with the difference between the demands of its super-ego and those of its real objects, with the result that it is constantly wavering between its introjected objects and its real ones—between its world of phantasy and its world of reality.

The attempt to effect an adjustment between the super-ego and id cannot be successful in early childhood, for the pressure of the id and the corresponding severity of the super-ego absorb as yet the whole energy of the ego. When, at the onset of the latency period, the development of the libido and the formation of the super-ego have reached completion, the ego is stronger and can approach the task of making an adjustment on a broader basis between the factors concerned. The strengthened ego joins with the super-ego in setting up a common aid which includes above all the subjection of the id and its adaptation to the demands of real objects and the external world At this period of its development the child's ego-ideal is the well-behaved, 'good' child that satisfies its parents and teachers.

This stabilization is, however, shattered in the period just before puberty and, more especially, at puberty itself. The resurgence of libido which takes place at this period strengthens the demands of the id, while at the same time the pressure of the super-ego is increased. The ego is once more hard pressed and finds itself faced with the necessity of arriving at some new adjustment; for the old one has failed and the instinctual impulses can no longer be kept down and restricted as they were before. The child's anxiety is increased by the fact that its instincts might now more easily break through in reality and with more serious consequences than in early childhood.

The ego, in agreement with the super-ego, therefore sets up a new aim. The original objects of his love need to be given up. We see the adolescent often at odds with those around him and on the look-out for new objects. Such a requirement is, however, to a certain extent, also in harmony with reality, which imposes different and higher tasks upon him at this age; and in the further course of his development this flight from the original object leads to a partial detachment from personal objects in general and to the substitution of principles and ideals in their stead.

The final stabilization of the individual is not achieved until he has passed through the period of puberty. At the termination of this period his ego and super-ego are able to agree in setting up adult aims. Instead of being dependent on his immediate environment the individual now adapts himself to the larger world about him; though he acknowledges the claims of the new reality, he sets them up as his own internal demands. As he successfully detaches himself from his original objects, he achieves a greater independence from objects in general. An adjustment of this kind rests in his recognition of a new reality and is effected with the assistance of a stronger ego. And once more, as in the first period of flowering of his sexual life, the pressure arising from the menacing situation between the exaggerated demands of the id and the super-ego contributes much towards this strengthening of his ego. The contrary, inhibiting effect of such a pressure is seen in the fresh limitation of his personality, usually a permanent one, which overtakes him at the close of this period. The flowering of his phantasy life which accompanies, though to a milder degree than in the first period of childhood, this second emergence of his sexuality is as a rule once again severely curtailed when he has passed the period of puberty. We now have before us the 'normal' adult.

One more point. We have seen that in early childhood the super-ego and the id cannot as yet be reconciled with each other. In the latency period stability is achieved by the ego and super-ego uniting in the pursuit of a common aim. At puberty, a situation similar to the early period is created, and this is once more followed by a mental stabilization of the individual. We have already discussed the differences between these two kinds of stabilization; and we can now see what they have in common. In both cases an adjustment is reached by the ego and super-ego agreeing upon a common aim and setting up an ego-ideal that takes into account the demands of reality.[1]

[1] In *Inhibitions, Symptoms and Anxiety* (1926), Freud says: 'Just as the ego controls the path to action in the external world, so it controls access to consciousness. In repression it exercises its power in both directions . . .' (*S.E.* **20,** p. 95). On the other hand he says: 'I drew a picture of its (the ego's) dependent relationship to the id and to the super-ego and . . . how powerless and apprehensive it was in regard to both.' (*ibid.* p. 95.) My theory of the growth of the ego is in agreement with these two statements, for it shows how the forces of the super-ego and ego react on each other and determine the whole course of the individual's development.

In the earlier chapters of this book I have tried to show that the development of the super-ego ceases, along with that of the libido, at the onset of the latency period. I would now like to emphasize as a point of central importance that what we have to deal with in the various stages that follow the decline of the Oedipus conflict are not changes in the super-ego itself, but a growth of the ego, which involves a consolidation of the super-ego. In the latency period the child's ego and super-ego share the aim of adapting themselves to the environment and of adopting ego-ideals belonging to that environment. This fact, and not the actual change of its super-ego may explain the general process of stabilization in the latency period.

We must now pass from our discussion of the development of the ego to a consideration of the relationship of this process to the mastering of anxiety-situations which I described as such an essential factor in development.

I have said that the small child's play activities, by bridging the gulf between phantasy and reality, help it to master its fear of internal and external dangers. Let us take the typical 'mother' games of little girls. Analysis of normal children shows that these games, besides being wish-fulfilments, contain the deepest anxiety belonging to early anxiety-situations, and that beneath the little girl's ever-recurring desire for dolls there lies a need for consolation and re-assurance. The possession of her dolls is a proof that she has not been robbed of her children by her mother, that she has not had her body destroyed by her and that she is able to have children. Moreover, by nursing and dressing her dolls, with whom she identifies herself, she obtains proof that she had a loving mother, and thus lessens her fear of being abandoned and left homeless and motherless. This purpose is also served to some extent by other games which are played by children of both sexes, as, for instance, games of furnishing houses and travelling, both of which spring from the desire to find a new home—in the final resort, to re-discover their mother.

A typical boys' game, and one which brings out the masculine components very clearly, is playing with carts, horses and trains. This symbolizes a way into the mother's body. In their play boys enact over and over again, and with every kind of variation, scenes of fighting with their father inside the mother's body and copulating with her. The boldness, skill and cunning with which they defend themselves against their enemies in their games of fighting assure them that they can successfully combat their castrating father, and this lessens their fear of him. By these means and by representing himself as copulating with his mother in various ways and showing his prowess in it, the boy tries to prove to himself that he possesses a penis and sexual potency—two things whose loss his deepest anxiety-situations have led him to fear. And, since along with his aggressive tendencies his restorative ones towards his mother come out as well in these games, he also proves to himself that his penis is not destructive; and in this way he relieves his sense of guilt.[1]

The intense pleasure which children who are not inhibited in their play get from games proceeds not only from the gratification of their wish-fulfilling trends, but also from the mastery of anxiety which they achieve in their games. But in my opinion it is not merely a question of two separate functions being carried out side by side; what happens is that the ego employs every wish-fulfilling mechanism to a large extent for the purpose of mastering anxiety as well. Thus by a complicated process which mobilizes all the forces of the ego, children's games effect a transformation of anxiety into pleasure. We will examine later how this fundamental process affects the economy of the mental life and ego-development of the adult.

Nevertheless, as far as small children are concerned, the ego can never fully achieve the aim of mastering anxiety by means of play. As long as anxiety remains latently operative, it makes itself felt as a constant incentive to play; but as soon as it becomes manifest it interrupts their game.

In the play of small children we can thus recognize that the early ego of the child only partially achieves the aim of mastering anxiety. With the onset of the latency period the child masters its anxiety better and at the same time shows a greater capacity to come up to the demands of reality. Its games lose their imaginative content and their place is gradually taken by schoolwork. The child's preoccupation with the letters of the alphabet, arithmetical numbers and drawing, which has at first the character of play, largely replaces its games with toys. The way in which letters are joined together, the child's zeal in getting their shape and order right and in making them of even size, and the delight in achieving correctness in each of these details, are all based on the same internal conditions as its former activity in building houses and playing with dolls. A beautiful and orderly exercise-book has the same symbolic meaning for the girl as house and home, namely, that of a healthy, unimpaired body. Letters and numbers represent parents, brothers and sisters, children, genitals and excrements to her and are vehicles for her original aggressive tendencies as well as for her reactive ones. The evidence for the refutation of her fears she obtains from successfully completed homework, which takes the place of playing with dolls and furnishing houses. Analyses of children in the latency period show that not only every detail of their homework, but all their various activities in

[1] This subject will be more fully discussed in Chapter XII.

handicrafts, drawing and so on, are utilized in phantasy to restore their own genitals and body, as well as their mother's body and its contents, their father's penis, their brothers and sisters, etc. In the same way, every single item of their own or their doll's clothing, such as collars, cuffs, shawl, cap, belt, stockings, shoes, has a symbolic significance.[1]

In the normal course of their development, the care which younger children lavish on the 'drawing' of letters and numbers is extended, as they grow older, to intellectual achievement as a whole. But even so, their satisfaction in such achievements is largely dependent on the appreciation they receive from the people about them; it is a means of gaining the approval of their elders. In the latency period, therefore, we see that the child finds a refutation of its danger-situations to a great extent in the love and approval of its real objects; the relationship to its objects and to reality is overemphasized.

In the boy, writing is the expression of his masculine components.[2] The stroke of the pen and the success with which he forms letters represent an active performance of coitus, and are a proof of his possession of a penis and of sexual potency. Books and exercise-books stand for the genitals or the body of his mother or sister.[3] To a six-year-old boy, for instance, the capital letter 'L' meant a man on a horse (himself and his penis) riding through an archway (his mother's genitals); 'i' was the penis and himself, 'e' his mother and her genitals, and 'ie' the union of himself and her in coitus. Capital letters and small ones represent in general parents and children.[4] The active copulation phantasies of boys come out also in active games and in sport, and we find the same phantasies expressed in the details of these games as in their homework. The boy's wish to surpass his rivals and so to obtain an assurance against the danger of being castrated by his father—a wish which corresponds to the masculine mode of dealing with anxiety-situations and which is of so much importance later on at the age of puberty—makes its appearance while he is still in the latency period. In general the boy is less dependent than the girl on the approval of his environment even in this period, and achievement for its own sake already plays a much greater part in his psychological life than in hers.

[1] Cf. Flugel, *The Psychology of Clothes* (1930).

[2] In girls, too, writing and other activities of the kind are mainly derived from masculine components.

[3] In connection with his feminine components, the boy's exercise-book stands for his own body, and the accomplishment of his school task an attempt to restore it.

[4] Cf. my paper, 'The Role of the School in the Libidinal Development of the Child' (1923, *Writings*, 1).

We have described the stabilization which takes place in the latency period as being based upon an adaptation to reality effected by the ego in agreement with the super-ego. The attainment of such an aim depends upon a combined action of all the forces engaged in keeping down and restricting the id-instincts. It is here that the child's struggle to break itself of masturbation comes in — a struggle which, to quote Freud, 'claims a large share of its energies' during the latency period and whose full force is directed against its masturbation phantasies as well. And these phantasies, as we have repeatedly seen, form an element not only in children's play, but in their learning activities and all their later sublimations as well.[1]

The reason why, in the latency period, the child stands in such great need of the approval of its objects is because it wants to lessen the opposition of its super-ego (which at this stage tends to adapt itself to its objects) to its desexualized masturbation phantasies. Thus in this period it has on the one hand to fulfil the demand of giving up masturbation and of repressing its masturbation phantasies, and on the other to fulfil the counter-demand of putting into effect successfully and to the satisfaction of its elders those same masturbation phantasies in their desexualized form of everyday interests and activities; for it is only with the help of such satisfactory sublimations that it can procure the comprehensive refutation of its anxiety-situations needed by its ego. On its successful escape from this dilemma will depend its stabilization in the latency period. The sanction of those in authority, which the latency child needs in order to master its anxiety, is also a precondition for this process.

This brief review of such very complicated and widely ramified processes of development must of necessity be a schematic one. In actual fact, the boundary between the normal and the neurotic child

---

[1] In my paper, 'The Role of the School in the Libidinal Development of the Child' (1923), I have discussed the unconscious significance of certain articles used at school and have examined the underlying causes of inhibitions in learning and in school life. In consequence of an excessive repression of its masturbation phantasies the child suffers from an inhibition of its imaginative life which affects both its play and work. During the latency period this inhibition is very conspicuous in the whole character of the child. In *The Question of Lay Analysis* (1926), Freud writes: 'I have an impression that with the onset of the latency period they (children) become mentally inhibited as well, stupider. From that time on, too, many lose their physical charm.' (*S.E.* **20,**, p. 215.) It is indeed true that the ego maintains its position of superiority over the id at great cost to the individual. In those periods of life when it is not so completely successful in subduing the id (i.e. during the first and second periods of the flowering of sexuality) it enjoys a much fuller imaginative activity, and this expresses itself in less stability of mind on the one hand and greater richness of personality on the other.

is not very sharply drawn, especially during the latency period. The neurotic child may be good at school. The normal child is not always eager to learn, since he often seeks to disprove his anxiety-situations in other ways, for example, by displaying physical prowess. In the latency period the normal girl will often master her anxiety in pre-eminently masculine ways, and the boy can still be described as normal even though he chooses more passive and feminine modes of behaviour for the same purpose.

Freud has brought to our notice the typical ceremonials which set in in the latency period and which are a result of the child's struggle against masturbation.[1] He says that this period 'is characterized by ... the erection of ethical and aesthetic barriers in the ego'. Owing to 'the reaction-formations in the ego of the obsessional neurotic, which we recognize as exaggerations of normal character-formation',[2] the line of demarcation between obsessional reactions and the characterological development of the normal child, fostered as it is by his educational environment, is not easily fixed in children in the latency period.

It will be remembered that I have put forward the view that the situation from which the obsessional neurosis originates lies in early childhood. But I have said that in this period of development, only isolated obsessional traits crop up. They do not in general become organized so as to form an obsessional neurosis until the latency period sets in. This systematization of obsessional traits, which goes along with a consolidation of the super-ego[3] and a strengthening of the ego, is achieved by the super-ego and ego[4] establishing a common aim. This common aim forms the keystone of their power over the id. And although the suppression of the child's instincts demanded by his objects is carried out with the assistance of his obsessional mechanisms, it will not be successful unless all the factors involved are acting in concert against the id. In this comprehensive process of organization, the ego manifests what Freud has called 'the tendency of the ego to synthesize'.[5]

Thus in the latency period the obsessional neurosis is adequate to

---

[1] Cf. *Inhibitions, Symptoms and Anxiety* (1926) (*S.E.* **20**, p. 116).

[2] *Ibid.*, pp. 114 and 115.

[3] In this process the child's various identifications become more integrated, the demands made by its super-ego more unified and its internalized objects better adjusted to the external situation. Cf. also my paper, 'Personification in the Play of Children' (1929, *Writings*, **1**).

[4] In *Inhibitions, Symptoms and Anxiety* (1926) (*S.E.* **20,**, p. 113) Freud says that in obsessional neurosis 'the ego and the super-ego have a specially large share in the formation of the symptoms'.

[5] *Ibid.*, p. 112.

satisfy the requirements of the child's ego, super-ego and objects. In general adults strongly reject a child's affects. This is often so successful because that rejection answers at this age to the child's internal requirements.[1] We often experience in analysis that a child is made to suffer and gets into conflict if the people in charge of it have identified themselves too strongly with its disobedience and aggressive trends. Its ego only feels equal to the task of keeping down the id and opposing forbidden impulses so long as its elders assist its efforts. The child needs to receive prohibitions from without, since these, as we know, support prohibitions from within. It needs, in other words, to have representatives of its super-ego in the outer world. This dependence upon objects in order to be able to master anxiety is much stronger in the latency period than in any other phase of development. Indeed it seems to me to be a definite prerequisite for a successful transition into the latency period that the child's mastery of anxiety should rest upon its object-relations and adaptation to reality.

Nevertheless it is necessary for the child's future stability that this mechanism of mastering anxiety should not predominate to excess. If the child's interests and achievements and other gratifications are too completely devoted to its endeavours to win love and recognition from its objects; if, that is, its object-relations are the pre-eminent means of mastering its anxiety and allaying its sense of guilt, its mental health in future years is not planted in firm soil. If it is less dependent on its objects and if the interests and achievements by means of which it masters its anxiety and allays its sense of guilt are done for their own sake and afford it interest and pleasure in themselves, its anxiety will undergo a better modification and a wider distribution—will be levelled down, as it were. As soon as its anxiety has thus been reduced, its capacity for libidinal gratification will grow, and this is a pre-condition for the successful mastering of anxiety. Anxiety can only be mastered where the super-ego and id

---

[1] The child's environment can also directly affect its neurosis. In some analyses I have found that the favourable influence exerted on the patient by a change in the environment was attributable to the fact that it had led him to exchange one set of symptoms, which had been very tiresome, for another which, though equally important in the structure of his neurosis, was less noticeable. Another thing which may make the child's symptoms disappear is an increase of his fear of his objects. I once had a boy patient, aged fourteen (cf. my paper, 'A Contribution to the Psychogenesis of Tics', 1925), who had done very well in his lessons at school but had been very inhibited in games and sport, until his father, who had been away for a long time, came home and brought pressure to bear on him to overcome his inhibition. The boy did in fact do so to some extent, out of fear of him; but at the same time he was overtaken by a severe inhibition in learning, which still persisted when he came to me for analysis at the age of fourteen.

have come to a satisfactory adjustment and the ego has attained a sufficient degree of strength.[1]

Since object relations in the latency period give so much mental support even to normal children it is not easy to detect those frequent cases in which this factor receives excessive significance. But in the period of puberty we can clearly do so, as the child's dependence upon its objects is no longer sufficient, if this is its chief means of mastering anxiety. This is one of the reasons why, I think, psychotic illnesses usually do not break out till later childhood, during or after the age of puberty. If we take as our yardstick the strength of the ego, based on a lessening of the severity of the super-ego, which includes a greater amount of instinctual freedom, together with an adaptation to the aims of this period of development—then we shall not run the risk of over-rating the adaptation to the demands of education and of reality in the latency period as a criterion of successful development and health.[2]

Freud says that 'the advent of puberty opens a decisive chapter in the history of an obsessional neurosis' and furthermore, at that time 'the early aggressive impulses [will] be re-awakened; but a greater or lesser proportion of the new libidinal impulses—in bad cases the

[1] If due attention is paid to the indications, we shall be able to observe the beginnings of later illnesses and impairments of development much more clearly in the first period of childhood than in the latency period. In a great many cases of people who have fallen ill at puberty or later, it has been found that they suffered from great difficulties in early childhood but were well adapted during latency, at which period they showed no marked difficulties and were amenable—often all too amenable—to their educational environment.—In cases where the anxiety belonging to the earliest stages is too intense or has not been properly modified, the process of stabilization in the latency period, which rests upon obsessional mechanisms, does not take place at all.

[2] If the requirements of the latency period have been too successfully imposed and the child's docility is too great, its character and its ego-ideals will remain in a state of subservience to its environment for the rest of its life. A weak ego—the result of maladjustment between super-ego and id—runs the risk of being unable to carry out the task of detaching the individual from his objects at the age of puberty and of setting up independent internal standards, so that he will fail from a characterological point of view. A lessened dependence upon its objects on the part of the child works in quite well with the educational demands made upon it at that time. In none of my latency-period analyses has a child become detached from its objects in the sense in which children at the age of puberty do. All that has happened is that its fixations become less strong and ambivalent. In this period of life, in becoming less dependent on its objects it becomes better able to find other objects, and thus prepares itself for the subsequent detachment it must make from its objects at puberty. Analysis does not increase but lessens the difficulties the child has in adapting itself to its environment and coming to terms with it; for the more internal freedom it has the better will it be able to do this.

whole of them—will have to follow the course prescribed for them by regression and will emerge as aggressive and destructive tendencies. In consequence of the erotic trends being disguised in this way and owing to the powerful reaction-formations in the ego, the struggle against sexuality will henceforward be carried on under the banner of ethical principles.'[1]

The erection of new principles and new idealized father-imagos and the heightened demands on himself are used by the child for the purpose of moving away from his original objects. By doing so he is able to call up his original positive attachment to his father and in-crease it with less risk of coming into collision with him. This event corresponds to a splitting of his father imago. The exalted and admired father can now be loved and adored while the 'bad' father— often represented by his real father or by a substitute such as a schoolmaster—summons very strange feelings of hatred which are common at this period of development. And in the aggressive rela-tionship to the hated father the boy reassures himself that he is his father's match and will not be castrated by him. In his relation to the admired father-imago he can satisfy himself that he possesses a powerful and helpful father, and can also identify himself with him; out of all this he draws a greater belief in his own constructive capacities and sexual potency.

It is here that his activities and achievements come in. By means of those achievements, whether physical or intellectual, which call for courage, strength and enterprise, among other things, he proves to himself that the castration he dreads so much has not happened to him, and that he is not impotent. His achievements also gratify his reactive trends and alleviate his sense of guilt. They show him that his constructive capacities outweigh his destructive tendencies, and they also represent restitution to his objects. By giving him these assurances they greatly add to the satisfaction they afford him.[2] The alleviation of his anxiety and sense of guilt, which in the latency period he has found in the successful accomplishment of his activities when they are made ego-syntonic by the approval of his environ-ment, must in the period of puberty to a much greater extent come from the value which his work and achievements have for him in themselves.

We must now give a brief consideration to the way in which the

---

[1] *Inhibitions, Symptoms and Anxiety* (1926) (*S.E.* **20**, p. 116).

[2] In many of his sublimations, particularly his intellectual and artistic efforts, the boy makes extensive use of the feminine mode of mastering anxiety. He utilizes books and work, in their significance of bodies, fertility, children, etc., as a refutation of the destruction of his body which, in the feminine position, he awaits at the hands of the mother who is his rival.

girl deals with her anxiety-situations at puberty. At this age she normally retains the aims of the latency period and the modes of mastering anxiety adequate to that phase longer than the boy does. Very often the young girl at puberty is dominated by the masculine mode of mastering anxiety. We shall see in the next chapter why it is more difficult for her to establish the feminine position than it is for the boy to establish the masculine one. The young girl makes higher demands on herself and on others too. Her standards and ideals adopt the form of abstract principles to a lesser extent, but instead are more related to admired people. Her desire to please extends to mental achievements as well and plays a part even when they reach the highest levels. Her attitude to her work, in so far as the masculine components are not predominantly involved, corresponds to her attitude towards her own body; and her activities in relation to these two interests are largely concerned with dealing with her specific anxiety-situations. A beautiful body or a perfect piece of work provide the growing girl with the same counter-proofs as she needed as a child—namely, that the inside of her body has not been destroyed, and that the children have not been taken out of it. As an adult woman, her relation to her own child, which often takes the place of her relation to her work, is a very great help to her in dealing with anxiety. To have it and nurse it and watch it grow and thrive— these things provide her, exactly as in the case of the little girl and her dolls, with ever-renewed proofs that her possession of a child is not endangered, and serve to alleviate her sense of guilt.[1] The danger-situations, both great and small, which she had to deal with in the process of bringing up her children are calculated, if things go well, to provide a constant refutation of her earliest fears. Similarly, her relation to her home, which is equivalent to her own body, has a special importance for the feminine mode of mastering anxiety, and has, besides, another and more direct connection with her early anxiety-situation. As we have seen, the little girl's rivalry with her mother finds utterance, among other things, in phantasies of driving her out and taking her place as mistress of the house. An important part of this anxiety-situation for children of both sexes, but more especially for girls, consists in the fear of being turned out of the house and being left homeless.[2] Their contentment with their own home is always partly based on its value as a refutation of this element in their anxiety-situation. It is indispensible to the normal

---

[1] Cf. the next chapter for a discussion of the more underlying factors in her relations to her child.

[2] The fear of becoming a beggar child or a homeless orphan appears in every child analysis. It plays a large part in fixating the child to its mother, and is one of the forms taken by its fear of loss of love.

stabilization of the woman that her children, her work, her activities, and the care and adornment of her person and home should furnish her with a complete refutation of her danger-situation.[1] Her relation to men, furthermore, is largely determined by her need to convince herself through their admiration of the intactness of her body. Her narcissism, therefore, plays a great part in her mastery of anxiety. It is as a result of this feminine mode of mastering anxiety that women are so much more dependent on the love and approval of men—and of objects in general—than men are upon women. But men, too, extract from their love-relations a tranquillization of their anxiety which contributes essentially to the sexual satisfaction they get from them.

The normal process of mastering anxiety seems to be conditional upon a number of factors, in which the specific methods employed act in conjunction with quantitive elements, such as the amount of sadism and anxiety present and the degree of the ego's capacity to tolerate anxiety. If these interacting factors attain a certain optimum, it appears that the child is able to modify quite successfully even very large quantities of anxiety, and can achieve a satisfactory or even outstanding development of its ego and a high level of mental health. The conditions under which he can master anxiety are as specific as the conditions under which he can love, and are, as far as can be seen, very intimately bound up with them.[2] In some cases, best typified in the age of puberty, the condition for mastering anxiety is that the individual shall overcome danger-situations under especially difficult circumstances which give rise to strong fear; in others, it is that he shall avoid as far as he can—and even, in extreme cases, in a phobic way—all such circumstances. Between these two extremes is situated what can be regarded as a normal incentive to obtain pleasure from the overcoming of anxiety-situations that are associated with not too much, and not too direct (and therefore more evenly apportioned) anxiety.

In this chapter I have tried to show that all activities and sublimations of the individual also serve to master his anxiety and alleviate his guilt. The motive force of all activities and interests is, besides the satisfaction of his aggressive impulses, the desire to make restitution towards his object and restore his own body and sexual parts. We have also seen[3] that in a very early stage of his development his sense of omnipotence is enlisted in the service of his destructive impulses. When his reaction-formations set in, this sense of

---

[1] In some women I have been able to establish the fact that when they have completed their morning toilet they have had a feeling of freshness and energy in contrast to a previous mood of depression. Washing and dressing stood for restoring themselves in many ways.

[2] Cf. Chapter XI.   [3] Cf. Chapter IX.

negative, destructive omnipotence makes it necessary for him to believe in his constructive omnipotence; and the stronger his sense of sadistic omnipotence has been, the stronger must his sense of positive omnipotence now be, in order that he may be able to come up to the demands of his super-ego for making restitution. If the restitution required of him necessitates a very strong sense of constructive omnipotence—as, for instance, that he shall make complete restitution towards both parents and towards his brothers and sisters, etc., and, by displacement, towards other objects and even the entire world—then, whether he will do great things in life and whether the development of his ego and of his sexual life will be successful,[1] or whether he will fall a victim to severe inhibitions, will depend upon the strength of his ego and the degree of his adaptation to reality which regulates those imaginary demands.

To sum up what has been said: I have tried to get some insight into the complicated process, involving all the energies of the individual, by means of which the ego attempts to master his infantile anxiety-situations. The success of this process is of fundamental importance for the development of his ego, and a decisive factor for his mental health. For with the normal person it is this manifold reassurance against his anxiety and guilt—a reassurance which constantly flows from many sources and which he derives from his activities and interests and from his social relations and erotic satisfactions—that enables him to leave his original anxiety-situations far behind and to distribute and weaken the full force of their impact upon him. Thanks to the general application of this mechanism in even unimportant actions, a way of mastering anxiety of no small economic importance for the normal individual emerges from the mere overcoming of everyday difficulties.[2]

Finally, I must examine how the account given in these pages of the normal method of dealing with anxiety-situations compares with Freud's view on the subject.[3] In his *Inhibitions, Symptoms and Anxiety* he writes: 'It must be, therefore, that certain determinants of anxiety are relinquished and certain danger-situations lose their significance as the individual becomes more mature.' This statement, however, is qualified by his subsequent remarks. After the sentence just quoted

---

[1] If the tasks laid upon him are too exacting and the discrepancy between his destructive and constructive omnipotence exceeds a certain limit, sublimations can become inhibited and productivity and sexual development can be disturbed. In Chapter XII we shall discuss a case in point.

[2] If even everyday activities are so much bound up with anxiety this will give the neurotic an additional reason for finding such actions burdensome and may make him unable to perform them.

[3] *Inhibitions, Symptoms and Anxiety* (S.E. **20,** p. 148).

he goes on: 'Moreover, some of these danger-situations manage to survive into later times by modifying their determinants of anxiety so as to bring them up to date.' I think that my theory of the modifications of anxiety helps us to understand by what means the normal person gets away from his anxiety-situations and modifies the conditions under which he feels anxiety. Analytic observation strongly inclines me to believe that even a wide removal from his anxiety-situations such as the normal individual achieves does not amount to a relinquishment of them. To all intents and purposes these anxiety-situations, it is true, have no direct effects upon him; but in certain circumstances such effects will reappear. If a normal person is put under a severe internal or external strain, or if he falls ill or fails in some other way, we may observe in him the full and direct operation of his deepest anxiety-situations. Since, then, every healthy person *may* succumb to a neurotic illness, it follows that he can never have entirely given up his old anxiety-situations.

The following remarks by Freud would seem to bear out this view. In the passage just quoted he writes: 'The neurotic will differ from the normal person in that his reactions to the dangers in question will be unduly strong. Finally, being grown-up affords no absolute protection against a return of the original traumatic anxiety-situation. Each individual has in all probability a limit beyond which his mental apparatus fails in its function of mastering the quantities of excitation which require to be disposed of.'

Chapter XI

THE EFFECTS OF
EARLY ANXIETY-SITUATIONS
ON THE SEXUAL DEVELOPMENT
OF THE GIRL

PSYCHO-ANALYTIC investigation has thrown much less light on the psychology of women than on that of men. Since the fear of castration was the first thing that was discovered as an underlying motive force in the formation of neurosis in men, analysts naturally began by studying aetiological factors of the same kind in women. The results obtained in this way held good in so far as the psychology of the two sexes was similar but not in so far as it differed. Freud has well expressed this point in a passàge in which he says: '. . . Furthermore, is it absolutely certain that fear of castration is the only motive force of repression (or defence)? If we think of neurosis in women we are bound to doubt it. For though we can with certainty establish in them the presence of a castration *complex*, we can hardly speak of a castration *anxiety* where castration has already taken place.'[1]

When we consider how important every advance in our knowledge of castration anxiety has been both for understanding the psychology of the man and for effecting a cure of his neurosis, we shall expect that a knowledge of whatever anxiety is its equivalent in the female child will enable us to perfect our therapeutic treatment of her, and help us to get a clearer idea of the lines along which her sexual development moves forward.

The Anxiety-Situation of the Girl

In my 'Early Stages of the Oedipus Conflict'[2] I have made a contribution to this still unsolved problem and have put forward the view that the girl's deepest fear is of having the inside of her body robbed and destroyed. As a result of the oral frustration she experiences from her mother, the girl turns away from her and takes her father's penis as her object of satisfaction. This desire urges her

[1] *Inhibitions, Symptoms and Anxiety* (1926), *S.E.* **20,** p. 123.
[2] (1921) *Writings*, **1.**

to make further important steps in her development. She evolves phantasies of her mother introducing her father's penis into her body and giving him the breast; and these phantasies form the nucleus of early sexual theories which arouse feelings of envy and hatred in her at being frustrated by both parents. At this stage of development children of both sexes believe that it is the mother, the source of nourishment, whose body contains all that is desirable, including their father's penis. This sexual theory increases the small girl's hatred of her mother on account of the frustration she has suffered from her, and contributes to the production of sadistic phantasies of attacking and destroying her mother's inside and depriving it of its contents. Owing to her fear of retaliation, such phantasies form the basis of the girl's deepest anxiety-situation.

In his paper on 'The Early Development of Female Sexuality' (1927), Ernest Jones gives the name *aphanisis* to the complete and lasting destruction of the capacity to obtain libidinal satisfaction which he considers an early and dominant anxiety-situation for children of both sexes.[1] This assumption is close to my own view. It seems to me that the destruction of the capacity to obtain libidinal gratification implies a destruction of those organs which are necessary for the purpose. And the girl expects to have those organs destroyed in the course of the attacks that will be made, principally by her mother, upon her body and its contents. Her fears concerning her genitals are especially intense, partly because her own sadistic impulses are very strongly directed towards her mother's genitals and the erotic pleasures she (the mother) gets from them, and partly because her fear of being incapable of enjoying sexual satisfaction serves in its turn to increase her fear of having had her own genitals damaged.

Early Stages of the Oedipus Conflict

According to my experience, the girl's Oedipus tendencies are ushered in by her oral desires for her father's penis. These desires are already accompanied by genital impulses. Her wish to rob her mother of her father's penis and incorporate it in herself, I have found, is a fundamental factor in the development of her sexual life. The resentment her mother has aroused in her by withdrawing the nourishing breast from her is intensified by the further wrong she has done her in not granting her her father's penis as an object of satisfaction; and this double grievance is the deepest source of the hatred the female child feels towards her mother as a result of her Oedipus trends.

[1] *Papers on Psycho-Analysis*, 4th and 5th editions.

These assumptions differ in some respects from accepted psycho-analytical theory. Freud has come to the conclusion[1] that it is the castration complex that introduces the girl's Oedipus complex, and that what makes her turn away from her mother is the grudge she bears her for having denied her a penis of her own. The divergence between Freud's view and the one put forward here, however, becomes less great if we reflect that they agree on two important points—namely, that the girl wants to have a penis and that she hates her mother for not giving her one. But, according to my assumption, what she primarily wants is not to possess a penis of her own as an attribute of masculinity, but to incorporate her father's penis as an object of oral satisfaction. Furthermore, I think that this desire is not an outcome of her castration complex but the most fundamental expression of her Oedipus trends, and that consequently the female child is brought under the sway of her Oedipus impulses not indirectly, through her masculine tendencies and her penis-envy, but directly, as a result of her dominant feminine instinctual components.[2]

When the girl turns to her father's penis as the wished-for object, several factors determine the intensity of her desire. The demands of her oral-sucking impulses, heightened by the frustration she has suffered from her mother's breast, create in her a phantasy picture of her father's penis as an organ which, unlike the breast, can provide her with a tremendous and never-ending oral gratification.[3]

[1] 'Some Psychical Consequences of the Anatomical Distinction between the Sexes' (1925), *S.E.* **19**.

[2] In her paper, 'On the Genesis of the Castration Complex' (1924), Karen Horney has supported the view that what gives rise to the girl's castration complex is the frustration she has suffered in the Oedipus situation, her desire to possess a penis springs primarily from her Oedipus wishes and not from her wish to be a man. She looks upon the desired penis as a part of her father and as a substitute for him.

[3] In her *Psychoanalyse der weiblichen Sexualfunktionen* (1925), Helene Deutsch has pointed out that already very early on in her life the small girl, in taking her father as the object of her affections next in order to her mother, directs towards him a great part of that true sexual libido, attached to the oral zone, with which she has cathected her mother's breast, since 'in one phase of her development her unconscious equates her father's penis with her mother's breast as an organ for giving suck'. I also agree with the writer in her view that in the equation of the penis with the breast, the vagina takes on the passive role of the sucking mouth 'in the process of displacement from above downwards', and that this oral, sucking activity of the vagina is implied by its anatomical structure as a whole (p. 54). But whereas according to Helene Deutsch these phantasies do not become operative until the girl has reached sexual maturity and has experienced the sexual act, in my opinion the early equation of the penis with the breast is ushered in by the frustration she has

To this phantasy her urethral-sadistic impulses add their contribution. For children of both sexes attribute far greater urethral capacities to the penis—where, indeed, they are more visible—than to the female urinary organ. The girl's phantasies about the urethral capacity and power of the penis become allied to her oral phantasies, in virtue of the equation which small children make between all bodily substances; and in her imagination the penis is an object which possesses magical powers of providing oral satisfaction. But since the oral frustration she has suffered from her mother has stimulated all her other erotogenic zones as well and has aroused her genital trends and desires in regard to her father's penis, the latter becomes the object of her oral, urethral, anal and genital impulses. Another factor which serves to intensify her desires in this direction is her unconscious sexual theory that her mother has incorporated her father's penis, and her consequent envy of her mother.

It is the combination of all these factors, I think, which endows her father's penis with such enormous powers in the eyes of the small girl and makes it the object of her most ardent admiration and desire.[1] If she retains a predominantly feminine position, this attitude towards her father's penis will often lead her to assume a humble and submissive attitude towards the male sex. But it can also cause her to have intense feelings of hatred for having been denied the things which she has so passionately adored and longed for; and if she takes up a masculine position it can give rise to all the signs and symptoms of penis-envy in her.

But since the small girl's phantasies about the enormous powers and huge size and strength of her father's penis arise from her own oral-, urethral- and anal-sadistic impulses, she will also attribute extremely dangerous properties to it. This aspect of it provides the substratum of her terror of the 'bad' penis, which sets in as a reaction to the destructive impulses which, in combination with libidinal ones, are directed towards it. If her oral sadism is dominant, she will regard her father's penis within her mother principally as

---

suffered from the breast in early childhood, and at once exerts a powerful influence on her and greatly affects the whole trend of her development. I also believe that this equation of penis and breast, accompanied as it is by a 'displacement from above downwards', activates the oral, receptive qualities of the female genital at an early age, and prepares the vagina to receive the penis. It thus clears the way for the little girl's Oedipus tendencies—though these, it is true, do not unfold their full power until much later—and lays the foundation of her sexual development.

[1] She invests her mother with some of this glory and will in some cases only value her as the possessor of her father's penis.

a thing to be hated, envied and destroyed;[1] and the hate-filled phantasies which she centres upon her father's penis as something that is giving her mother satisfaction will in some cases be so intense that they will cause her to displace her deepest and most powerful anxiety—her fear of her mother—on to her father's penis as a hated appendage of her mother. If this happens, the adult woman will suffer severe impairments in her development and will be led into a distorted attitude towards the male sex. She will also have a more or less defective relationship to her objects and be unable to overcome, or overcome completely, the stage of partial love.[2,3]

In virtue of the omnipotence of thoughts, the [girl's] oral desire for her father's penis makes her feel that she has in fact incorporated it; hence her ambivalent feelings towards her father's penis become extended to this internalized one. As we know, in the stage of partial incorporation the object is represented by a part of itself; so that the father's penis stands for his whole person. That is why, I think, the child's earliest father-imagos—the nucleus of the paternal super-ego—are represented by his penis. As I have tried to show, the terrifying and cruel character of the super-ego in children of both sexes is due to the fact that they have begun to introject their objects at a period of development when their sadism is at its height. Hence, their earliest imagos assume the phantastic aspect which their own dominant pre-genital impulses have im-

---

[1] She will have the same attitude towards the children in her mother's body. We shall later on return to this subject and consider in what way her hostility to the children inside her mother affects her relations to her own brothers and sisters, to her own imaginary children, and, in after years, to her real ones.

[2] Cf. Abraham, 'A Short Study of the Development of the Libido' (1924).

[3] My patient Erna, whose case-history has been related in Chapter III, was a typical instance. Her father was in her eyes mainly the bearer of the penis which satisfied her mother and not herself. It turned out that her penis-envy and her castration wishes, which were exceedingly strong, were ultimately based upon the frustration she had experienced in regard to his penis in her oral position. Since, in focussing her hatred on his penis, she imagined that her mother had possession of it, the feeling she entertained towards her mother, though filled with hatred, was a more personal one than what she felt for her father. It is true that another reason why she turned away from him was to protect him from her own sadism. And the concentration of her hatred on his penis also helped to make her spare him as an object (cf. Abraham). Analysis was able to bring out in her a more friendly and human attitude towards her father, and this advance was accompanied by favourable changes in her relations with her mother and her objects in general. Concerning this relationship to the father's penis and father himself, I should like to draw attention to the points of similarity that exist between my patient and two cases that Abraham has reported on p. 483 of his above-mentioned work.

parted to them.[1] But this drive to introject the father's penis, that is, the Oedipus object, and to keep it inside is much stronger in the girl than in the boy. For the genital tendencies which coincide with her oral desires have a receptive character too, so that under normal circumstances the girl's Oedipus trends are to a far greater extent under the dominance of oral impulses than are those of the boy. It is a matter of decisive importance for the formation of the super-ego and the development of sexual life whether the prevailing phantasies are those of a 'good' penis or a 'bad' one. But in either case, the girl, being more subordinated to her introjected father, is more at the mercy of his powers for good or evil than the boy is normally in relation to his super-ego.[2] And her anxiety and sense of guilt in regard to her mother serve to complicate still further her divided feelings about her father's penis.

In order to simplify our survey of the whole situation I will first of all follow the development of the girl's attitude to her father's penis and then try to discover how far her relationship to her mother affects her relationship with her father. In favourable circumstances the girl believes in the existence of a dangerous, introjected penis, as well as of a beneficent and helpful one. As a result of this ambivalent attitude, anxiety is generated which drives the very young child as well as the adult to seek sexual experiences. This impetus which strengthens, and is added to her libidinal desires for a penis arises in the following way. Her fear of the introjected 'bad' penis is an incentive to her continually introjecting a 'good' one in coitus.[3] Moreover, her sexual acts, whether in the form of *fellatio, coitus per anum* or normal coitus, help her to ascertain whether the fears which play such a dominant and fundamental role in her mind in connection with copulation are well grounded or not. The reason why copulation has become fraught with so much peril in the imagination of children of both sexes is that their sadistic wish-phantasies have transformed that act, as done between their father and mother, into a very threatening danger-situation.[4]

[1] Cf. Chapter VIII and my paper 'Early Stages of the Oedipus Conflict' (1928, *Writings*, 1).

[2] The girl's super-ego is consequently more potent than the boy's; and we shall later on discuss the effect this has upon her ego-development and object-relations.

[3] As we have already seen in an earlier part of this book, the child's fear of the 'bad' things inside itself, such as its internalized 'bad' objects, dangerous excrements and bodily substances, usually encourages it to try every kind of process of introjection and ejection and is thus a fundamental factor in its development.

[4] The child's wish that its parents should copulate in a sadistic way is in my

I have already gone into the nature of these sadistic masturbation phantasies in some detail, and have found that they fall into two distinct, though interconnected, categories. In those of the first category the child employs various sadistic means to make a direct onslaught upon its parents either combined in coitus or separately; in those of the second, which are derived from a somewhat later period of the phase when sadism is at its height, its belief in its sadistic omnipotence over its parents finds expression in a more indirect fashion. It endows them with instruments of mutual destruction, transforming their teeth, nails, genitals, excrements and so on, into dangerous weapons and animals, etc., and pictures them, according to its own desires, as tormenting and destroying each other in the act of copulation.

Both categories of sadistic phantasies give rise to anxiety from various sources. In connection with the first category the girl is afraid of being counter-attacked by one or both parents, but more particularly by her mother as the more hated one of the two. She expects to be assailed from within as well as from without, since she has introjected her objects at the same time as she has attacked them. Her fears on this score are very closely connected with sexual intercourse,[1] because her primary sadistic actions have to a very great extent been directed against her parents as she imagined them copulating together. But it is more especially in phantasies belonging to the second category that copulation, in which, according to her sadistic desires, her mother is utterly destroyed, becomes an act fraught with immense danger to herself. On the other hand, the sexual act, which her sadistic phantasies and wishes have transformed into a situation of such extreme danger, is for this very reason also the most powerful method of mastering anxiety—the more so because the libidinal gratification that accompanies it affords her the highest attainable pleasure and thus lessens her anxiety on its own score.

This view throws a new light, I think, on the motives which urge the individual to perform the sexual act and on the psychological sources which contribute to the libidinal satisfaction he obtains from that act. As we know, the libidinal satisfaction of all his

experience an important factor in the production and maintenance of its sexual theories, so that the latter not only owe their character to the influence which its pre-genital impulses have upon the formation of its phantasies but are the result of the destructive wishes it directs against its copulating parents. In analysing the child's sexual theories, therefore, I have found it important from a therapeutic point of view to pay attention to the fact that they spring from its sadistic desires and so give rise to a strong sense of guilt in its mind.

[1] These phantasies also give rise to danger-situations which are not in themselves attached to the sexual act.

erotogenic zones implies a satisfaction of his destructive components as well, owing to the fusion of his libidinal and destructive impulses that has taken place in those stages of his development which are dominated by his sadistic trends. Now, in my opinion, his destructive impulses have aroused anxiety in him as early as in the first months of his life. In consequence, his sadistic phantasies become bound up with anxiety, and this tie between the two gives rise to specific anxiety-situations. Since his genital impulses set in while he is still in the phase when sadism is at its height—or so I have found—and copulation represents, in his sadistic phantasies, a vehicle of destruction for his parents, these anxiety-situations which are aroused in the early stages of his development become connected with his genital activities as well. The effect of such a fusion is that, on the one hand, his anxiety intensifies his libidinal needs, and, on the other, the libidinal satisfaction of all erotogenic zones is used in the service of mastering anxiety. Libidinal satisfaction diminishes his aggressiveness and with it his anxiety. In addition, the pleasure he gets from such satisfaction seems in itself to allay his fear of being destroyed by his own destructive impulses and by his objects, and to militate against *aphanisis* (Jones), i.e. his fear of losing his capacity to achieve libidinal satisfaction. Libidinal satisfaction, as an expression of Eros, reinforces his belief in his helpful imagos and diminishes the dangers which threaten him from his death instinct and his super-ego.

The more anxiety the individual has and the more neurotic he is, the more the energies of his ego and his instinctual forces will be absorbed in the endeavour to overcome anxiety; and then too, the libidinal satisfaction will primarily be employed for the purpose of mastering anxiety. In the normal person, who is further removed from his early anxiety-situations and has modified them more successfully, the effect of those situations upon his sexual activities is, of course, far less; but as I see it, it is never entirely absent.[1] The normal person too, feels an impulsion to test his specific anxiety-situations in his relations to his partner in love, which strengthens and gives colour to his libidinal fixations; thus the sexual act always helps the normal person to master anxiety. The dominant anxiety-situations and the quantities of anxiety present are specific elements of the conditions for love which apply to everyone.

If the girl, who tests her anxiety-situations by means of the sexual act which corresponds to a test by reality, is supported by feelings of a confident and hopeful kind, she will be led to take as her object a person who represents the 'good' penis. In this case, the relief of anxiety which is achieved by the sexual act will give

[1] Cf. Chapter X.

her a strong enjoyment and considerably add to the purely libidinal satisfaction she experiences; and beyond this, it lays the foundations for lasting and satisfactory love relationships. But if the circumstances are unfavourable and her fear of the introjected 'bad' penis predominates, the necessary condition for her ability to love will be that she shall make this reality-test by means of a 'bad' penis— i.e. that her partner in love shall be a sadistic person. The test she makes in this case is meant to inform her of what kind of damage her partner will inflict on her through the sexual act. Even her anticipated injuries in this respect serve to allay her anxiety and are of importance in the economy of her mental life.[1] The impulsion to relieve the fear of internal and external dangers by means of proofs in the external world appears to me to be an essential factor in repetition compulsion.[2] The more neurotic the individual is, the more are these proofs bound up with the need for punishment. The stronger the anxiety of the earliest anxiety-situations and the weaker the hopeful currents of feeling, the less favourable are the conditions with which these counterproofs are bound up. In such cases only severe punishment, or rather unhappy experiences (which are taken as punishment), can replace the dreaded punishment which is anticipated in phantasy. Her choice of a sadistic partner is also based upon a drive to incorporate once more a sadistic 'bad' penis (for that is how she views the sexual act) which will destroy the dangerous objects within her. Thus the deepest root of feminine masochism would seem to be the woman's fear of the dangerous objects she has internalized; and her masochism would ultimately be none other than her sadistic instincts turned inwards against those internalized objects.[3]

According to Freud,[4] sadism, although it first becomes apparent in relation to an object, was originally a destructive instinct directed against the organism itself (primal sadism) and was only later diverted from the ego by the narcissistic libido; and erotogenic masochism is that portion of the destructive instinct which has not been able to be turned outward in this way and has remained

[1] The reason for this phenomenon lies in the fact that no suffering inflicted by outside sources can be as great as that inflicted in phantasy by continuous and overwhelming fear of internal injuries and dangers.

[2] See Chapter VII.

[3] In her paper, 'The Significance of Masochism in the Mental Life of Women' (1930), Helene Deutsch expresses views on the origins of masochism which differ widely from my own and which are based on the assumption, equally at variance with mine, that the Oedipus complex of the girl is introduced by her castration-wishes and castration-fears.

[4] Cf. *Beyond the Pleasure Principle* (1920), *S.E.* **18,** and 'The Economic Problem in Masochism' (1924), *S.E.* **19.**

within the organism and been libidinally bound there. He furthermore thinks that in so far as any part of the destructive instinct which has been directed outward is once more turned inwards and drawn away from its objects, it gives rise to secondary or feminine masochism. As far as I can see, however, when the destructive instinct has reverted in this way it still adheres to its objects; but now they are internalized ones, and in threatening to destroy them, it also threatens to destroy the ego in which they are situated. In this way in feminine masochism the destructive instinct is once more directed against the organism itself. Freud says[1] '. . . a sense of guilt, too, finds expression in the manifest content of masochistic phantasies; the subject assumes that he has committed some crime (the nature of which is left indefinite) which is to be expiated by these painful and tormenting procedures'. There seem to me to be certain points in common between the self-tormenting behaviour of the masochist and the self-reproaches of the melancholiac, which, as we know, are in fact directed towards his introjected object. It would seem, therefore, that feminine masochism is directed towards the ego as well as towards the introjected objects. Moreover, in destroying his internalized object the individual is acting in the interests of self-preservation; and in extreme cases his ego will no longer be able to turn his death-instinct outwards, for both life and death-instincts have united in a common aim and the former has been withdrawn from its proper function of protecting the ego.

We will now briefly consider one or two other typical forms which may be assumed by the sexual life of women in whom fear of the introjected penis is paramount.[2] Women, who, besides having strong masochistic inclinations, harbour more hopeful currents of feeling, often tend to entrust their affections to a sadistic partner and at the same time to make endeavours of every kind—endeavours which often take up all the energies of their ego—to turn him into a 'good' object. Women of this kind, in whom fear of the 'bad' penis and belief in the 'good' one are evenly balanced, often fluctuate between the choice of a 'good' external object and a 'bad' one.

Not infrequently the woman's fear of the internalized penis urges her to test her anxiety-situation again and again, with the result that she will be under a constant compulsion to perform the sexual

[1] 'The Economic Problems in Masochism' (1924), *S.E.* **19**, p. 162.
[2] Of course, these various forms overlap in many cases. In dealing with such a wealth and complexity of material I can do no more than give a schematic account of one or two such forms, my main object being to describe a few of the consequences that arise from this most fundamental anxiety in the female individual.

act with her object, or as a variant to this, to exchange that object for another. In differently constituted cases, again, the same fear will have an opposite outcome and the woman will become frigid.[1] As a child, her hatred of her mother made her change her father's penis from a desirable and bountiful object into a dangerous and evil one; whilst, in her imagination, she had transformed the vagina into an instrument of death, and the whole of her mother into a source of danger to her father having sexual intercourse with her. Her fear of the sexual act is thus based both on the injuries she will receive from the penis and on the injuries she will herself inflict on her partner. Her fear that she will castrate him is due partly to her identification with her sadistic mother and partly to her own sadistic trends.

As I have already shown, if the girl adopts a masochistic attitude, her sadistic trends are directed towards her internalized objects. But should her fear of the internalized penis impel her to defend herself against its threats from within by projection, she will direct her sadism towards the external object—towards the penis which is being introjected afresh in the act of coitus, and thus towards her sexual partner. In such cases, the ego has once more succeeded in turning the destructive instinct away from itself and now too from the internalized objects, and is again directing it towards an external object. If the girl's sadistic trends predominate, she will still regard copulation as a test by reality of her anxiety, but in an opposite way. Her phantasies that her vagina and body as a whole are destructive to her partner and that in *fellatio* she will bite off his penis and tear it to pieces are now the means of overcoming her fear of the penis she has incorporated and of her real object. In employing her sadism against her external object she is in phantasy also waging a war of extermination against her internalized objects.

The Omnipotence of Excreta

In the sadistic phantasies of both boy and girl the excreta play a large part. The omnipotence of the function of the bladder and

[1] Such an outcome depends greatly, it would seem, upon the extent to which the ego is able to overcome anxiety. As we learnt in the last chapter, it sometimes happens that the individual can master his anxiety (or rather, transform it into pleasure) only on condition that the reality-situations which he has to surmount are of a particularly difficult or dangerous nature. We sometimes find similar conditions laid down for his love-relations, in which case copulation itself represents the danger-situation. Hence frigidity in women would in part be due to a phobic avoidance of an anxiety-situation. As far as can be seen, there is a close relation between specific conditions of mastering anxiety and of obtaining sexual satisfaction.

the bowels[1] is closely connected with paranoid mechanisms.[2] These mechanisms are most effective in that phase in which, in its sadistic masturbation phantasies, the child destroys its copulating parents in secret ways by means of its urine, faeces and flatus;[3] these primary means and ways of attack become secondarily reinforced on account of its fear of being counter-attacked and are employed for defensive purposes.[4]

As far as I can judge, the girl's sexual life and ego are more strongly and enduringly influenced in their development than are those of the boy by this sense of omnipotence of the function of the bladder and bowels. The attacks they make with their excreta are levelled at their mother, in the first instance at her breast and then at the inside of her body. Since the girl's destructive impulses against her mother's body are more powerful and enduring than the boy's, she will evolve stronger clandestine and cunning methods of attack, based upon the magic of excrements and other excretions[5] and upon the omnipotence of her thoughts, in conformity with the hidden and mysterious nature of that world within her mother's body and her own; whereas the boy will concentrate his feelings of hatred on his father's penis, which he assumes to be inside his mother,

[1] Cf. Freud, *Totem and Taboo* (1913), *S.E.* **13**, p. 85; also, Ferenczi, 'Stages in the Development of a Sense of Reality' (1913), and Abraham, 'The Narcissistic Evaluation of Excretory Processes in Dreams and Neurosis' (1917).

[2] For the connection between paranoia and anal functions, cf. Freud, Ferenczi, Von Ophuijsen, Stärcke and others.

[3] Cf. Chapter X.

[4] Sadistic omnipotence of this kind, used primarily to destroy the parents or one of them by means of the excreta, becomes modified in the course of the child's development and is often employed to inflict moral pain on the object or to control and dominate it intellectually. Owing to this modification and because the child now makes its attacks in a secret and insidious fashion and has to display an equal watchfulness and mental ingenuity in guarding against counter-attacks of a corresponding character, its original sense of omnipotence becomes of fundamental importance for the growth of its ego in both sexes. In his paper referred to above, Abraham takes the view that the omnipotence of the functions of the bladder and bowels is a precursor of the omnipotence of thoughts; and in his paper, 'The Madonna's Conception through the Ear' (1923), Ernest Jones has shown that thoughts are equated to flatus. I too think that the child equates its faeces, and more especially its invisible flatus, with that other secret and invisible substance, its thoughts, and furthermore that it imagines that in its covert attacks on its mother's body it has put them inside her by magic means. (Cf. Chapter VIII of this book.)

[5] The fact that the woman attaches her narcissism to her body as a whole must be in part due to her connecting her sense of omnipotence with her various bodily functions and excretory processes, and thus distributing it to a greater extent over the whole of her body, whereas the man focusses it more upon his genitals. After all, in the last analysis it is through her body that she captures and controls her real objects by magic means.

and on his real one, and thus directs them to a larger extent towards the external world and what is tangible and visible. He also makes greater use of the sadistic omnipotence of his penis, with the result that he has other modes of mastering anxiety as well,[1] while the woman's mode of mastering anxiety remains under the dominion of her relation to an inner world, to what is concealed, and therefore to the unconscious.[2]

As has already been said, when the [girl's] sadism is at its greatest height she believes that the sexual act is a means of annihilating the object and at the same time she is also carrying on a war of extermination against the internalized objects. By means of the omnipotence of her excrements and thoughts she endeavours to overcome the terrifying objects inside her own body and originally inside her mother's. If her belief in her father's 'good' penis inside her is strong enough she will make it the vehicle of her sense of omnipotence.[3] If her belief in the magical power of her excreta and thoughts preponderates, it will be through their power that she will govern and control both her internalized and her real objects in phantasy. Not only do these different sources of magical power operate at the same time and reinforce one another, but her ego makes use of them and plays them off against one another for the purpose of mastering anxiety.

Early Relation to the Mother

The [girl's] attitude to the introjected penis is strongly influenced by her attitude to her mother's breast. To summarize the primary elements: the first objects that she introjects are her 'good' mother and her 'bad' one,[4] as represented by the breast. Her desire to suck

[1] In this chapter and in the next we shall consider how the anatomical differences between the sexes contribute to separate out the lines along which the sense of omnipotence and consequently the modes of mastering anxiety develop in each sex.

[2] In my 'Contribution to the Theory of Intellectual Inhibition' (1931, Writings, 1), I have shown that in his unconscious the individual regards his penis as the representative of his ego and his conscious, and the interior of his body—what is invisible—as the representative of his super-ego and his unconscious.

[3] In her paper, 'The Role of Psychotic Mechanisms in Cultural Development' (1930), Melitta Schmideberg has shown that the introjection of his father's penis (= his father) greatly enhances the individual's narcissism and sense of omnipotence.

[4] In Chapter VIII we saw how the 'good' breast becomes turned into a 'bad' one in consequence of the child's imaginary attacks upon it, for the child directs all the resources of its sadism in the first instance against the breast for not giving it enough satisfaction so that a primary introjection of both a good and a bad mother-imago takes place before any other imagos are formed.

or devour the penis is directly derived from her desire to do the same to her mother's breast so that the frustration she suffers from the breast prepares the way for the feelings which her renewed frustration in regard to the penis arouses. Not only do the envy and hatred she feels towards her mother colour and intensify her sadistic phantasies against the penis, but her relations to the mother's breast affect her subsequent attitude towards men in other ways as well. As soon as she begins to be afraid of the 'bad' introjected penis she also begins to run back to her mother who, both as a real person and as an introjected figure, should give help to her. If her primary attitude to her mother has been dominated by the oral-sucking position, so that it contains strong positive and hopeful elements, she will be able to take shelter to some extent behind her 'good' mother-imago against her 'bad' mother-imago and against the 'bad' penis; if not, her fear of her introjected mother will increase her fear of the internalized penis and of her terrifying parents united in copulation, too.

The importance which the girl's mother-imago has for her as a 'helping' figure and the strength of her attachment to her mother are very great, since in her phantasy her mother is the possessor of the nourishing breast and the father's penis and children and thus has the power to satisfy all her needs. For when the small girl's early anxiety-situations set in, her ego makes use of her need for nourishment in the widest sense to assist her in overcoming anxiety. The more she is afraid that her body is poisoned and exposed to attack, the more she craves for the 'good' milk, 'good' penis and children[1] over which, as her phantasy tells her, her mother has unlimited command. She needs these 'good' things to protect her against the 'bad' ones, and to establish a certain equilibrium inside her. In her phantasy her mother's body is therefore a kind of store-house which contains the means of satisfying all her desires and of allaying all her fears. It is these phantasies, leading back to her mother's breast as her earliest source of satisfaction and as the one most fraught with consequences, which are responsible for her immensely strong attachment to her mother. And the frustration she suffers from her mother gives rise, under the pressure of her anxiety, to renewed complaints against her and to strengthened sadistic attacks upon her body.

At a somewhat later stage of her development, however, at a time when her sense of guilt is making itself felt in every quarter,[2] this

[1] We shall presently enquire in greater detail into the deeper significance attached to the possession of children. It suffices here to remark that the imaginary child inside the body represents a helpful object.

[2] It must be remembered that in her imagination, besides having attacked

very desire to get possession of the 'good' contents of her mother's body, or rather her feeling that she has done so and thus exposed her mother, as it were, to its 'bad' contents, arouses a most severe sense of guilt and anxiety in her. The act of having demolished the child [inside her mother] is equated in her phantasy with the complete demolition of that reservoir from which she draws the satisfaction of all her mental and physical needs. This fear, which is of such tremendous importance in the mental life of the small girl, goes to strengthen still further the ties that bind her to her mother. It gives rise to an impulsion to make restitution and give her mother back all that she has taken from her—an impulsion which finds expression in numerous sublimations of a specifically feminine kind.

But this impulsion runs counter to another impulsion, itself strengthened by the same fear, to take away everything her mother has got in order to save her own body. At this stage of her development, therefore, the girl is governed by a compulsion both to take away and to give back, and this compulsion, as has elsewhere been said,[1] is essential for the origin of obsessional neurosis. For instance, we see small girls drawing little stars or crosses, which signify faeces and children, or older ones writing letters and numbers on a sheet of paper that stands for their mother's body or their own, and taking great care to leave no empty spaces. Or else they will pile up pieces of paper neatly in a box until it is quite full. Very frequently they will draw a house to represent their mother, and then put a tree in front of it for their father's penis and some flowers beside it for children. Older girls will draw or sew or make dolls and dolls' dresses or books, etc.; and these things typify their mother's re-constituted body (either as a whole or each damaged part individually), their father's penis and the children inside her, or their father and brothers and sisters in person.

While they are engaged in these activities or after they have completed them, children will often show rage, depression or disappointment, or even reactions of a destructive kind, which are determined by the fear of not being able to make restitution. Anxiety of this kind, which is an underlying obstacle to all constructive trends, arises from various sources.[2] The girl has in phantasy taken

---

her parents, the girl has injured or killed her brothers and sisters inside her mother. Her fear of retaliation and her sense of guilt on account of this give rise to disturbances in her relation to her real brothers and sisters and consequently in her capacity for social adaptation in general.

[1] Cf. Chapter IX.

[2] If anxiety is so strong that it cannot be bound by obsessional mechanisms, the violent mechanisms belonging to earlier stages will be brought into play, together with the more primitive defensive mechanisms employed by the ego.

possession of her father's penis and faeces and children, and then, owing to the fear of penis, children and excrements that sets in with her sadistic phantasies, she loses faith in their good qualities. The questions in her mind now are: will the things she gives back to her mother be 'good', and can she give them back correctly as regards quality and quantity and even as regards the order in which they should be arranged inside (for that, too, is a part of the pre-condition of restitution)? Again, if she does believe that she has well and truly given her mother back the 'good' contents of her body she becomes afraid of having endangered her own person by doing so.

These sources of anxiety give rise, furthermore, to a special distrust in the girl towards her mother. From time to time girls will wrap up their drawings or paper patterns, or whatever is symbolizing the penis or children for them at the time, tie them up and carefully deposit them in their drawer of toys, with every sign of the deepest suspicion towards me. On these occasions I am not allowed to come near the parcel or even the drawer and must move away or not look on while it is being done up. On entering my room many of my girl patients will look suspiciously at the stock of paper and pencils in the drawer reserved for them, in case they should not belong to them or be smaller in size or fewer in number than on the day before; or they will want to make sure that the contents of their drawer have not been disarranged, and that all is in good order and no article is missing or exchanged for something else.[1] Analysis shows that the drawer and the parcels inside represent their own body and that they are afraid not only that their mother will attack and despoil it but will put 'bad' things inside it in exchange for the 'good' ones.

In addition to these many sources of anxiety a further element is added which aggravates the feminine position and the relationship of the girl to her mother—the anatomy of her body. Compared to the boy who enjoys the support of the male position and who has the possibility of reality-testing thanks to his possession of a penis, the girl child cannot get any support against anxiety from her feminine position[2] since her possession of children which would be a complete confirmation and fulfilment of that position, is, after all, only a prospective one.[3] Nor does the structure of her body afford

---

[1] I may mention that each child has a drawer of its own in which the toys, paper and pencils, etc., which I put out for it at the beginning of its hour and renew from time to time, are put away, together with the things it brings from home.

[2] Cf. my 'Early Stages of the Oedipus Conflict' (1928, *Writings*, 1).

[3] In her paper, 'The Significance of Masochism in the Mental Life of Women' (1930), Helene Deutsch points out this fact as an obstacle to the maintenance of the feminine position.

her any possibility of knowing what the actual state of affairs inside her is. It is this inability to know anything about her condition which aggravates what, in my opinion, is the girl's deepest fear—namely that the inside of her body has been injured or destroyed[1] and that she has no children or only damaged ones.

The Role of the Vagina in Infantile Sexual Development

The fact that the female child's anxiety concerns the inside of her body explains to a large extent, I think, why in her early sexual organization the part played by the vagina should be overshadowed by the activity of the clitoris. Even in her very earliest masturbation phantasies, in which she transforms her mother's vagina into an instrument of destruction, she shows an unconscious knowledge about the vagina. For although, owing to the predominance of her oral and anal tendencies, she likens it to the mouth and to the anus, she nevertheless thinks of it in her unconscious, as many details of her phantasies clearly demonstrate, as a cavity in the genitals which is meant to receive her father's penis.

But beyond this general unconscious realization of the existence of the vagina the small girl also often possesses a quite conscious knowledge of it. Analysis of a number of small girls has convinced me that, in addition to those quite special cases mentioned by Helene Deutsch[2] in which the patient has undergone sexual assault and defloration and has in consequence obtained a knowledge of this sort and been led to indulge in vaginal masturbation, many small girls are consciously aware that they have an opening in their genitals. In some instances they have got this knowledge from mutual investigations made during sexual games with other children, whether boys or girls; in others, they have discovered the vagina for themselves. However, they undoubtedly have a specially strong inclination to deny or repress such knowledge—an inclination which springs from the anxiety they feel in regard to this organ and to the inside of their body. Analyses of women have shown that the fact that the vagina is a part of the interior of their body, to which so much of their deepest anxiety is attached, and that it is the organ which they regard as pre-eminently dangerous and endangered in their sadistic phantasies about copulation between their parents, is of fundamental importance in giving rise to sexual disturbances and frigidity in them and, in particular, in inhibiting vaginal excitability.

[1] This is partly the reason why female narcissism extends over the whole body. Male narcissism is focussed upon the penis because the boy's chief fear is of being castrated.
[2] *Loc. cit.*

There is a good deal of evidence to show that the vagina does not enter upon its full functions until the sexual act has been performed.[1] And, as we know, it often happens that the woman's attitude to copulation is completely altered after she has experienced it and that her inhibition in regard to it—and, before the event, such an inhibition is so usual as to be practically normal—is often replaced by a strong desire for it. We may infer from this that her previous inhibition was in part maintained by anxiety and that the sexual act has removed that anxiety.[2] I should be inclined to attribute this reassuring effect of sexual intercourse to the fact that the libidinal satisfaction which she receives from copulation confirms her in the belief that the penis she has incorporated during the act is a 'good' object and that her vagina does not have a destructive effect upon it. Her fear of the internalized and external penis—a fear which has been all the greater from being unverifiable—is thus removed by the real object. In my view, the girl's fears concerning the inside of her body contribute, in addition to the operation of biological factors, to prevent the emergence of a clearly discernible vaginal phase in her early childhood. Nevertheless, I am convinced, on the strength of a number of analyses of small girls, that the mental representation of the vagina exerts its full share of influence, no less than the mental representation of all the other libidinal phases, upon the infantile genital organization of the female child.

The same factors which tend to conceal the mental function of the vagina in the girl go to intensify her fixation on the clitoris. For the latter is a visible organ and one which can be submitted to reality tests. I have found that clitoral masturbation is accompanied by phantasies of various descriptions. Their content changes extremely rapidly, in accordance with the violent fluctuations which take place between one position and other in the early stages of the girl's development. They are at first for the most part of a pregenital kind; but as soon as the child's desires to incorporate her father's penis in an oral and genital manner grow stronger they assume a genital and vaginal character (being often already accompanied, it would seem, by vaginal sensations) and thus, to begin with, take a feminine direction.[3]

---

[1] Helene Deutsch supports this view in her book, *Psychoanalyse der weiblichen Sexualfunktionen* (1925).

[2] We have already considered the structure of those cases in which the sexual act fails to reduce anxiety and even increases it.

[3] In his paper, 'One of the Motive Factors in the Formation of the Super-Ego in Women' (1928), Hanns Sachs has suggested the possibility that, since a vaginal phase cannot establish itself at that age, the girl displaces her obscure sensations in the vagina on to the mouth.

Since the little girl begins to identify herself with her father very soon after she has identified herself with her mother, her clitoris rapidly takes on the significance of a penis in her masturbation phantasies. All her clitoral masturbation phantasies belonging to this early stage are dominated by her sadistic trends, and that appears to me decisive for the fact that they, and her masturbatory activities in general, diminish or cease altogether when her phallic phase comes to an end, at a period when her sense of guilt emerges more strongly. Her realization that her clitoris is no substitute for the penis she desires is, in my opinion, only the last link in a chain of events which determines her future life and in many cases condemns her to frigidity for the rest of her days.

The Castration Complex

The identification with her father which the girl displays so clearly in the phallic phase, and which bears every sign of penis-envy and castration complex,[1] is, as far as my own observations go, the outcome of a process comprising many stages.[2] In examining some of the more important of these steps we shall see in what way her identification with her father is affected by anxiety arising from her feminine position and how the masculine position she adopts in each of her phases of development is superimposed upon a masculine position belonging to an earlier phase.

When the female infant gives up her mother's breast and turns to her father's penis as an object of satisfaction she identifies herself with her mother. But as soon as she suffers frustration in this position too, she very speedily identifies herself with her father, who, in her phantasy, obtains satisfaction from her mother's breast and entire body, that is, from those primary sources of satisfaction which she herself has been so painfully forced to relinquish. Feelings of hatred and envy towards her mother as well as libidinal desires

---

[1] Cf. Abraham, 'Manifestations of the Female Castration Complex' (1921).

[2] Karen Horney was the first psycho-analyst to bring the castration complex of the woman into relation with her early feminine position as a small girl. In her paper, 'On the Genesis of the Castration Complex in Women' (1923), the writer has pointed out certain factors which she believes are material in establishing in the girl an envy of the penis based on pre-genital cathexes. One of these is the satisfaction of scoptophilic and exhibitionistic tendencies which she notices that the boy obtains from urinating; another is her belief that possession of a penis affords a greater amount of satisfaction of urethral erotism; while others are derived from the difficulties that beset her in regard to her feminine position—such as envy of her mother for having children—and increase her tendency to identify herself with her father as well as intensifying her penis-envy. Dr Horney believes, moreover, that the same factors which induce the girl to take up a homosexual attitude lead, though in a minor degree, to the production of a castration complex in her.

for her, go to create this earliest identification of the girl with her sadistic father, and in this identification enuresis plays an important role.

Children of both sexes regard urine in its positive aspect as equivalent to their mother's milk, as they unconsciously equate all bodily substances with one another. My observations go to show that wetting, in its earliest meaning in the sense of a positive giving act and of a sadistic inversion, is an expression of a feminine position in boys as well as in girls.[1] It would seem that the hatred children feel towards their mother's breast for having frustrated their desires arouses in them, either simultaneously with their cannibalistic impulses or closely following them, phantasies of injuring and destroying her breast with their urine.[2]

As has already been said, in the sadistic phase the girl puts her greatest belief in the magical powers of her excreta, while the boy makes his penis the principal executant of his sadism. But in her, too, belief in the omnipotence of her urinary functions leads her to identify herself—though to a lesser extent than does the boy—with her sadistic father, to whom she attributes special urethral-sadistic powers in virtue of his possession of a penis.[3] Thus wetting very soon comes to represent a masculine position for children of both sexes; and in connection with the girl's earliest identification with

[1] According to Helene Deutsch enuresis is the expression of a feminine position in the boy and a masculine one in the girl. *Psychoanalysis of the Neuroses*, 1930, (p. 51).

[2] In doing this they make use of a mechanism which is, I think, of general importance in the formation of sadistic phantasies. They convert the pleasure they give their object into its opposite by adding destructive elements to it. As a revenge for not getting enough milk from their mother they will produce in imagination an excessive quantity of urine and so destroy her breast by flooding it or melting it away; and as a revenge for not getting 'good' milk from her they will produce a harmful fluid with which to burn up or poison her breast and the milk it contains. This mechanism also gives rise to phantasies of tormenting and injuring people by giving them too much good food. In this case the subject may suffer, as I have found in more than one instance, from the retaliatory anxiety of being suffocated or of being too full, etc., in connection with taking food. One patient of mine could hardly control his rage if he was offered, even in the friendliest way, food, drink or cigarettes a second time. He would immediately feel 'stuffed up' and would lose all desire to eat, drink or smoke any more. Analysis showed that his behaviour was ultimately caused by phantasies of the early sadistic character described above.

[3] In her paper, 'On the Genesis of the Castration Complex in Women' (1923), Karen Horney states that one of the factors which encourage the girl's primary penis-envy in connection with her urethral-erotic impulses is that her sadistic phantasies of omnipotence which are based on urinary functions are especially closely associated with the stream of urine which the boy is able to produce.

her sadistic father it becomes a means of destroying her mother; while at the same time she appropriates her father's penis in her imagination by castrating him.

The girl's identification with her father on the basis of his introjected penis[1] follows closely, in my experience, upon the primary sadistic identification she has made with him by means of wetting. In her earliest masturbation phantasies she has identified herself alternately with each of her parents. The feminine position which is associated with the internalization of her father's penis makes her afraid of her father's 'bad' penis which she has internalized. But this anxiety leads to a strengthening of the identification with her father, for in order to counter this fear she activates the defensive mechanisms of identification with the anxiety-object.[2] Her possession of the penis she has stolen from him arouses a sense of omnipotence which increases her faith in her destructive magic through her excreta. In this position her hatred and sadism against her mother becomes intensified and she has phantasies of destroying her with the help of her father's penis; while at the same time she satisfies her feelings of revenge against the father who has frustrated her and finds in her sense of omnipotence and in her power over both parents a defence against anxiety. I have found this attitude especially strongly developed in some patients in whom paranoid traits predominated;[3] but it is also very powerful in women whose homosexuality is deeply coloured by feelings of a hostile rivalry with the male sex. It would thus apply to that group of female homosexuals, described by Ernest Jones, to which I referred earlier.

[1] In considering the origins of homosexuality in women, Ernest Jones in his paper, 'The Early Development of Female Sexuality' (1927), has come to certain very fundamental conclusions which my own findings fully endorse. Briefly, they are to the effect that the presence of very strong phantasies of *fellatio* in the female, allied to a powerful oral sadism, prepares the way for a belief that she has taken forcible possession of her father's penis and puts her into a special relation of identification with him. In her homosexual attitude, derived in this way, she will show a lack of interest in her own sex and a strong interest in men. Her endeavour will be to win recognition and respect from men, and she will have strong feelings of rivalry, hatred and resentment against them. As regards character-formation, she will exhibit in general marked oral-sadistic traits; and her identification with her father will be employed to a great degree in the service of her castration wishes.

[2] Cf. Chapter VII.

[3] The reader may be referred in general to the case-history of Erna in Chapter III; but one characteristic point may be cited from it here. At the age of six Erna suffered from severe insomnia. She had a terror of burglars and thieves which she could only overcome by lying on her stomach and banging her head on the pillows. This meant having sadistic coitus with her mother, in which she played the part of her supposedly sadistic father.

The possession of an external penis would help to convince the girl in the first place that in reality she has that sadistic power over both her parents without which she cannot master her anxiety,[1] and in the second place that the penis, as a means of sadistic power over her objects, is evidence that the internalized dangerous penis and the introjected objects can be overcome; so that having a penis ultimately serves to protect her own body.

While her sadistic position, reinforced as it is by her anxiety, thus forms the basis of a masculinity complex in her, her sense of guilt also makes her want to have a penis. The real penis she desires will now be used to make restitution towards her mother. As Joan Riviere has observed,[2] the girl's wish to compensate her mother for having deprived her of her father's penis furnishes important additions to her castration complex and penis-envy. When the girl is obliged to give up her rivalry with her mother out of fear of her, her desire to placate her and make up for what she has done leads her to long intensely for a penis as a means of making restitution. In Joan Riviere's opinion the intensity of her sadism and the extent of her capacity to tolerate anxiety are factors which will help to determine whether she will take up a heterosexual line or a homosexual one.

We must now examine more closely why it is that in some cases the masculine position and the possession of a penis are an indispensible condition without which the girl cannot make restitution to her mother. Early analysis has demonstrated the existence in the unconscious of a fundamental principle governing all reactive and sublimatory processes, which demands that restitutive acts must adhere in every detail to the damage that has been done in phantasy. Whatever wrongs the child has done in phantasy in the way of stealing, injuring and destroying it must make good by giving back, putting to rights and restoring, one by one. This principle also requires that the same sadistic instruments (i.e. penis, excrements, etc.) that have been used to damage and destroy shall be once more turned into 'good' things and be used as a means of making well. Whatever harm the 'bad' penis or 'bad' urine have done, the 'good' penis[3] or 'good' urine must put right again.

[1] In her paper, 'Womanliness as a Masquerade' (1929), Joan Riviere has pointed out that in her anger and hatred against her parents for giving one another sexual satisfaction the girl has phantasies of castrating her father and taking possession of his penis and thus getting her father and mother into her power and killing them.

[2] *Loc. cit.*

[3] In her 'Psychotic Mechanisms in Cultural Development' (1930) Melitta Schmideberg traces the part played in the history of medicine by a belief in the magical qualities of the 'good' penis, as symbolized by medicine, and of the

Let us consider the case of a girl who has centred her sadistic phantasies more especially around the indirect destruction of her mother by her father's dangerous penis and who has identified herself very strongly with her sadistic father. As soon as her reactive trends and her desires to make restitution set in in force, she will feel urged to restore her mother by means of a penis with healing powers and thus her homosexual trends will become reinforced. An important factor in this connection is the extent to which she feels that her father has been incapacitated from making restitution, either because she believes that she has castrated him or has put him out of the way or has transformed his penis into a 'bad' one, and that she must therefore give up hope of restoring him.[1] If she believes this very strongly she will have to play his part herself, and this again will tend to make her adopt a homosexual position.

The disappointment and doubts and the sense of inferiority which overtake the girl when she realizes that she has no penis, and the fears and feelings of guilt which her masculine position give rise to (in the first place towards her father because she has deprived him of his penis and of the possession of her mother, and in the second place towards her mother because she has taken her father away from her), combine to break down that position. Moreover, her original grievance against her mother for having prevented her from getting her father's penis as a libidinal object joins forces with her new grievance against her for having withheld from her the possession of a penis of her own as an attribute of masculinity; and this double grievance leads her to turn away from her mother as an object of genital love. On the other hand, her feelings of hatred against her father and her envy of his penis, which arise from her masculine position, stand in the way of her once more adopting a feminine role.

According to my experience, the girl, after having left the phallic phase, passes through yet another phase, a post-phallic one, in which she makes her choice between retaining the feminine position

---

'bad' one, as symbolized by the demon of illness. She attributes the psychological effects of physical remedies to the following causes. The person's original attitude of aggression against his father's penis—an attitude which has turned that organ into an extremely dangerous one—is succeeded by an attitude of obedience and submission towards him. If he takes the medicines he is given in this latter spirit, they, as representing the 'good' penis, will counteract the 'bad' objects inside him.

[1] If her homosexuality emerges in sublimated ways only, she will, for instance, protect and take care of other women (i.e. her mother), adopting in these respects a husband's attitude towards them, and will have little interest in the male sex. Ernest Jones has shown that this attitude develops in female homosexuals in whom the oral-sucking fixation is very strong.

or abandoning it. I would say that by the time she has entered upon the latency period, her feminine position which has attained the genital level and is passive[1] and maternal in character and which involves the functioning of her vagina with reference to its psychical representative, has been established in all its fundamentals. That this is so becomes evident when we consider how frequently small girls take up a genuinely feminine and maternal position. A position of this kind would be unthinkable unless the vagina was behaving as a receptive organ. As has already been pointed out, important alterations take place in the function of the vagina as a result of the biological changes the girl undergoes at puberty[2] and of her experience of the sexual act; and it is these alterations which bring the girl's psycho-sexual development to its final stage and which make her a woman in the full sense of the word.

I find myself in agreement on many points with Karen Horney's paper, 'The Flight from Womanhood',[3] in which she comes to the conclusion that the vagina as well as the clitoris plays a part in the early life of the female child. [She points out that] it would be reasonable to infer from the later aspects of frigidity in women that the vaginal zone is more likely to be strongly cathected with anxiety and defensive affects than the clitoris. She believes that the girl's 'incestuous wishes are unerringly aimed by her unconscious at the vagina'. According to this approach, frigidity [in later life] ought to be considered as a manifestation of defence against those phantasies which so greatly threaten the ego.

I also share Karen Horney's opinion that the girl's inability to obtain any certain knowledge about her vagina or, unlike the boy who can inspect his genitals, to submit it to a reality test in order to find out whether it has been overtaken by the dreaded consequences of masturbation tends to increase her genital anxiety and makes her more likely to adopt a masculine position. Karen Horney furthermore distinguishes between the girl's secondary penis-envy, which emerges in the phallic phase, and her primary penis-envy, which rests upon certain pre-genital cathexes such as scoptophilia and urethral erotism. She believes that the girl's secondary penis-envy is used to repress her feminine desires; with the dissolution of her Oedipus complex she invariably—though to varying degrees—

---

[1] Helene Deutsch also believes that the true passive feminine attitude of the vagina is to be found in its oral and sucking activity (*Psychoanalyse der weiblichen Sexualfunktionen*, 1925).

[2] In the small boy, too, the psychical representation of the functions of the penis which set in only in the period of reproduction is the precondition of the masculine position.

[3] *Loc. cit.*

not only relinquishes her father as a sexual object but at the same time also moves away from the feminine role, regressing to her primary penis-envy.

The views I put forward in my paper 'The Early Stages of the Oedipus Conflict'[1] concerning the final stage of the girl's genital organization agree in many essentials with those which Ernest Jones came to at about the same time. In his paper, 'The Early Development of Female Sexuality',[2] he suggests that the vaginal functions were originally identified with the anal, and that the differentiation of the two—a still obscure process—takes place in part at an earlier stage than is generally supposed. He assumes the existence of a mouth-anus stage which forms the basis of the girl's heterosexual attitude founded on an identification with her mother. According to his view, the normal girl's phallic phase is only a weakened form of the identification made by homosexual females with the father and his penis, and is, like it, pre-eminently of a secondary and defensive character.

Helene Deutsch is of a different opinion.[3] She assumes, it is true, the existence of a post-phallic phase during which the final outcome of the girl's later genital organization is prepared. But she believes that the girl does not have any such thing as a vaginal phase at all, and that it is the exception for her to know anything about the existence of her vagina or to have any sensations there, and that therefore when she has finished her infantile sexual development she cannot take up a feminine position in the genital sense. In consequence, her libido, even in so far as a feminine position is being maintained, is obliged to retrogress to earlier positions dominated by her castration complex (which in Helene Deutsch's view precedes her Oedipus complex); and a backward step of this kind would be a fundamental factor in the production of feminine masochism.

Restitutive Trends and Sexuality

I have already examined the part played by the girl's restitutive tendencies in consolidating her homosexual position. But, the consolidation of her heterosexual position, too, depends upon that position being in conformity with the demands of her super-ego.

As we saw in an earlier part of this chapter, even where the normal individual is concerned, the sexual act, in addition to its libidinal motivation, helps him to master anxiety. I shall now add that his genital activities have yet another motive force, which is

[1] (1927) *Writings*, 1.
[2] (1927) In *Papers on Psychoanalysis* 4th and 5th edns.
[3] Helene Deutsch, 'The Significance of Masochism in the Mental Life of Women' (1930).

his desire to make good by means of copulation the damage he has done in his sadistic phantasies.[1] When, as a result of the stronger emergence of genital impulses, his ego reacts to his super-ego with less anxiety and more guilt, he finds in the sexual act a pre-eminent means of making reparation to the object, because of its connection with his early sadistic phantasies. The nature and extent of his restitutive phantasies, which are equivalent to the imaginary damage, will not only be an important factor in his various activities and in the formation of his sublimations but will very greatly influence the course and outcome of his sexual development.[2]

Turning to the girl, we find that such considerations as the contents and composition of her sadistic phantasies, the magnitude of her reactive trends and the structure and strength of her ego will affect her libidinal fixations and help to decide whether the restitution she makes shall have a masculine or a feminine character or be a mixture of the two.[3]

Another thing which seems to me to be of importance for the final outcome of the girl's development is whether the restitutive phantasies which she builds up upon her specific sadistic ideas can decisively influence the development of her ego as well as her sexual life. Ordinarily they are interwoven and thus help to establish a certain libido-position and a corresponding ego-position. If, for instance, the small girl's sadism has been strongly centred in phantasies of damaging her mother's body and stealing children and her father's penis from it, she may be able, when her reactive trends set in in force, to maintain her feminine position under certain conditions. In her sublimations she will give effect to her desire to restore her mother and give her back her father and children, say, by becoming a nanny, a hospital nurse or a masseuse, or by pursuing intellectual interests;[4] and if at the same time she

[1] In her paper, 'Some Unconscious Mechanisms in Pathological Sexuality and their Relation to Normal Sexual Activity' (1933), Melitta Schmideberg has also come to the conclusion that restitutive tendencies are of great importance as an incentive to heterosexual and homosexual activities. The paper must be consulted for details.

[2] If his sense of guilt is excessive, the fusion of his sexual activities and his reactive tendencies may give rise to severe disturbances of his sexual life. We shall reserve for the next chapter a discussion of the effect which the desire to make restitution has upon the sexual development and potency of the male individual.

[3] Even where her sadism remains dominant, the means she employs to master her anxiety will influence her sexual life and may either lead her to maintain a homosexual attitude or adopt a heterosexual one, both positions being based upon her sadistic tendencies.

[4] In my 'Infantile Anxiety-Situations Reflected in a Work of Art and in the Creative Impulse' (1929), I have analysed an account by Karen Michaelis

has sufficient belief in the possibility of her own body being restored by having children or performing the sexual act with a penis having 'healing' powers, she will also employ her heterosexual position as an aid to mastering anxiety. Moreover, her heterosexual position strengthens her sublimatory trends which aim at the restoration of her mother's body, for it shows her that copulation between her parents has not injured her mother, or at any rate that it can restore her; and this belief, in turn, helps to consolidate her in her heterosexual position.

What the girl's final position is going to be will also depend, given the same underlying conditions, upon whether her belief in her own constructive omnipotence comes up to the strength of her reactive trends. If it does, her ego can set up a further aim to be fulfilled by her restitutive trends. This is that both her parents should be restored and should once more be united in amity. It is now her father who, in her phantasies, makes restitution to her mother and gratifies her by means of his health-giving penis; whilst her mother's vagina, originally a dangerous thing in phantasy, restores and heals her father's penis which it has injured. In thus looking upon her mother's vagina as a health- and pleasure-giving organ, the girl is not only able to call up once more her earliest view of her mother as the 'good' mother who gave her suck, but can think of herself, in identification with her, as a healing and giving person and can regard the penis of her partner in love as a 'good' penis. Upon an attitude of this kind will rest the successful development of her sexual life and her ability to become attached to her object by ties of sex no less than of affection and love.

As I have tried to show in these pages, the final outcome of the infantile sexual development of the individual is the result of a long-drawn-out process of fluctuation between various positions and is built up upon a great number of interconnected compromises between his ego and his super-ego and between his ego and his id. These compromises, being the result of his endeavour to master anxiety, are themselves to a great extent an achievement of his ego. Those which, in the girl, go to maintain her feminine role and which find typical expression in her later sexual life and general behaviour

---

of a young woman who suddenly developed a great talent for painting portraits of women without ever having handled a brush before. I have tried to show that what caused this sudden burst of artistic productivity was anxiety emanating from her most profound danger-situations, and that painting female portraits symbolized a sublimated restoration both of her mother's body, which she had attacked in phantasy, and of her own, destruction of which she anticipated out of dread of retaliation; so that in this way she was able to allay fears arising from the deepest levels of her mind.

are, to mention only a few, that her father's penis shall gratify herself and her mother alternately;[1] that a certain number of the children shall be allocated to her mother, and the same number, or rather fewer, to herself; that she shall incorporate her father's penis, while her mother shall receive all the children—and so on. Masculine components enter into such compromises as well. The small girl will sometimes imagine that she appropriates her father's penis in order to carry out a masculine role towards her mother, and then gives it back to him again.

In the course of an analysis it becomes apparent that every change for the better which takes place in the individual's libido position springs from a diminution of his anxiety and sense of guilt and at once takes effect in the production of fresh compromises. The more the anxiety and guilt which the girl feels is decreased and the more her genital stage comes to the fore, the more easily is she able to acknowledge her mother's feminine and maternal role, or rather to return it to her, and at the same time to take a similar role herself and sublimate her male components.

External Factors

We know that the child's early instinctual life on the one hand and the pressure of reality upon it on the other interact upon each other and that their combined action shapes the course of its mental development. In my judgment, reality and real objects affect its anxiety-situations from the very earliest stages of its existence, in the sense that it regards them as so many proofs or refutations of its anxiety-situation which it has displaced into the outer world, and they thus help to guide the course of its instinctual life. The behaviour of its objects and the nature of its experiences contribute in this way to the strengthening and also to the weakening of the child's dominant anxiety-situations. And since, owing to the inter-action of the mechanisms of projection and introjection, the external factors influence the formation of its super-ego and the development of its object-relationship and instincts, they will also assist in determining what the outcome of its sexual development will be.

If, for instance, the small girl looks in vain to her father for the love and kindness which shall confirm her belief in the 'good' penis

---

[1] Phantasies with this content play a part in the homosexuality of women similar to that played in the homosexuality of men by phantasies of meeting their father's penis, as an object of satisfaction or of hatred, inside their mother's body. This may be because, where the girl's attitude is predominantly sadistic, they represent the destruction, undertaken in common by herself and her mother, of her father's penis; or, where it is predominantly positive, a libidinal satisfaction obtained in common with her from his penis.

inside her and be a counter-weight to her belief in the 'bad' penis there, she will often grow more firmly entrenched in her masochistic attitude and the 'sadistic father' may even become an actual condition of love for her; or his behaviour to her may increase her feelings of hatred and anxiety against his penis and impel her to abandon the feminine role or to become frigid.

Actually, whether the outcome of her development is to be favourable or unfavourable will depend upon the interaction of a whole number of external factors. Her father's attitude to her is not the only thing which helps to decide what type of person she will fall in love with. It is not only a question, say, of whether he favours or neglects her too much in comparison with her mother or her sisters, but of his direct relations with them. How far she will be able to maintain her feminine position and in that position evolve a wish for a kindly father-imago also depends very greatly upon her sense of guilt towards her mother and thus upon the nature of the relations between her mother and father.[1] Furthermore, certain events, such as the illness or death of one of her parents or of a brother or sister, can assist in strengthening in her either the one sexual position or the other, according to the way in which they affect her sense of guilt.

Another thing which plays a very important part in the development of the child is the presence in its early life of a person, besides its father or mother, whom it looks upon as a 'helping' figure and who gives it support in the external world against its phantastic fears. In dividing its mother into a 'good' mother and a 'bad' one and its father into a 'good' father and a 'bad' one, it attaches the hatred it feels for its object to the 'bad' one or turns away from it, while it directs its restorative trends to its 'good' mother and 'good' father and, in phantasy, makes good towards them the damage it has done its parent-imagos in its sadistic phantasies.[2] But if, because its anxiety is too great or for realistic reasons, its Oedipus objects have not become good imagos, other persons, such as a kindly nurse, brother or sister, a grandparent or an aunt or uncle can, in certain circumstances, take over the role of the 'good' mother or

---

[1] Since the way in which each child will receive the impressions of reality is already largely determined by his or her early anxiety-situations, the same events will have different effects on different children. But there can be no doubt that the existence of happy and harmonious relations between their parents and between themselves and their parents is of underlying importance for their successful sexual development and mental health. Of course, a happy family life of this kind presupposes in general that the parents are not neurotic; so that a constitutional factor enters into the situation as well.

[2] Cf. Chapter IX.

the 'good' father.[1] In this way its positive feelings, whose growth has been inhibited owing to its excessive fear of its Oedipus objects, can come to the fore and attach themselves to a love-object.

As has been pointed out more than once, the existence of sexual relations between children in early life, especially between brothers and sisters, is a very common occurrence. The libidinal craving of small children, intensified as it is by their Oedipus frustrations, together with the anxiety emanating from their deepest danger-situations, impel them to indulge in mutual sexual activities, since these, as I have more particularly tried to show in the present chapter, not only gratify their libido but enable them to search for manifold confirmations and refutations of their various fears in connection with the sexual act. I have repeatedly found that if such sexual objects have acted in addition as 'helping' figures, early sexual relations of this kind exert a favourable influence upon the girl's relations to her objects and upon her later sexual development.[2] Where an excessive fear of both parents, together with certain external factors, would have produced an Oedipus situation which would have prejudiced her attitude towards the opposite sex and greatly hampered her in the maintenance of her feminine position and in her ability to love, the fact that she has had sexual relations with a brother or brother-substitute in early childhood and that that brother has also shown real affection for her and been her protector, has provided the basis for a heterosexual position in her and developed her capacity for love. In some of the cases I have in mind the girl had had two types of love-object,[3] one representing the stern father and the other the kind brother. In other cases, she had developed an imago which was a mixture of the two types; and here, too, her relations to her brother had lessened her masochism.

In serving as a proof grounded upon reality of the existence of the 'good' penis, the girl's relations with her brother fortify her belief in the 'good' introjected penis and moderate her fear of 'bad'

---

[1] A pet animal may also play the part of a 'helping' object in the imagination of children and thus assist in diminishing their anxiety. And so may a doll or a toy animal, to which they often assign the function of protecting them while they are asleep.

[2] Cf. Chapter VII.

[3] Each type had become important at different periods of her life. Analysis showed that whenever her anxiety increased in amount and certain external factors became operative she was led to choose the more sadistic type of person or at least to be unable to resist his advances; while, as soon as she had succeeded in detaching herself from that sadistic object, the other, kindly type, representing her brother, emerged and she became less masochistic and was able to choose a satisfactory object.

introjected objects. They also help her to master her fear of these objects, since in performing sexual acts with another child she gets a feeling of being in league with him against her parents. Their sexual relations have made the two children accomplices in crime, by reviving in them sadistic masturbation phantasies that were originally directed against their father and mother and causing them to indulge in them together. In thus sharing in that deepest guilt each child feels relieved of some of the weight of it and is also less frightened, because it believes that it has an ally against its dreaded objects. As far as I can see, the existence of a secret complicity of this sort, which, in my opinion, plays an essential part in every relationship of love, even between grown-up people, is of special importance in sexual attachments where the individual is of a paranoid type.[1]

The girl also regards her sexual attachment to the other child, who represents the 'good' object, as a disproof by means of reality of her fear of her own sexuality and that of her object as something destructive; so that an attachment of this sort may prevent her from becoming frigid or succumbing to other sexual disturbances in later life.

Nevertheless, although, as we see, experiences of this kind can have a favourable effect upon the girl's sexual life and object-relationships, they can also lead to grave disorders in that field.[2] If her sexual relations with another child serve to confirm her deepest fears—either because her partner is too sadistic or because performing the sexual act arouses yet more anxiety and guilt in her on account of her own excessive sadism—her belief in the harmfulness of her introjected objects and her own id will become still stronger, her super-ego will grow more severe than ever, and, as a result, her neurosis and all the defects of her sexual and characterological development will gain ground.[3]

Development at Puberty

The mental upheavals which the child undergoes during the age of puberty are, as we know, to a large extent due to the intensification of its impulses which accompanies the somatic changes that are taking place in it. In the girl the onset of menstruation gives additional reinforcement to her anxiety. In her *Zur Psychoanalyse weiblichen Sexualfunktionen*[4] Helene Deutsch has discussed at length

[1] For a fuller discussion of this point see the following chapter.
[2] Cf. Chapter VII on this head.
[3] This is still more the case where the child has been seduced or raped by an adult. Such an experience as is well known, can have very serious effects upon the child's mind.
[4] *Loc. cit.*

what the onset of menstruation means to the girl and the trial it imposes on her; she has come to the conclusion that the first flow of blood is equivalent in the unconscious to having actually been castrated and having forfeited the possibility of having a child, and is, therefore, a double disappointment. Helene Deutsch points out that menstruation also signifies a punishment for having indulged in clitoral masturbation and, in addition, that it regressively revives the girl's infantile view of copulation according to which it is nearly always a sadistic act involving cruelty and the flow of blood.[1]

My own data fully bear out Helene Deutsch's view that the disappointments and shocks to her narcissism which the girl receives when she begins to menstruate make a great impact. But I think that their pathogenic effect is due to the circumstances that they reactivate past fears in her. They are only a few items in a whole chain of anxiety-situations which menstruation brings to the surface once more. These fears, as we have seen earlier in the present chapter, are, briefly, the following:

1. Because the unconscious equates all bodily substances with one another in phantasy, she identifies her menstrual blood with her dangerous excreta.[2] Since she has learned early on to associate bleeding with injury, her fear that these dangerous excreta have damaged her own body seems to her to have been borne out by reality.

2. The menstrual flow increases her terror that her body will be attacked. In this connection various fears are at work: (a) Her fear of being attacked and destroyed by her mother partly out of revenge, partly so as to get back her father's penis and the children which she (the girl) has deprived her of. (b) Her fear of being attacked and damaged by her father through his copulating with her in a sadistic way,[3] either because she has had sadistic masturbation phantasies about her mother or because he wants to get back the penis she has taken from him. Her phantasy that in thus forcibly

---

[1] Cf. *loc. cit.*, S. 36.

[2] Cf. Lewin, 'Kotschmieren, Menses und weibliches Über-Ich' (1930).

[3] In her paper, 'Psychoanalytisches zur Menstruation' (1931), Melitta Schmideberg has pointed out that the girl regards menstruation, among other things, as the result of having been copulated with sadistically by her father and that she is all the more terrified since she believes that this action on his part was done in retaliation for her aggression towards both him and her mother. Just as in her sadistic phantasies as a child he was the executive of her aggressive desire against her mother, so now he is the one to carry out the punishment her mother metes out to her. In addition, his sadistic coitus with her represents his own punishment of her for the castration-wishes she harbours against the male sex in connection with copulation.

recovering his penis from her he will injure her genitals underlies, I think, the idea she has later on that her clitoris is a wound or scar where her penis once was. (c) Her fear that the interior of her body will be attacked and destroyed by her introjected objects either directly or indirectly as a consequence of their fight with one another inside her. Her phantasy that she has introjected her violent parents in the act of performing sadistic coitus and that they are endangering her own inside in destroying each other there is a source of acute fears. She regards the bodily sensations which menstruation often gives rise to within her, and which her anxiety augments, as a sign that all the dreaded injuries and all her hypochondriacal fears have come true.

3. The flow of blood from the interior of her body convinces her that the children inside her have been injured and destroyed. In some analyses of women I have found that their fear of being childless (i.e. of having had the children inside them destroyed) had been intensified since the onset of menstruation and had not been removed until they actually did have a child. But in many cases menstruation in adding to their fear of having damaged or abnormal children, causes them, consciously or unconsciously, to reject pregnancy altogether.

4. Menstruation, by confirming the girl in the knowledge that she has no penis and in the belief that her clitoris is the scar or wound left by her castrated penis,[1] makes it harder for her to maintain a masculine position.

5. In being a sign of sexual maturity, menstruation activates all those sources of anxiety, mentioned earlier on in this chapter, which are connected with her ideas that sexual behaviour has a sadistic character.

Analyses of female patients at the age of puberty shows that for the reasons given above the girl feels that her feminine position as well as her masculine one has become untenable. Menstruation has a much greater effect in activating sources of anxiety and conflicts in the girl than do the parallel developmental processes in the boy. This is partly why she is sexually more inhibited than he is at puberty.

The effects of menstruation on the girl's mind are in part responsible for the fact that at this age the girl's neurotic difficulties often increase very greatly. Even if she is normal menstruation resuscitates

[1] In my opinion, the girl's primary phantasy, mentioned under 2(b), to the effect that her genitals (clitoris) have been damaged through her having had her introjected penis forcibly taken from her, or her fear that this will happen, forms the basis of her phantasy that her genitals have been damaged by castration.

her old anxiety-situations, though, since her ego and her methods of mastering anxiety have been adequately developed, she is better able to modify her anxiety than she was in early childhood. Ordinarily, too, she obtains a strong satisfaction from the onset of menstruation. Provided that her feminine position has been well established during the first expansion of her sexual life, she will regard menstruation as a proof of being sexually mature and a woman, and as a sign that she may put still greater confidence in her expectation of receiving sexual gratification and having children. If this is so, she will look upon menstruation as definite evidence against various sources of anxiety.

Relations to her Children

In describing the early sexual development of the female individual I did not go very fully into her desire to have children, since I wanted to deal with her infantile attitude to her imaginary children at the same time as I dealt with her attitude in later life, during pregnancy, to the real child inside her.

Freud has stated that the girl's desire to have a child takes the place of her wish to possess a penis;[1] but according to my observations, it is her desire for her father's penis in an object-libidinal sense originating from her oral position, that precedes the wish for a child. In some cases the principal equation she makes is between children and faeces, in others between child and penis. In the first case her relation to the child seems to develop mainly on narcissistic lines. It is more independent of her attitude to the man and closely connected with her own body and with the omnipotence of her excrements. In the second case her attitude to her child rests more strongly upon her relations to her father or to his penis. There is a universal infantile sexual theory to the effect that the mother incorporates a new penis every time she copulates and that these penises, or a part of them, turn into children. In consequence of this theory the girl's relations to her father's penis influence her relations first of all to her imaginary children and later on to her real ones.

In the book which I have already quoted, *Zur Psychoanalyse der weiblichen Sexualfunktionen*, Helene Deutsch, in discussing the attitude of the pregnant woman to the child inside her, puts forward the following view. The woman looks upon her child both as a part of her self and as an object outside it 'in regard to which she repeats all the positive and negative object-relationships which she has had

---

[1] Cf. Freud, 'Some Psychical Consequences of the Anatomical Distinction between the Sexes' (1927), *S.E.* **19**.

towards her own mother'. In her phantasies her father has been turned into her child in the act of copulation, 'which, ultimately, represents to her unconscious the oral incorporation of her father', and he 'retains this role in the real or imaginary pregnancy which ensues'. After this process of introjection has taken place her child becomes 'the incarnation of the ego-ideal which she has already developed earlier' and also represents 'the embodiment of her own ideals which she has not been able to attain'. The ambivalent attitude she has towards her child is partly due to this fact that it stands for her super-ego—often in strong opposition to her ego— and revives in her those ambivalent feelings towards her father which arose out of her Oedipus situation. But it is also partly due to her making a regressive cathexis of her earlier libidinal positions. Her identification of children with faeces, of which she has a narcissistic valuation, becomes the basis of a similar narcissistic valuation of her child; and her reaction-formations against her original over-estimation of her excrements awakens feelings of disgust in her and makes her want to expel her child.

My own view goes beyond what Helene Deutsch has said in one or two points. The equation which the girl has made in the early stages of her development between her father's penis and a child leads her to give to the child inside her the significance of a paternal super-ego, since his internalized penis forms the nucleus of that super-ego. This early equation not only determines her ambivalence to her imaginary child, and later in life, as a mother, to her real one, but also determines the quantity of anxiety which decisively influences her relations to her child. The equation she has made between faeces and children has also, I have found, affected her relation to her imaginary child when she is still quite small. And the anxiety which she feels on account of her phantasies about her poisonous and burning excreta, and which, in my opinion, reinforces her trends to expel, belonging to the earlier anal stage, forms the basis for her feelings of hatred and fear later on towards the real child inside her.

As I have already pointed out, the girl's fear of her 'bad' introjected penis induces her to strengthen her introjection of a 'good' penis, since it offers her protection and assistance against the 'bad' penis inside her, and her bad imagos which she experiences as dangerous excrements. It is this friendly 'good' penis, often conceived of as a small one, which takes on the significance of a child. This imaginary child, which affords the small girl protection and help, primarily represents in her unconscious the 'good' contents o⸱ her body. The support it gives her against her anxiety is, of course, purely phantastic, but then the objects she is afraid of are equally phantastic; for in this stage of her development she is mostly governed by psychic reality.[1]

It is because the possession of children is a means of overcoming her anxiety and allaying her sense of guilt that I see in the little girl's normal and intense need for children, the deepest reason for this desire which is greater than any other. As we know, grown-up women often have a stronger desire to have a child than to have a sexual partner.

The small girl's attitude towards the child is also of great importance for the development of her sublimations. The imaginary attacks she makes upon her mother's inside by means of her poisonous and destructive excreta bring on misgivings about the contents of her own body. Owing to her equation of faeces with children her phantasies about the 'bad' faeces inside her lead her to have phantasies about having a 'bad' child[2] there, and that is equivalent to having an 'ugly' abnormal one. The girl's reaction-formations to her sadistic phantasies about dangerous faeces give rise, it seems to me, to sublimations of a specifically feminine type. In analysing small girls we can see very clearly how closely their longing to possess a 'beautiful' (i.e. 'good' and healthy) child and their indefatigable efforts to beautify their imaginary baby and their own body are connected with their fear of having produced in themselves and put inside their mother 'bad' and ugly children whom they liken to poisonous excrement.

Ferenczi has described the changes[3] which the child's interest in faeces undergoes in the various stages of its development, and has come to the conclusion that its coprophilic tendencies are early sublimated in part into a pleasure in shining things. One element in this process of sublimation is, I think, the child's fear of 'bad' and dangerous pieces of stool. From this there is a direct sublimatory path leading to the theme of 'beauty'.[4] The very strong need which women feel to have a beautiful body and a lovely home and for beauty in general is based on their desire to possess a beautiful interior to their body in which 'good' and lovely objects and innocuous excrements are lodged. Another line of sublimation from

[1] Recognition of internal reality is the foundation of adaptation to external reality. The child's attitude to its phantasy-objects, which, in this stage of its life, are phantastic imagos of its external, real objects will determine its relations to those objects later on.

[2] The equation of a 'bad' penis or bad pieces of stool with a child, has already been discussed. The two equations exist side by side and reinforce each other.

[3] Ferenczi, 'The Origin of Interest in Money' (1914).

[4] Probably also for the purpose of disfiguring her mother or making her ugly.

the girl's fear of 'bad' and 'dangerous' excrements leads to the idea of 'good' products in the sense of health-giving ones (though, incidentally, 'good' and 'beautiful' often mean the same thing to the small child), and in this way goes to strengthen in her those original maternal feelings and desires to give which spring from her feminine position.

If the small girl's hopeful feelings predominate she will believe not only that her internalized penis is a 'good' one but that the children inside her are helpful beings. But if she is filled with fear of a 'bad' internalized penis and of dangerous excrements, her relation to her real child in later life will often be dominated by anxiety. Despite this, where her relations to her sexual partner do not satisfy her, she will establish a relation to her child which will afford her gratification and mental support. In these cases, in which the sexual act itself has received the significance of an anxiety-situation too strongly and her sexual object has become an anxiety-object to her, it is her child which attracts the quality of a 'good' and helpful penis to itself. Again, a woman who overcomes anxiety precisely by means of her sexual activities may have a fairly good relation to her husband and a bad one to her child. In this case she has displaced her anxiety concerning the enemy inside her for the most part on to her child; and it is her fears resulting from this which, I have found, are at the bottom of her fear of pregnancy and child-birth and which add to her physical sufferings while she is pregnant and may even render her psychologically incapable of conceiving a child.

We have already seen in what way the woman's fear of the 'bad' penis can increase her sadism. Women who have a strong sadistic attitude to their husband usually look upon their child as an enemy. Just as in phantasy they regard the sexual act as a means of destroy-ing their object, so do they want to have a child mainly in order to get it into their power as though it were something hostile to them. They can then employ the hatred which they feel for their internal, dreaded foe against external objects—against husband and child. There are also, of course, women who have a sadistic attitude to their husband and a relatively friendly one to their children, and vice versa. But in every case it is the woman's attitude to her introjected objects, especially her father's penis, which will determine her attitude to her husband and child.

The attitude of the mother to her children is based, as we know, upon her early relations to her objects. Those emotional relation-ships which she had in early childhood towards her father and uncles and brothers, or towards her mother and aunts and sisters, will be reflected to a greater or lesser degree in her relationship to the child according to its sex. If she has principally equated the idea of a child with that of a 'good' penis, it will be the positive elements of those relationships which she will carry over to her child.[1] She will condense a number of friendly imagos in its person,[2] and it will represent the 'innocence' of infancy and will be in her eyes what she would like to picture herself as having been in early childhood. And one of the ultimate motives for the hopes she places upon its growing up well and happily is that she may be able to recreate her own unsatisfactory childhood as a time of happiness.

There are, I think, a whole number of factors which help to strengthen the emotional relationship which the mother has towards her child. In bringing it into the world she has produced the strongest refutation in reality of all the fears that arise from her sadistic phantasies. The birth of her child not only signifies in her unconscious that the interior of her own body and the imaginary children there are unharmed or have been made well again but invalidates all sorts of fears associated with the idea of children. It shows that the children inside her mother—her brothers and sisters—and her father's penis (or her father) which she has attacked there, and also her mother, are all unharmed or made whole again. Giving birth to a baby thus represents restoring a number of objects—even, in some cases, recreating a whole world.

Giving suck to her child is very important too, and forms a very close and special tie between her and it. In giving her child a product of her own body which is essential to its nourishment and growth she is enabled finally to disprove and put a happy end to that vicious circle which was started in her as an infant by her attacks upon her mother's breast as the first object of her destructive impulses and which contained phantasies of destroying the breast by biting it to pieces and dirtying, poisoning and burning it by means of her excreta. For in her unconscious she regards the fact that she is giving her child nourishing and beneficial milk as a proof that

---

[1] The girl often identifies her phantasy-child in her unconscious with a small and innocuous penis. It is partly in this connection that her relations with her brother or some other child help her to confirm her belief in the 'good' penis. As a small child she ascribes an enormous amount of sadism to her father's penis and finds her brother's small penis, if less worthy of admiration, at any rate not so dangerous.

[2] In *Civilization and its Discontents* (1930) (*S.E.* **21**, p. 113), Freud says: 'It (aggressiveness) forms the basis of every relation of affection and love among people (with the single exception, perhaps, of the mother's relation to her male child).' Where the woman is strongly affected by the equation between the child and the 'good' penis, she is especially liable to concentrate all the positive elements of her feeling upon her child, should it be a boy.

her own early sadistic phantasies have not come true or that she has succeeded in restoring the objects of them.[1]

As has already been pointed out, the individual loves his 'good' object the more since, by being the aim and object of his restitutive tendencies, it affords him gratification and lessens his anxiety. No other object possesses this qualification to such an eminent degree as does the helpless little child. Furthermore, in expending her maternal love and care upon her child she not only fulfils her earliest desires but, as she identifies herself with it, shares the pleasures she gives it. In thus reversing the relationship of mother and child she is able to experience a happy renewal of her earliest attachment to her own mother and to let her primal feelings of hatred for her recede into the background and her positive feelings come to the fore.

All these factors contribute to give children a tremendous importance in the emotional life of women. And we can readily see why it is that their mental balance should be so much upset if their child does not turn out well and, especially, if it is abnormal. Just as a healthy and thriving child is a refutation of a whole number of fears so is an abnormal, sickly, or merely rather unsatisfactory one a confirmation of them, and may even come to be regarded as an enemy and a persecutor.

Ego Development

We shall now only consider briefly the relation between the formation of the girl's super-ego and the development of her ego. Freud has shown that some of the differences that exist between the super-ego formation of the girl and that of the boy are associated with anatomical distinctions between the sexes.[2] These anatomical distinctions affect, I think, both the development of the super-ego and the ego in various ways. In consequence of the structure of the female genitals, which marks their receptive function, the girl's Oedipus trends are more largely dominated by her oral impulses, and the introjection of her super-ego is more extensive than in the

---

[1] She also takes this as a proof by reality that her urine, which she likens to milk, is not harmful; just as, on the other hand, she often looks upon her menstrual blood as a proof by reality that her urine and other excreta are dangerous substances. Moreover, the fact that her supply of milk does not give out is a refutation not only of her fear, arising from her sadistic phantasies, that her breast has been destroyed, but convinces her that her excrements are not harmful to her own body. These were the weapons she used to attack her mother's breast in her imagination and now she sees that they have done no harm.

[2] 'Some Psychical Consequences of the Anatomical Distinction between the Sexes' (1927), S.E. 19.

boy. In addition there is the absence of a penis as an active organ. The girl's greater dependence upon her super-ego which is the result of her stronger introjective tendencies is further increased by the fact that she has no penis.

I have already put forward the view in earlier pages of this book that the boy's primary sense of omnipotence is associated with his penis, which is also the representative in his unconscious of activities and sublimations proceeding from his masculine components. In the girl, who does not possess a penis, the sense of omnipotence is more profoundly and extensively associated with her father's introjected penis than it is in the case of the boy. This is the more so because the picture which she has formed as a child of his penis inside her and which determines the standards she sets up for herself has been evolved out of extremely highly coloured phantasies and is thus more exaggerated than the boy's both in the direction of 'goodness' and of 'badness'.

This view that the super-ego is more strongly operative in women than in men seems at first sight to be out of keeping with the fact that, compared to men, women are often more dependent upon their objects, more easily influenced by the outer world and more variable in their moral standards—that is, apparently less guided by the requirements of a super-ego. But I think that their greater dependence upon objects, associated with the greater significance of loss of love,[1] is actually closely related to a greater efficacy of the super-ego. Both characteristics have a common origin in the greater

---

[1] In his paper, 'One of the Motive Factors in the Formation of the Super-Ego in Women' (1928), Hanns Sachs has pointed out the curious fact that although women are in general more narcissistic than men, they feel the loss of love more. He has sought to explain this apparent contradiction by supposing that when her Oedipus conflict comes to an end the girl tries to cling to her father either through her desire to have a child by him or by means of oral regression. His view agrees with mine in stressing the significance that her oral attachment to her father has for the formation of her super-ego. But according to him this attachment comes about through a regression after she has been disappointed in her hopes of having a penis and of obtaining genital satisfaction from her father; whereas in my view her oral attachment to her father, or, more correctly, her desire to incorporate his penis, is the foundation and starting-point of her sexual development and of the formation of her super-ego.

Ernest Jones attributes the greater effect which the loss of her object has upon the woman to her fear that her father will not give her sexual satisfaction (cf. his paper, 'The Early Development of Female Sexuality', 1927). According to him, the reason why the frustration of sexual satisfaction is so intolerable to her—and in this matter, of course, the woman is more dependent than the man on the other party—is because it stirs up her deepest anxiety, which is her fear of aphanisis, i.e. of having her capacity for experiencing sexual pleasure entirely abolished.

propensity women have to introject their object and set it up in themselves, so that they erect a more powerful super-ego there. This propensity, moreover, is increased precisely by their greater dependence upon their super-ego and their greater fear of it. The girl's most profound anxiety, which is that some unascertainable damage has been done to her inside by her internalized objects, impels her, as I have already shown, to be continually testing her fears by means of her relations to real objects. It impels her, that is, to reinforce her introjective trends in a secondary way. Again, it would seem that her mechanisms of projection are stronger than the man's, in conformity with her stronger sense of the omnipotence of her excrements and thoughts; and this is another factor which induces her to have stronger relations with the outer world and with objects in reality, partly for the purpose of controlling them by magic.

This fact that the processes of introjection and projection are stronger in the woman than in the man not only affects, I think, the character of her object-relationships but is of importance for the development of her ego. Her dominating and deep-seated need to give herself up in complete trust and submission to the 'good' internalized penis is one of the things that underlies the receptive quality of her sublimations and interests. But her feminine position also strongly impels her to obtain secret control of her internalized objects by means of the omnipotence of her excrements and of her thoughts; and this fosters in her a sharp power of observation and great psychological understanding, together with a certain artfulness, cunning and inclination towards deceit and intrigue. This side of her ego-development is brought out in the main with reference to her maternal super-ego, but it also colours her relation to her paternal imago.

In *The Ego and the Id* Freud writes:[1] 'If they' [the object-identifications] 'obtain the upper hand and become too numerous, unduly powerful and incompatible with one another, a pathological outcome will not be far off. It may come to a disruption of the ego in consequence of the different identifications becoming cut off from one another by resistances; perhaps the secret of cases of what is described as "multiple personality" is that the different identifications seize hold of consciousness in turn. Even when things do not go so far as this, there remains the question of conflicts between the various identifications into which the ego comes apart, conflicts which cannot after all be described as entirely pathological.' A study of the early stages of the formation of the super-ego and their relation to the development of the ego fully confirms this last statement. And, as far as can be seen, any further investigation of

[1] *S.E.* **19**, p. 30.

personality as a whole, whether normal or abnormal, will have to proceed along the lines Freud has indicated. It seems that the way to extend our knowledge of the ego is to learn more about the various identifications it makes and the attitudes it has to them. Only by pursuing this line of enquiry can we discover in what ways the ego regulates the relations that exist between those identifications, which, as we know, differ according to the stage of development in which they have been made and according to whether they refer to the subject's mother or father or a combination of the two.

The girl is more hampered in the formation of a super-ego in respect of her mother than the boy is in respect of his father, since it is difficult for her to identify herself with her mother on the basis of an anatomical resemblance, owing to the fact that the internal organs which subserve female sexual functions—both her mother's and her own—and the possession of [internal] children do not admit of any investigation or test by reality. This obstacle, the significance of which for female sexual development I have already mentioned, increases the power of her terrifying mother-imago—that product of her own imaginary sadistic attacks upon her mother—who endangers the inside of her body and calls her to account for having deprived her of her children, her faeces and the father's penis.

The methods of attack, based on the omnipotence of her excrements and of thoughts, which the girl employs against her mother influence the development of her ego not only directly, as it seems, but indirectly too. Her reaction-formations against her own sadistic omnipotence and the transformation of the latter into constructive omnipotence enable her to develop sublimations and qualities of mind which are the direct opposite of those traits which we have just described and which are allied to the primary omnipotence of her excrements. They incline her to be frank and trustful, capable of making sacrifices, ready to devote herself to the duties before her and willing to undergo much for their sake and for the sake of other people. These reaction-formations and sublimations tend once more to make her sense of omnipotence, based upon her internalized 'good' objects, and her attitude of submission to her paternal super-ego the dominating forces in her feminine attitude.[1]

---

[1] As has already been seen, the different kinds of magic act in conjunction and are interchangeable. They are also played off against one another by the ego. The girl's fear of having 'bad' children (faeces) inside her as a result of the magical powers of her excrements acts as an incentive to her to overemphasize her belief in the 'good' penis. Her equation of the 'good' penis with a child makes it possible for her to hope that she has incorporated 'good' children and these are an offset to the children inside her which she likens to 'bad' faeces.

Moreover, an essential part in her ego-development is played by her desire to employ her 'good' urine and 'good' faeces in rectifying the effects of her 'bad' and harmful excrements and in giving away good and beautiful things—a desire which is of overwhelming importance in childbirth and the act of suckling the child, for the 'beautiful' child and the 'good' milk which she produces counterbalance the fear of her harmful faeces and dangerous urine. Indeed this desire forms a fruitful and creative basis for all those sublimations which arise out of the psychical representatives of childbirth and suckling at the breast.

The characteristic thing about the development of the woman's ego could be formulated thus: the girl's super-ego becomes raised to very great heights and much magnified and her ego looks up to it and submits itself to it. And because her ego tries to live up to this exalted super-ego it is spurred on to all kinds of efforts which result in an expansion and enrichment of itself. Thus whereas in the man it is the ego and, with it, reality-relations which mostly take the lead, so that his whole nature is more objective and matter of fact, in the woman it is the unconscious which is the dominating force. In her case, no less than in his, the quality of her achievements will depend upon the quality of her ego, but they receive their specifically feminine character of intuitiveness and subjectivity from the fact that her ego is submitted to a loved internal spirit. They represent the birth of a spiritual child, conceived by its father; and this spiritual procreation is attributed to her super-ego. It is true that even a markedly feminine line of development exhibits numerous features which spring from masculine components, but it seems as if it was the woman's dominating belief in the omnipotence of her father's incorporated penis and of the growing child inside her which renders her capable of achievements of a specifically feminine kind.

At this point we cannot help comparing the mental situation of women with that of children, who, as I maintain, are to a much greater degree under the dominion of their super-ego and, at the same time, in need of their objects than the adult. We all know that the woman is much more akin to the child than is the man; and yet in many aspects of her ego-development she differs quite as much from the child as he. I see the explanation for these differences in this: in her development the woman introjects her Oedipus objects more strongly than the man, which leads to a fuller ego-development, although two limiting factors have to be considered: the unconscious retains a wider hold on her personality, to some extent analogous to the situation of the child; and she leans on the powerful super-ego within partly in order to dominate or to outdo it.

If the girl clings in the main to the imaginary possession of a penis as a masculine attribute, her development will be radically different. In reviewing her sexual history I have already discussed the various reasons which oblige her to adopt a masculine position. As regards her activities and sublimations—which she regards in her unconscious as reality-evidence of her possession of a penis or as substitutes for it—these are not only used to compete with her father's penis but invariably serve, in a secondary way, as a defence against her super-ego and in order to weaken it. In girls of this type, moreover, the ego takes a stronger lead and their pursuits are for the most part an expression of male potency.

As far as the girl's sexual development is concerned, I have already emphasized the significance of a good mother-imago for the formation of a good father-imago. If she is in a position to entrust herself to the internal guidance of a paternal super-ego which she believes in and admires, it always means that she has good mother-imagos as well; for it is only where she has sufficient trust in a 'good' internalized mother that she is able to surrender herself completely to her paternal super-ego. But in order to make a surrender of this kind she must also believe strongly enough in her possession of 'good' things inside her body—of friendly internalized objects. Only if the child which, in her phantasy, she has had, or expects to have, by her father is a 'good' and 'beautiful' child—only, that is, if the inside of her body represents a place where harmony and beauty reign (a phantasy which is also present in the man) can she give herself without reserve, both sexually and mentally, to her paternal super-ego and to its representatives in the external world. The attainment of a state of harmony of this kind is founded on the existence of a good relationship between her ego and its identifications and between those identifications themselves, and especially of a peaceful union of her father-imago and her mother-imago.

The girl-child's phantasies in which she tries to destroy both her parents out of envy and hatred are the fountain-head of her deepest sense of guilt; at the same time they also form the basis of her most overpowering danger-situations. They give rise to a fear of harbouring in herself hostile objects which are engaged in deadly combat (i.e. in destructive copulation) with each other or which, because they have discovered her guilt, are allied in enmity against her ego. If her father and mother live a happy life together the immense gratification she obtains from this fact is to a great extent due to the relief which their good relations with each other afford the sense of guilt she feels on account of her sadistic phantasies. For in her unconscious the good understanding between them is a confirmation in reality of her hope of being able to make restitution in every possible way. And if her restitutive mechanisms have been successfully established she will not only be in harmony with the external world, but—and this is, I think, a necessary condition for the attainment of such a state of harmony and of a satisfactory object-relationship and sexual development—she will be at one with her internal world and with herself. If her menacing imagos fade into the background and her kindly father-imago and mother-imago emerge to act in friendly co-operation and give her a guarantee of security and harmony within her own body, she can work out her feminine and her masculine components in the sense and spirit of her introjected parents, and she will have secured a basis in herself for the full development of a harmonious personality.

Postscript

Since writing the above I note that a paper by Freud has appeared[1] in which he more especially discusses the long period of the girl's attachment to her mother, and endeavours to isolate that attachment from the operation of her super-ego and her sense of guilt. This, in my judgment, is not possible, for I think that the girl's anxiety and sense of guilt which arise from her aggressive impulses go to intensify her primary libidinal attachment to her mother at a very early age. Her multifarious fears of her phantastic imagos (her super-ego) and of her 'bad', real mother forces the still quite small girl to find protection in her 'good' real mother. And in order to do this she has to over-compensate for her primary aggression towards the latter.

Freud also emphasizes that the girl feels hostility, too, towards her mother and is afraid of being 'killed (eaten up?) by her'. In my analysis of children and adults I have found that the girl's fear of being devoured, cut to bits or destroyed by her mother springs from the projection of impulses of her own of the same sadistic kind against her, and that those fears are at the bottom of her earliest anxiety-situations. Freud also states that girls and women who are strongly attached to their mother used more especially to react with rage and anxiety to enemas and colonic irrigations which she had administered to them. Expressions of affect of this sort are, as far as my experience goes, caused by their fear of sustaining anal attacks from her—a fear which represents the projection of their anal-sadistic phantasies on to her. I am in agreement with Freud's view that in females the projection in early childhood of hostile impulses against their mother is the nucleus of paranoia in later

[1] 'Female Sexuality' (1932), *S.E.* **21**, p. 225.

life.[1] But, according to my observations, it is the imaginary attacks they have made upon the interior of their mother's body by means of destructive excrements that poison, burn and explode, which more particularly give rise to their fears of pieces of stool as persecutors and of their mother as a terrifying figure as a result of projection.

Freud believes that the girl's long attachment to her mother is an exclusive one and takes place before she has entered the Oedipus situation. But my experience of analysis of small girls has convinced me that their long-drawn-out and powerful attachment to their mother is never exclusive and is bound up with Oedipus impulses. Moreover, their anxiety and sense of guilt in relation to their mother also affects the course of those Oedipus impulses; for in my view, the girl's defence against her feminity springs less from her masculine trends than from her fear of her mother. If the small girl is too frightened of her mother she will not be able to attach herself strongly enough to her father and her Oedipus complex will not come to light. In those cases, however, in which a strong attachment to the father has not been established until the post-phallic stage, I have found that the girl has nevertheless had positive Oedipus impulses at an early stage, though these often did not emerge clearly. These early stages of her Oedipus conflict still bear a some-what phantastic character, since they are centred round the penis of her father; but in part they are already concerned with her real father.

In some of my papers I have adduced as the earliest factors in the withdrawal of the girl from her mother, the grudge she feels against her for having subjected her to oral frustration (a factor which Freud also mentioned in the paper under discussion) and her envy of the mutual oral satisfaction which, on the strength of her earliest sexual theories, she imagines that her parents obtain from copulation. These factors, based on the equation of breast with penis, incline her to turn towards her father's penis in the second half of her first year; this is the cause of her attachment to her father being fundamentally affected by her attachment to her mother. Freud also points out that the one is built upon the other, and that many women repeat their relation to their mother in their relation to men.

[1] Cf. my papers, 'Early Stages of the Oedipus Conflict' (1928) and 'The Importance of Symbol-Formation in the Development of the Ego' (1930) [both in Writings, 1] and Chapter III of this book.

Chapter XII

THE EFFECTS OF
EARLY ANXIETY-SITUATIONS
ON THE SEXUAL DEVELOPMENT
OF THE BOY

THE analysis of the very small child shows that in its earliest stages the boy's sexual development runs on the same lines as that of the girl.[1] In the boy, the oral frustration he experiences reinforces his destructive trends against his mother's breast. As in the girl, too, the period when sadism is at its height, introduced by the oral-sadistic impulse, sets in with the withdrawal of the mother's breast—a phase in which the aim is to attack the inside of her body.

The Feminine Phase

In this phase the boy has an oral-sucking fixation on his father's penis, just as the girl has. This fixation is, I consider, the basis of true homosexuality in him. This view would agree with what Freud has said in *Leonardo da Vinci and a Memory of his Childhood*,[2] where he comes to the conclusion that Leonardo's homosexuality goes back to an excessive fixation upon his mother—ultimately upon her breast—and thinks that this fixation became displaced on to the penis as an object of satisfaction. In my experience every boy moves on from an oral-sucking fixation upon his mother's breast to an oral-sucking fixation upon his father's penis. It is this which forms the basis of homosexuality.

In the phantasy of the boy, his mother incorporates his father's penis, or rather, a number of them, inside herself; side by side with his relations to his real father, or, to be more precise, his father's penis, he develops a relation in phantasy to his father's penis inside his mother's body. Since his oral desires for his father's penis are one of the motives of his attacks on his mother's body—for he wants to take by force the penis which he imagines as being *inside his mother* and

---

[1] In so far as this is so those stages will be only very briefly alluded to here. For a more detailed discussion of them the reader is referred to Chapters VIII and IX of this book.

[2] *S.E.* **11**.

to injure her in doing so—his attacks also represent, among other things, his earliest situations of rivalry with her, and thus form the basis of the boy's femininity complex.[1]

The forcible seizure of his father's penis and of the excrements and children out of his mother's body gives rise to an intense fear of retaliation. His having destroyed the interior of his mother's body in addition to robbing it becomes, furthermore, a source of deepest fear of her. And the more sadistic his imaginary destruction of her body has been the greater will be his dread of her as a rival.

Early Stages of the Oedipus Conflict

The boy's genital impulses, which, though at first overlaid by his pre-genital ones and made to serve their ends, do nevertheless substantially affect the course of his sadistic phase and lead him to take his mother's body and genitals as a sexual object. He thus desires to have sole possession of her in an oral, anal and genital sense and attacks his father's penis within her with all the sadistic means at his disposal. His oral position, too, gives rise to much hatred against his father's penis as a consequence of the frustration he has experienced from his father. Ordinarily his destructive impulses towards his father's penis are very much stronger than the girl's, since his longing for his mother as a sexual object induces him to concentrate his hatred more intensely upon it. Moreover, it has already been the outstanding object of anxiety to him in the earliest stages of his development, for his direct aggressive impulses towards it have aroused a proportionate fear of it. This fear once again reinforces his hatred of it and his desire to destroy it.

As we have seen in the last chapter, the girl retains her mother's body as the direct object of her destructive impulses for a much longer time and to a much more intense degree than the boy; and her positive impulses towards her father's penis—both the real one and the imaginary one inside her mother's body—are normally much stronger and more enduring than his. In his case, it is only during a certain period of that early stage in which his attacks upon his mother's body dominate the picture that his mother is the actual object of destruction. It is very soon his father's penis, supposedly inside her, which to an even greater extent draws to itself his aggressive tendencies against her.

Early Anxiety-Situations

Besides the fears which the boy feels in consequence of his rivalry with his mother, his fear of his father's dangerous internalized penis stands

[1] For a detailed account of the phenomena that make their appearance in connection with the feminine phase in the male, I may refer the reader to my

in the way of his maintaining a feminine position. This latter fear, together with the growing strength of his genital impulses in particular, cause him to give up his identification with his mother and to fortify his heterosexual position. But if his fear of his mother as a rival and his fear of his father's penis are excessive, so that he does not properly overcome the feminine phase, a decisive bar to his becoming established in a heterosexual position will have arisen.

It is, furthermore, of great importance for the final outcome of the boy's development whether or not his early mental life has been dominated by a fear of his parents combined in copulation and forming an inseparable unit hostile to himself.[1] Anxiety of this kind makes it more difficult for him to maintain any position, and brings on danger-situations which I consider as the deepest sources of sexual impotence. These specific danger-situations arise from the boy's fear of being castrated by his father's penis inside his mother—that is, of being castrated by his combined, 'bad' parents—and his fear, often strongly evinced, of having his own penis prevented from retreating and of its being shut inside his mother's body.[2]

I have more than once pointed out that the anxiety-situations resulting from sadistic attacks made by children of both sexes on their mother's body fall into two categories. In the first, the mother's body becomes a place filled with dangers which give rise to all sorts of terrors. In the second, the child's own inside is turned into a place of a similar kind, by virtue of the child's introjection of its dangerous objects, especially its parents combined in copulation, and it becomes afraid of the perils and threats within itself. The anxiety-situations belonging to these two categories exert an influence upon one another, and are present in the girl as well as in the boy; and I have already examined elsewhere in this book the methods of mastering anxiety which are common to both. Briefly put, they are as follows: the child contends with its internalized 'bad' objects by means of the omnipotence of its excrements and also receives protection against them from its 'good' objects. At the same time it displaces its fear of internal dangers into the outer world by projection and finds evidence there to disprove them.

---

paper 'Early Stages of the Oedipus Conflict' (1928, *Writings*, **1**). Cf. also Karen Horney, 'The Flight from Womanhood' (1926), and Felix Boehm, 'The Femininity Complex in Men' (1929).

[1] The aetiological significance of such fears in the psychoses has been pointed out in Chapters VIII and IX.

[2] This fear has a bearing, I think, on various forms of claustrophobia. It seems certain that claustrophobia goes back to the fear of being shut up inside the mother's dangerous body. In the particular dread of not being able to extricate the penis from the mother's body it would seem that this fear has been narrowed down to a fear on behalf of the penis.

But besides this, each sex has its own essentially different modes of mastering anxiety. The boy develops his sense of the omnipotence of excreta less strongly than the girl, replacing it in part by the omnipotence of the penis; and in connection with this his projection of internal dangers is different from the girl's. The specific mechanism he employs for overcoming his fear both of internal and external dangers, at the same time as he obtains sexual satisfaction, is determined by the fact that his penis, as an active organ, is used to master his object and that it is accessible to tests by reality. In gaining possession of his mother's body by means of his penis he proves to himself his superiority not only over his dangerous external objects but over his internal ones as well.

Sadistic Omnipotence of the Penis

In the male child the omnipotence of excrements and thoughts is partly concentrated in the omnipotence of the penis, and especially in the case of excrements, partly replaced by it. In his imagination he endows his own penis with destructive powers and likens it to devouring and murderous beasts, firearms, and so on. His belief that his urine is a dangerous substance and his equation of his poisonous and explosive faeces with his penis go to make the latter the executive organ of his sadistic tendencies. Furthermore, certain physiological processes demonstrate that his penis really can change its appearance and he takes this as a proof of its omnipotence. Thus his penis and his sense of omnipotence become linked together in a way which is of fundamental importance for the man's activity and his mastery of anxiety. In child analysis we generally come across the idea of the penis as a 'magic wand', of masturbation as magic and of erection and ejaculation[1] as a tremendous heightening of the sadistic powers of the penis.[2]

The interior of the mother's body, which succeeds to the breast as the child's object, soon takes on the significance of a place which contains many objects (at first represented by the penis and excrements). In consequence the boy's phantasies of taking possession of his mother's body by copulating with her form the basis of his attempts to conquer the external world and to master anxiety along masculine

[1] Cf. Abraham, 'Ejaculatio Praecox' (1917).
[2] In his 'Beiträge zur Analyse des Sadismus und Masochismus' (1913), Federn has discussed the question of how the phenomena of active sadism arise in the male and has come to the conclusion that 'the active male organ-component that is awaking becomes transformed by means of unconscious mechanisms, of which symbolic representation is an important one, into sadism; or more correctly, the trends which flow from that component are turned into sadistic desires. At the same time all the active trends that have already been unfolded in the child become reactivated.'

lines. Both as regards the sexual act and sublimations he displaces his danger-situations into the outer world and overcomes them there through the omnipotence of his penis.

In the case of the girl, her belief in her father's 'good' penis and her fear of his 'bad' one fortify her introjective trends. Thus the test by reality against her 'bad' objects, carried out by the woman, is ultimately situated within herself once again. In the boy, belief in an internalized 'good' mother and fear of 'bad' objects assist him to displace his reality-tests outwards (i.e. into his mother's body). His internalized 'good' mother adds to the libidinal attraction which his real mother has for him and increases his wishes and hopes of combating and overcoming his father's penis inside her by means of his own penis. A victory of this kind would also be proof that he is able to get the better of the internalized assailants in his own body as well.[1]

This concentration of sadistic omnipotence in the penis is of fundamental importance for the masculine position of the boy. If he has a strong primary belief in the omnipotence of his penis he can pit it against the omnipotence of his father's penis and take up the struggle against that dreaded and admired organ. In order for a process of concentration of this kind to take effect it seems that his penis must be strongly cathected by the various forms of his sadism;[2] and the capacity of his ego to tolerate anxiety and the strength of his genital[3] impulses (which ultimately are libidinal ones) appear to have a decisive share in accomplishing this process. But if, when the genital impulses come to the fore, the ego should make too sudden and forcible a defence against the destructive impulses,[4] this process of focussing sadism in the penis will be interfered with.

---

[1] In some instances I have been able to ascertain that the boy uses his own penis as a weapon against his father's internalized penis as well by turning it inwards. He likens his stream of urine to his penis, and looks upon it as a stick or whip or sword with which he vanquishes his father's penis inside himself. I have also frequently come across a phantasy in which the boy pulls out his own penis to such a length that he can take it into his mouth — in one instance, into his anus. This phantasy is once again actuated by his wish to engage his penis in a direct struggle with his super-ego.

[2] According to Ferenczi (1922) pre-genital erotisms are displaced on to genital activities in virtue of a process of amphimixis.

[3] Reich has pointed out that the constitutional strength of the genital erotism of the individual is an important factor in the final outcome of his development (cf. his *The Function of the Orgasm*, 1927).

[4] Should genital feelings set in too soon and thus lead the ego to make a premature and over-strong defence against the destructive impulses, severe developmental inhibitions may result (cf. my paper, 'The Importance of Symbol-Formation in the Development of the Ego', 1930).

Incentives to Sexual Activity

The boy's hatred of his father's penis and the anxiety arising from the above-mentioned sources incite him to get possession of his mother in a genital way and so to increase his libidinal desires to copulate with her.[1] Moreover, as he gradually overcomes his sadism towards her he looks upon his father's penis inside her more and more not only as a source of danger to his own penis but as a source of danger to her body as well and feels that he must destroy it inside her for that reason. Another factor which acts as an incentive to having coitus with her (and which, in the girl, fortifies her homosexual position) is his desire for knowledge, which has been intensified by anxiety.[2] The desire for knowledge arises simultaneously with the destructive trends and is very soon pressed into the service of mastering anxiety. By means of the penetrating penis which is equated with an organ of perception, to be more precise, with the eye,[3] the ear or a combination of the two he wants to discover what sort of destruction has been done inside his mother by his own penis and excrements and by his father's, and to what kind of perils his penis is exposed there.

Therefore even at a time when the boy is still under the dominance of his sadism and when the means he employs are wholly of a destructive nature the drive to master anxiety becomes a stimulus to obtain genital satisfaction and a factor that promotes development. Furthermore, in this phase already those destructive measures themselves become in part pressed into the service of his restitutive tendencies in so far as his mother is to be rescued from his father's 'bad' penis inside her, although in doing so they still act in a forcible and injurious way.

'The Woman with a Penis'

The child's belief that its mother's body also contains the penis of its father leads, as I have tried to show, to the idea of the 'woman with a penis'. The sexual theory that the mother has a female penis of her own is, I think, the result of a modification by displacement of more deeply seated fears of her body as a place which is filled with a number of dangerous penises and of the two parents engaged in dangerous copulation. 'The woman with a penis' always means, I should say, the woman with the father's penis.[4]

[1] If the positive feelings for his mother cannot be sufficiently maintained, his mother's body, too, remains an object of hatred as the result of his aggression against his father's penis which he assumes to be inside her; he then turns away from his mother.

[2] Cf. Chapter VIII.

[3] Cf. Mary Chadwick, 'Über die Wurzel der Wissbegierde' (1925).

[4] In his 'Homosexualität und Ödipuskomplex' (1927), Felix Boehm has

Normally, the boy's fear of his father's penises inside his mother decreases as his relationship to his objects develops and as he goes forward in the conquest of his own sadism. Since his fear of the 'bad' penis is to a great extent derived from his destructive impulses against his father's penis, and since the character of his imagos depends largely on the quality and quantity of his own sadism, the reduction of that sadism and with it the reduction of his anxiety will lessen the severity of his super-ego and will thus improve the relations of his ego both towards his internalized, imaginary objects and towards his external, real ones.

Later Stages of the Oedipus Conflict

If, side by side with the imago of the combined parents, imagos of the single father and mother, especially the 'good' mother, are sufficiently strongly operative, the boy's growing relationship to objects and adaptation to reality will have the result that his phantasies about his father's penis inside his mother will lose their power, and his hatred, already reduced in any case, will be more strongly directed to his real object. This will have the effect that his imago of the combined parents is still more completely separated [into single figures]; and his mother will become pre-eminently the object of his libidinal impulses, while his hatred and anxiety will in the main go to his real father (or father's penis) or, by displacement, to some other object, as in the case of animal phobias. The separate imagos of his mother and father will then stand out more distinctly and the importance of his real objects will be increased; and he will now enter upon a phase in which his Oedipus trends and his fear of being castrated by his real father come into prominence.[1]

Nevertheless, the earliest anxiety-situations are, I have found, still latent in him to a greater or lesser degree, in spite of all the modifications they have undergone in the course of his development;[2] and

---

come to the conclusion that the phantasies which men often have that the woman's vagina conceals a big, 'dangerous' and moving penis — a female penis — receive their pathogenic value from the fact that they are unconsciously connected with ideas of the hidden presence in the mother's vagina of the father's huge and terrifying penis. In an earlier paper, 'Homosexualität und Polygamie' (1920), Boehm has also pointed out that men often have a desire to meet their father's penis inside their mother and that this desire is based on aggressive impulses against their father's penis.] Their impulse to attack his penis inside their mother's vagina and the repression of that aggressive impulse are important factors, Boehm thinks, in making them homosexual.

[1] When this happens it is a sign that the separation of his combined parent-imago has been successfully achieved, and that his infantile psychotic anxiety has been modified. Cf. Chapter IX.

[2] Cf. Chapters IX and X.

so, too, are all the defensive mechanisms and mechanisms belonging to later stages, which arise from those anxiety-situations. In the deepest layers of his mind, therefore, it is always by the 'bad' father's penis belonging to his mother that he expects to be castrated. But so long as his early anxiety-situations are not too powerful and, above all, so long as his mother stands for the 'good' mother to a sufficient extent, her body will be a desirable place, though a place which can only be conquered with greater or less risk to himself, according to the magnitude of the anxiety-situations involved. This element of danger and anxiety, which in every normal man allies itself to copulation, is an incentive to sexual activity and increases the libidinal satisfaction he gets from copulating; but if this incentive exceeds a certain limit it will have a disturbing effect and even prevent him from being able to perform the sexual act at all. In his deepest unconscious phantasies copulation involves overpowering or doing away with his father's penis supposed to be inside the woman. To this struggle with his father inside his mother are attached, I think, those sadistic impulses which are normally present when he takes possession of the woman in a genital way. Thus, while his original displacement of his father's penis to the inside of his mother's body makes her a permanent anxiety-object for him—though the degree to which this is so varies very greatly from person to person—it also increases the sexual attraction which women have for men very considerably, because it is an incentive to him to overcome his anxiety.

In the normal course of things, as the boy's genital trends grow stronger and he overcomes his sadistic impulses, his phantasies of making restitution begin to occupy a wider field. As has already been seen, restitutive phantasies in regard to his mother already exist while his sadism is still dominant and take the form of destroying his father's 'bad' penis inside her. Their first and main object is his mother, and the more she has stood for the 'good' object to him the more readily do his restitutive phantasies attach themselves to her imago.[1] This is especially clearly seen in play analysis. When the boy's reactive trends become stronger he begins to play in a constructive way. In games of building houses and villages, for instance, he will symbolize the restoration of his mother's body and his own[2] in a way that cor-

---

[1] That the boy's restitutive tendencies are directed to the 'good' object, and his destructive ones to the 'bad' object, has already been made clear in another connection.

[2] Since the boy's anxiety-situations in regard to his mother's inside and his anxiety concerning his own body are inter-related and interdependent, his phantasies of restoring his mother's body apply in every particular to the restoration of his own. We shall presently go on to consider this aspect of his phantasies of restitution.

responds in every detail with the acts of destruction he has played at in an earlier stage of his analysis, or still plays at in alternation with his constructive games. He will then build a town by putting houses together in all sorts of ways, and will set up a toy man—representing himself—as a policeman to regulate the traffic and this policeman will always be on the look-out to see that cars do not run into one another, or houses get damaged or pedestrians run over; whereas in former games the town was frequently being damaged by colliding vehicles, and the people knocked down. In a still earlier period, perhaps, his sadism took a more direct form and he used to wet, burn and cut up all sorts of articles which symbolized his mother's insides and its contents, i.e. his father's penis and children, while at the same time these destructive acts represented the damage his father's penis did and which he also wanted him to do there. As a reaction to these sadistic phantasies in which the violent and overpowering penis (his father's and his own), as represented by the moving cars, destroys his mother and injures the children inside, as represented by the toy people, he now has phantasies of restoring her body—the town—in all the respects in which he previously damaged it.

Restitutive Tendencies and Sexual Activities

It has repeatedly been said in these pages that the sexual act is a very important means of mastering anxiety for both sexes. In the early stages of the child's development the sexual act, in addition to its libidinal purposes, serves to destroy or injure the object (though positive tendencies are already at work behind the scenes). In later stages besides the libidinal satisfaction it provides the sexual act serves to restore the mother's injured body and thus to master anxiety and guilt.

In discussing the underlying sources of the girl's homosexual attitude, I pointed out how important to her is the idea of possessing a penis with healing powers and constructive omnipotence in the sexual act. What has been said there applies equally to the heterosexual attitude of the man. Under the supremacy of the genital stage he attributes to his penis in copulation the function not only of giving the woman pleasure, but of restoring all the damage which it and his father's penis have done in her. In analysing boys we find that the penis is supposed to perform all kinds of curative and cleansing functions. If, during his period of sadistic omnipotence, the boy has used his penis in imagination for sadistic purposes—such as flooding, poisoning or burning things with his urine—he will, in his period of making restitution, regard it as a fire-extinguisher, a scrubbing-brush or a container of healing medicines. Just as his former belief in the sadistic qualities of his own penis involved a belief in the sadistic power of his father's penis, so now his belief in his good 'penis' involves a belief in his father's 'good' penis; and just as then his sadistic phantasies went to transform his father's penis into an instrument of destruction for his mother, so now his restitutive phantasies and sense of guilt go to turn it into a 'good' organ with healing powers.[1] As a result, his fear of his 'bad' super-ego derived from his father becomes lessened, and he can reduce his identification with his 'bad' father in relation to his real objects (an identification which is in part based on his identification of himself with his anxiety-object) and enables him to identify himself more strongly with his 'good' father. If his ego is able to tolerate and modify a certain quantity of destructive feeling against his father and if his belief in his father's 'good' penis is strong enough, he can maintain both his rivalry with his father (which is essential for the establishment of a heterosexual position) and his identification with him. His belief in his father's 'good' penis increases the sexual attraction he feels for women, for in his phantasy they will then contain objects which are not so very dangerous and objects which—on account of his homosexual attitude in which the 'good' penis is a love-object—are actually desirable.[2] His destructive impulses will retain his father's rival penis as their object (experienced as a 'bad' object) and his positive impulses will be mainly directed to his mother.

Significance of the Feminine Phase in Heterosexuality

This result of the boy's development depends essentially on the favourable course of his early feminine phase. As I earlier emphasized it is a condition for a firm establishment of the heterosexual position that the boy should succeed in overcoming this phase. In an earlier paper[3] I pointed out that the boy often compensates the feelings of

[1] The boy's sense of guilt towards his mother and his fear that his father's 'bad' penis may do her harm contribute in no small degree to his endeavour to restore his father's penis as well and give it back to her, and to unite the two in an amicable fashion. In certain instances this desire can become so dominating that he will relinquish his mother as a love-object and make her over to his father entirely. This situation disposes him to go over to a homosexual position; in which case his homosexuality would serve the purpose of making restitution towards his father's penis, whose function it would then be to restore his mother and give her gratification.

[2] Where the boy's fear of the 'bad' penis or, not infrequently, his inability to tolerate his own sadism heighten his belief in the 'good' penis to an exaggerated degree, not only in regard to his father's penis inside his mother, but in regard to his super-ego, his attitude towards women may become quite distorted. The heterosexual act will serve first and foremost to satisfy his homosexual desires, and the womb will be nothing more than something which contains the 'good' penis.

[3] 'Early Stages of the Oedipus Conflict' (1928) *Writings*, I.

hate, anxiety, envy and inferiority that spring from his feminine phase by reinforcing his pride in the possession of a penis and that he displaces that pride on to intellectual activities.[1] This displacement forms the basis of a very hostile attitude of rivalry towards women and affects his character-formation in the same way as envy of the penis affects theirs. The excessive anxiety he feels on account of his sadistic attacks on his mother's body becomes the source of very grave disturbances in his relations to the opposite sex. But if his anxiety and sense of guilt becomes less acute it will be those very feelings which give rise to the various elements of his phantasies of restitution that will enable him to have an intuitive understanding of women.

This early feminine phase has yet another favourable effect on the boy's relations to women in later life. The difference between the sexual trends of the man and the woman necessitates, as we know, different psychological conditions of satisfaction for each and leads each to seek the fulfilment of different and mutually incompatible requirements in their relations to one another. Usually, the woman wants to have the object of her love always with her—in the last analysis, inside her; whereas the man, owing to his outwardly-orientated psycho-sexual tendencies and his method of mastering anxiety, is inclined to change his love-object frequently (though his desire to keep it, in so far as it represents his 'good' mother, goes against that tendency). Should he, in spite of these difficulties, nevertheless be able to be in touch with the mental needs of the woman, it will be to a large extent because of his earliest identification with his mother. For in that phase he introjects his father's penis as a love-object, and it is the desires and phantasies he has in this connection which, if his relation to his mother is a good one, help him to understand the woman's tendency to introject and preserve the penis.[2] In addition, the wish to have children by his father, which

[1] In her paper, 'Über die Wurzel der Wissbegierde' (1925), Mary Chadwick considers that the boy is reconciled to his inability to have a child by the exercise of his desire for knowledge and that scientific discovery and intellectual achievements take the place for him of having a child. It is, according to her, this displacement on to the mental plane of his envy of women for being able to have a child which makes him take up an attitude of rivalry to them in matters of intellect.

[2] Edoardo Weiss, in his paper, 'Über eine noch unbeschriebene Phase der Entwicklung zur heterosexuellen Liebe' (1925), states that the heterosexual choice of object made by the adult male results from the projection of his own femininity, and he believes that it is owing to this mechanism of projection that the adult man retains in part a maternal attitude towards his female partner. He also points out that the woman attains her final heterosexual position in a corresponding way, by giving up her masculinity and situating it in the man she loves.

springs from that phase, leads him to regard the woman as his child; and he plays the part of the bountiful mother towards her.[1] In this way he also satisfies his partner's love-wishes arising from her strong attachment to her mother. Thus, and only thus, by sublimating his feminine components and overcoming his feelings of envy, hatred and anxiety towards his mother,[2] which originated in his feminine phase, will the boy be able to consolidate his heterosexual position in the stage of genital dominance.

I have already mentioned why it is that, when the genital stage has been fully attained, a necessary condition for sexual potency should be that the boy believes in the 'goodness' of his penis—that is, in his capacity to make restitution by means of the sexual act.[3] This belief is ultimately bound up with a concrete condition—concrete from the point of view of psychic reality—namely the belief that the inside of his body is in a good state. In both sexes the anxiety-situations which arise from dangerous events, attacks and encounters inside one's own body and which dovetail with anxiety-situations relating to similar events inside the mother's body, constitute the most profound danger-situations. Fear of castration, which is only a part—though an important part—of the anxiety felt about the whole body, becomes, in the male individual, a dominating theme that overshadows all his other fears to a greater or lesser extent. But this is precisely because one of the deepest sources to which disturbances in his sexual potency go back is his anxiety about the interior of his body. The house or town which the boy is so keen to build up again in his play signifies not only his mother's renewed and intact body[4] but also his own.

Secondary Reinforcement of Penis-Pride

In describing the development of the boy, I have drawn attention to certain factors which tend, as I think, to increase yet more the

---

[1] Reich has shown that in many patients the penis assumes the role of the mother's breast, and semen, that of milk (cf. his *The Function of the Orgasm*, 1927).

[2] In an analogous manner by the successful overcoming of her penis envy and by the sublimation of her masculine components the girl creates the precondition for a well established heterosexual position.

[3] Such a conviction grows steadily stronger in analysis in proportion as the severity of his super-ego, anxiety and sadism diminish and the genital stage emerges more clearly, with an accompanying improvement in his relation to his object and in the relations between his super-ego, ego and id.

[4] The 'pure' and untouched woman then, is ultimately the woman who has not been sullied (destroyed) by his father's penis and his dangerous excrements, who can therefore give to the man good, healing—pure—substances out of her intact interior.

central significance which the penis possesses for him. They may be summed up as follows: (1) The anxiety arising from his earliest danger-situations—his fears of being attacked in all parts of his body and inside it—which include all his fears deriving from the feminine position, are displaced on to the penis as an external organ, where they can be more successfully mastered. The increased pride the boy takes in his penis, and all that this involves, may be said to be a method of mastering those fears and disappointments which his feminine position lays him open to more particularly.[1] (2) The fact that the penis is a vehicle first of the boy's destructive and then of his creative omnipotence, enhances its significance as a means of mastering anxiety. Moreover in thus fulfilling all these functions—i.e. in promoting his sense of omnipotence, his reality-testing and his relation to objects, and, by means of those functions, in serving the dominating function of mastering anxiety—the penis, or rather its psychic representative, is brought into specially close relation with the ego and is made into a representative of the ego and the conscious;[2] while the interior of the body, the imagos and the faeces—what is invisible and unknown, that is—are compared to the unconscious. Moreover, in analysing male patients, whether boys or men, I have found that as their fear of their bad imagos and faeces (i.e. the unconscious) that were supreme inside them diminished, their belief in their own sexual potency was strengthened and the development of their ego gained ground.[3] This latter effect is partly due to the fact that the boy's lessened fear of his 'bad' super-ego and the 'bad' contents of his body enables him to identify himself better with his 'good' introjected objects, and thus permits a further enrichment of his ego.

As soon as his confidence in the constructive omnipotence of his penis is firmly established, his belief in the power of his father's 'good' penis inside him will form the basis of a secondary belief in his omnipotence which will support and strengthen the line of development already laid down for him by his own penis. And, as has been said, the result of his growing relationship to objects will be that his unreal imagos recede into the background, while his feelings of hatred and fear of castration come into sharper relief and fix themselves on to his real father. At the same time his restitutive tendencies are increasingly directed towards external objects and his methods of mastering anxiety become more realistic. All these advances in his

---

[1] Cf. my 'Early Stages of the Oedipus Conflict' (1928, *Writings*, 1).

[2] This view is supported by a well-established fact of analytic observation, namely, that the penis and male potency stand for masculine activity in general.

[3] Cf. my paper, 'A Contribution to the Theory of Intellectual Inhibition' (1931, *Writings*, 1).

development run parallel with the growing supremacy of his genital stage and characterize the later stages of his Oedipus conflict.

Disturbances of Sexual Development

Stress has already been laid on the child's phantasy of its parents perpetually joined in copulation as a source of intense anxiety-situations. Under the influence of such a phantasy its mother's body represents above all a union of mother and father which is extremely dangerous and which is directed against the child. If the separation of this combined parent-imago does not take place to a sufficient degree in the course of its development, the child will be overtaken by severe disturbances both of its object-relationships and of its sexual life. A predominance of the combined parent-imago goes back, as far as my experience goes, to disturbances in the earliest relations of small children to their mother, or rather, to her breast.[1] This situation, while very fundamental in children of both sexes, is already different for each in the earliest stages of development. In the following pages I shall confine my attention to the boy and examine how these terrifying phantasies gain their predominance[2] and in what way they influence his sexual development.

In my analyses of boys and adult men I have found that when strong oral-sucking impulses have combined with strong oral-sadistic ones, the infant has turned away very early on from his mother's breast with hatred.[3] His early and intense destructive trends against her breast have led him to introject a 'bad' mother for the most part; and his concomitant and sudden giving up of her breast has been followed by an exceedingly strong introjection of his father's penis. His feminine phase has been governed by feelings of hatred and envy towards his mother, and at the same time, as a result of his powerful oral-sadistic impulses, he has come to have an intense hatred[4] and a correspondingly intense fear of his internalized father's penis. His extremely strong oral-sucking impulses have

[1] Cf. Chapter VIII.

[2] For a description of their application to the girl see the previous chapter.

[3] In some of these cases the sucking period has been short and unsatisfactory; in others the child had only been given the bottle. But even where the period of sucking has to all appearances been satisfactory, the child may nevertheless have turned away from the breast very soon and with feelings of hatred and may have introjected his father's penis very strongly. In this case, his behaviour must have been determined by constitutional factors. See Chapter VIII.

[4] The boy's over-strong hatred of his father's penis is based on excessively strong destructive phantasies directed towards his mother's breast and body; so that here, too, his early attitude to his mother influences his attitude to his father.

brought on phantasies of an uninterrupted and everlasting process of taking nourishment; but at the same time the receiving of nourishment and sexual satisfaction (both of them through copulation with the father's penis) have been transformed into torture and destruction. This leads him to the assumption that the interior of her body is filled to bursting point with his enormous 'bad' penises which are destroying her in all sorts of ways. In his imagination she has become not only the 'woman with a penis' but a kind of container for his father's penises and for his dangerous excrement which is equated with them.[1] In this way he has displaced on to his mother great quantities of hatred and anxiety which attached to his father and his father's penis.[2] Thus a strong and premature oral sadism on the one hand encourages the child to make attacks upon his parents joined in copulation and to be terrified of their imago in that aspect and on the other prevents him from forming a good mother-imago which could sustain him against his early anxiety-situations, and lay the foundation of a good super-ego in him (in the form of helping figures)[3] as well as becoming the basis of a heterosexual position.

To this must be added the consequence of a feminine phase which in such cases is too much governed by sadism. The boy's inordinately strong introjection of his father's monstrous 'bad' penis makes him believe that his body is exposed to the same dangers from within as his mother's is. And his introjection of his hostile combined parents, together with his very feeble introjection of a 'good' mother, work in the same direction. In giving rise to an excess of anxiety concerning his own inside, these introjective processes pave the way not only for serious mental ill-health but for severe disturbances in his sexual development. As I pointed out earlier in this chapter, the possession of 'good' contents in the body and with it, on the genital level, the

[1] The imagos which have arisen from these phantasies are usually not only quite at variance with the real picture of the boy's mother but entirely obscure it. Here cause and effect reinforce one another. Owing to the too strong operation of the boy's earliest anxiety-situations, the growth of his object-relationship and adaptation to reality have been arrested. As a consequence of this, his world of objects and reality cannot mitigate the anxiety belonging to those earliest anxiety-situations, so that these continue to dominate his mind. I have found that in such cases the child's relation to reality has remained permanently impaired; and consequently the reality continues to be received and evaluated later on predominantly according to his phantasized anxiety-situations.

[2] In the previous chapter we have traced an analogous process of displacement in the girl. Where her hatred and envy are mainly concerned with her father's penis which her mother has incoporated, she displaces those feelings, which were originally mostly directed to her mother, on to his penis, with the result that her attitude to men is open to severe disturbances.

[3] Cf. my paper, 'Personification in the Play of Children' (1929) *Writings*, I.

possession of a 'good' penis are a pre-condition of sexual potency. If the boy's attacks on his mother's breast and body have been exceptionally intense, so that, in his imagination, she has been destroyed by his father's penis and his own, he will have all the more need of a 'good' penis with which to restore her; and he will have to have especial confidence in his potency in order to dissipate his terrors of his mother's dangerous and endangered body, filled with his father's penises. Yet it is precisely his fear on account of his mother and the contents of his own body which prevents him from believing in his possession of a 'good' penis and sexual potency. The cumulative effect of all these factors may be to make him turn away from women as objects of love, and, according to what his early experiences have been, either to suffer from disturbances of potency in his heterosexual position or to become homosexual.[1]

Case History:

The patient was a thirty-five year old homosexual (Mr A) who suffered from a severe obsessional neurosis with paranoid and hypochondriacal traits and whose potency was severely disturbed. His feelings of distrust and aversion which dominated his relations to women in general, could in his analysis ultimately be traced to phantasies that his mother was continuously united with his father in intercourse when he could not see her. He assumed that the inside of her body was filled with his father's dangerous penises.[2] In the transference situation, his hatred and fear of his mother, which in various ways covered up the guilt which he felt in relation to her,[3] was always closely connected to the coital situation of his parents. A fleeting glance at my dress and appearance, when he felt very anxious, would always prove to Mr A that I looked ill or unkept and that I was not well. This in fact meant that I was internally poisoned and destroyed. These feelings could be traced back to the testing and anxious looks with which, as a small boy, he had eyed his mother in the morning in order to find out whether she had been poisoned or destroyed by intercourse with his father.[4] Every morning he expected

---

[1] In extreme cases his libido will be unable to maintain any position whatever.

[2] Owing to this displacement his mother acquired the qualities of his father's penis to such an extent that very little of her own personality remained. Mr A unconsciously identified her with his father's penis (consciously with a boy). As a result of these multiple displacements the patient had even consciously great difficulties in distinguishing between the sexes.

[3] Ernest Jones has pointed to this mechanism in his paper, 'Fear, Guilt and Hate' (1929).

[4] When Mr A's anxiety was particularly severe, the street and my house (and, as we found, the whole world) appeared to be drowned in dirt. In this

to find his mother dead. In this frame of mind, any detail, however insignificant, in his mother's appearance and behaviour, any difference of opinion between the parents, any minute change in his mother's attitude to him—in short, everything that occurred around him—became a piece of evidence that the ever-waited catastrophe had actually happened. His masturbation phantasies (wish-fulfilment) in which he imagined that his parents had destroyed each other in many ways, became a source of much worry,[1] fear and guilt. This anxiety made him watch his environment without interruption and increased his obsessional desire for knowledge. The constant desire to observe his parents during intercourse and to discover their sexual secrets absorbed all his ego-energy. At the same time this desire was reinforced by his wish to prevent his mother from having sexual intercourse and to protect her from the harm which his father's dangerous penis would cause her.[2]

His feelings with regard to his parents' intercourse were reflected in the transference situation in, among other things, the great interest which Mr A took in my cigarette smoking. If for instance, he noticed that there was a cigarette end still in the ashtray from the preceding session, or if there was a smell of smoke in the room he wondered whether I smoked a lot, whether I smoked before breakfast, if I smoked a good brand, and so on. These questions and their allied affects were connected with his fear for his mother. They were determined by his wish to hear how often and in which way his parents had intercourse during the night and what effect this had on his mother. His feelings of frustration, jealousy and hatred which were intimately connected with the primal scene found an outlet in those

state of mind Mr A identified me frequently with the charwoman who cleaned the stairs and who appeared to him so disgusting. This woman was so unpleasant in his eyes because she roused his sense of guilt and anxiety. She represented his mother who was degraded and impoverished through his fault and who tried in vain to clean the soiled and poisoned inside of her body —the house. As a consequence of his phantasies of having attacked his copulating parents and the inside of his mother's body with his poisonous excrements he felt responsible for her state.

[1] As I wish to illustrate that certain early anxiety situations may be at the root of severe sexual disturbances, I shall only pick out two factors from the wealth of early impressions and influences which had contributed to the outcome of his development: His mother was an ailing woman and his father was a harsh and tyrannical man who was feared by the whole family.

[2] The primary jealousy of the small child which leads the child to disturb the sexual satisfaction and intimacies of his parents receives in general a secondary and essential re-inforcement through anxiety. The child fears—in fulfilment of his sadistic phantasies—that his parents will injure or even kill each other in intercourse; and this fear impels the child to observe and disturb his parents.

affects with which Mr A reacted at times when for instance, I lit a cigarette at a moment which he considered inappropriate. He became furious and blamed me for lacking interest in him and thought that I was only concerned with smoking while I ignored the disturbance which it created for him, and so on. Then again, he suggested that I should give up smoking altogether. At other times he waited with impatience until I lit a cigarette; he almost asked me to do so, and could scarcely wait for the noise of the matches, but insisted that I should not strike the match when he was unprepared for it. It became clear that this state of tension was a repetition of the situation when, as a small boy, he listened at night for the noises which came from his parent's bed. He could scarcely contain himself until at last he heard the first signs of intercourse (the striking of the match) in order to be sure that the whole event would soon be over. But sometimes he had a real desire that I should smoke. This could be traced back to his fear as a small boy that both his parents were dead and to his longing for the noises of his parents in intercourse which would tell him that they were alive. In a later stage of analysis when he had less fear about the consequences of intercourse, the wish that I should smoke was determined in the following way: the trends of a later phase of development led to the wish for his parents to have intercourse because it was now equated with reconciliation and with an action that satisfied and healed them both. He also wished to be relieved of his feeling of guilt at having subjected his parents to deprivation.

So far as his own smoking was concerned, Mr A gave it up from time to time in the hope that this would remove his hypochondriacal complaints. He never persisted in this endeavour for very long because unconsciously smoking was also a remedy for these complaints. As the cigarette stood for his father's 'bad' penis, he imagined annihilating the 'bad' objects inside his body by smoking;[1] but as the cigarette also represented his father's 'good' penis, he smoked to restore his body and his objects inside him.

Mr A's obsessional symptoms were closely related to his numerous fears. By way of displacement they originated as 'charm and countercharm';[2] they served the purpose of confirming or refuting questions

[1] This phantasy may also provide an impetus towards alcoholism. Alcohol representing the bad penis or bad urine, serves to destroy the bad internalized penis. Melitta Schmideberg in her paper: 'The Role of Psychotic Mechanisms in Cultural Development' (1930) has pointed out that the drugs represent the 'good' penis which offers protection against the 'bad' introjected objects. Owing to the ambivalence [of the addict] the incorporated drug very soon receives the meaning of a 'bad' penis, and this fact lends a further impetus to addiction.

[2] Freud, *Totem and Taboo*, S.E. **13**.

as to whether his parents were having intercourse at the time, whether certain dangerous events connected with their intercourse had occurred as he expected, whether the injuries resulting from these events could be remedied, and so forth. The obsessional neurosis in all its elements was based on the destructive and constructive omnipotence which originated in him in relation to his parents combined in intercourse, and which had been enlarged and developed in relation to his wider surroundings.

Mr A's sexuality, which had a thoroughly obsessional character and was severely disturbed, served the same purpose of proof and counter-proof. His excessive fear of his father's penis interfered not only with the maintenance of his heterosexual position, but also with the establishment of his homosexuality.

As a result of his very strong identification with his mother and of his dominant phantasy of having incorporated his copulating parents, Mr A related to his own body dangers which threatened his mother from the incorporation of the penis. In the transference situation Mr A's hypochondriacal complaints often became more pronounced when his negative transference increased.[1] If for instance, whether for external or internal reasons, there was an increase in the strength of his phantasies that his mother was engaged in dangerous intercourse with his father, or that, as a consequence of intercourse, she was harbouring his father's dangerous penis inside herself—then his hatred of me, and at the same time his fears for the inside of his own body, also grew stronger. Because of this identification with his mother, he took everything that made him think that a catastrophe was happening inside her as an indication that the inside of his own body was also being destroyed. But the main reason for the hatred of his mother for copulating with his father was the danger to which she exposed not only herself but indirectly him too, since in his phantasy the internal parents were copulating inside his body.

In addition, when he imagined that his mother was joined with his father in intercourse she always became an enemy. For instance, he sometimes felt a very strong aversion to my voice and words. This aversion was not only based on an equation of my words with dangerous and poisonous excrements, but also on the phantasy that it was his father or rather his father's penis in me that spoke through me. This penis influenced my words and actions against him in a

---

[1] The details of the hypochondriacal complaints are generally determined by the structure and details of the sadistic phantasies. For example, I repeatedly found that sensations of burning are connected with urethral phantasies. As the urine was meant to scald the objects, it scalded the inside of his own body too. In these cases, furthermore, the father's internalized penis and its urine was given the capacity for scalding, poisoning and eroding.

hostile manner in the same way that his father within him made him act badly against his mother. He was also afraid that his father's penis could, when I spoke, jump out of my mouth and attack him. My words and my voice were therefore also equated with his father's penis.

If his mother was destroyed there was no longer a 'good' helpful mother. His phantasies in which his mother's breast was bitten and torn to pieces, or poisoned by means of urine and faeces led him very early to introject a poisoning and dangerous mother-imago who impeded the development of a 'good' mother-imago. This factor favoured the development of his paranoid traits too, in particular his ideas of being poisoned and persecuted. Both in the external world (originally in his mother's body) as well as inside his own body, the patient did not succeed in getting sufficient support against his father's penis and the pieces of stool representing persecutors. In this way not only were his fear of his mother and his castration anxiety increased, but also his faith in the 'good' inside of his body and his own 'good' penis was suppressed. This was an essential factor that contributed to the severe disturbance of his sexual development. The fear of damaging the woman with his 'bad' penis (or rather, of not being able to restore her in intercourse) was, apart from his fear of his mother's dangerous body, the basis for Mr A's disturbed potency.

The fact that his faith in the 'good' mother was not sufficiently established had a significant effect when he fell ill. During the war Mr A fought for a longish period in the front line and came through the dangers and troubles of the war relatively well. His severe breakdown occurred some time later on a journey in a small remote place where he fell ill with dysentery. His analysis revealed that the symptoms had reactivated the old hypochondriacal anxiety which was based on the anxiety situation, namely the fear of the 'bad' internal penis, poisoning excrements, and so on. The precipitating factor was the behaviour of his landlady in whose nursing care my patient was left for some time. The woman nursed him badly, treated him unkindly and did not even give him enough milk and food. This experience reactivated the trauma of being weaned with all its associated affects of hatred and anxiety. Over and above this, Mr A unconsciously took the landlady's behaviour as a full confirmation of his anxiety that there was no longer a 'good' mother and that he was hopelessly delivered over to internal destruction and to external enemies. His faith in the 'good' mother, which had never been sufficiently established, could not be maintained against the simultaneous and excessive activation of all his anxiety-situations. This lack of a good and helpful mother-imago which could act against his anxieties was the last, decisive element in bringing about his break-down.

As I have tried to show in the example of Mr A, the consequence of a displacement of hatred and fear from the father's penis to the mother is that the fears associated with the woman's body become excessively increased and the sources of heterosexual attraction excessively diminished.

Adoption of Homosexuality

With the displacement of everything that is frightening and un-canny onto the invisible inside of a woman's body, there is often an-other associated process, which appears to be a pre-condition for the full establishment of the homosexual position. In the normal attitude the boy's penis represents his ego and his conscious, as opposed to his super-ego and to the contents of his body which represent his uncon-scious. In his homosexual attitude this significance is extended by his narcissistic choice of object to the penis of another male, and this penis now serves as a counter-proof against all his fears concerning the penis inside him and the interior of his body. Thus in homo-sexuality one mode of mastering anxiety is that the ego endeavours to deny, control or get the better of the unconscious by over-emphasiz-ing reality and the external world and all that is tangible, visible and perceptible to consciousness.

In such cases I have found that where the boy has had a homo-sexual relation in early childhood he has had a good opportunity of moderating his feelings of hatred and fear of his father's penis and of strengthening his belief in the 'good' penis. Upon such a relation, moreover, all his homosexual affairs in later life will rest. These are designed to provide him with a number of assurances, of which I will mention a few of the most common: (1) that his father's penis, both internalized and real, is not a dangerous persecutor either (a) for him or (b) for his mother; (2) that his own penis is not destructive; (3) that his fears, as a small child, lest his sexual relations with his brother or brother-substitute should be discovered and he should be turned out of the house, castrated or killed[1] have no foundation and, even as an adult, are to be disproved, since his homosexual acts are followed by no evil consequences; (4) that he has got secret con-federates and accomplices, for in early life his sexual relations with his brother (or brother-substitute) meant that the two were banded together to destroy their parents separately or combined in copula-tion. In his phantasy his partner in love will sometimes take on the role of his father, with whom he undertook secret attacks upon his

[1] Behind this fear lurks the fear of his mother as a rival who tries to make him responsible for the castration and theft of his father's penis.

mother during the sexual act and by means of it (one of the parents being thus played off against the other); sometimes he will play the part of his brother who, with himself, set upon and destroyed his father's penis inside his mother and himself.

The feeling (based upon having sadistic masturbation phantasies in common) of being in league with another against the parents by means of the sexual act, a feeling which is, I think, of general importance for the sexual relations of small children,[1] is closely bound up with paranoic mechanisms. Where such mechanisms are very strongly operative the child will have a strong bias towards finding allies and accomplices in his libidinal position and object-relationship. The possibility of getting his mother on to his side against his father—ultimately, that is, of destroying his father's penis inside her by copulating with her—may become a necessary condition for his adoption of a heterosexual position; and it may enable him when he is grown up to maintain the heterosexual position in spite of his having marked paranoid traits. On the other hand, if his fear of his mother's dangerous body is too strong and his good mother-imago has not been able to develop, his phantasies of allying himself with his father against his mother and of joining with his brother against both parents, will incline him to establish a homosexual position.

The child's impulse to play off his objects against one another and to get power over them by securing secret allies has its roots, as far as I can see, in phantasies of omnipotence in which, by means of the magical attributes of excrements and thoughts, poisonous faeces and flatus are introduced into the bodies of his objects in order to dominate or destroy them. In this connection the child's faeces are the instruments of his secret attacks upon the inside of his objects and are regarded by him as evil-doing objects or animals who are acting in the interest of his ego. These phantasies of grandeur and omnipotence play a great part in delusions of persecution and reference and in delusions of being poisoned. They take the place of fears of similar secret attacks by his objects as persecutors,[2] and, in addition, sometimes make the patient afraid of his own excrements, in case they should turn upon his ego in a hostile and treacherous way. In analysing both children and adults I have also come across a fear that their faeces have in some way assumed an independent existence and are no longer under their control, and are doing harm to their internal and external objects against the will of the ego. In such instances the faeces were equated with all sorts of small animals such as rats, mice, flies, fleas and so on.[3]

[1] Cf. Chapter VII.   [2] Cf. Chapter VIII.

[3] My five-year-old patient Franz, for instance, who revealed marked psychotic traits in his analysis, was afraid in the dark of a multitude of rats and

In those individuals in whom paranoid anxiety in regard to stool and penis as persecutors predominates, the homosexual love-object will represent first and foremost an ally against their persecutors. The individual's libidinal desire for a 'good' penis will be strongly over-compensated and will serve the purpose of concealing his feelings of hate and fear towards the 'bad' penis. Should such a compensation fail, his hatred and fear of his love-object will prevail and effect a paranoic transformation of the beloved person into the persecutor.[1]

These mechanisms, which are dominant in cases of paranoic character, enter, though to a lesser degree, into every homosexual activity. The sexual act between men always in part serves to satisfy sadistic impulses and to confirm the sense of destructive omnipotence; and behind the positive libidinal relation to the 'good' penis as an external love-object there lurk, to a greater or lesser extent, according to the amount of hatred present, not only hatred of the father's penis but also destructive impulses against the sexual partner and the fear of him that they give rise to.

In his 'Homosexualität und Ödipuskomplex' Felix Boehm has turned his attention to 'the part played by that aspect of the Oedipus-complex which consists of the child's hatred of his father and of his death-wishes and active castration-wishes against him'.[2] He has shown that in performing homosexual acts the male individual very frequently has two aims: (1) to make his partner impotent for the heterosexual act, in which case it is mostly merely a question of keeping him away from women, and (2) to castrate him, in which case he wants to get possession of his partner's penis as well so as to increase his own sexual potency with women. (As regards the first aim), my own observations lead me to believe that in addition to the primary jealousy of his father which gives rise to his wish to keep other men away from women (i.e. his mother or sister) there is a fear of the risks his mother incurs in copulating with him. Since those risks arise not only from his father's penis but from his own sadistic penis, he is pro-vided with a very strong motive for adopting a homosexual position.[3]

---

mice who would come out of the next-door room into his bedroom and advance upon him as he lay in bed, one lot attacking him from above, the other from below. They represented faeces coming from his parents and entering his anus and the other openings of the body as a result of his own anal-sadistic attacks upon his parents.

[1] Cf. Chapter IX.

[2] *Int. Z. f. Psychoanal.* (1926), **12**.

[3] Freud has drawn attention to the fact that in some cases what contributes to a homosexual choice of object are feelings of rivalry that have been sur-mounted and aggressive tendencies that have been repressed. (Cf. 'Certain Neurotic Mechanisms in Jealousy, Paranoia and Homosexuality', 1922, *S.E.* **18**.) Sadger has emphasized the boy's rivalry with his father and his desire to

In this position, as I have found from analyses both of boys and men, he has made a pact in his unconscious with his father and brothers by which they shall all abstain from having intercourse with his mother (and sisters) so as to spare her and shall seek compensation for that abstention in one another. As regards the second aim, I am in full agreement with Boehm's view. The child's desire to castrate his father so as to get his penis and be potent in sexual intercourse with his mother urges him towards a homosexual position. In some instances I have ascertained that his aim was not only to get possession of an especially potent penis but to store up an enormous amount of semen which, according to the small child's phantasies, is necessary in order to give his mother sexual gratification.[1] In addition to this, he wants to put 'good' penises and 'good' semen inside himself so as to make the interior of his body whole and well. And this wish is heightened in the genital stage by his belief that if his inside is unimpaired he will be able to give his mother 'good' semen and children as well—a situation which goes to increase his potency in the heterosexual position. If, on the other hand, his sadistic trends predominate, his desire to get possession of his father's penis and semen by means of the homosexual act will also in part have a heterosexual aim. For in identifying himself with his sadistic father he will have all the more power to destroy his mother by copulating with her.

It has been said more than once that the desire for knowledge provides a motive force in general for the performance of the sexual act. But where the individual obtains satisfaction of his desire for knowledge in connection with homosexual activities he employs it in part to increase his efficiency in the heterosexual position. The homosexual act is designed to realize his early childhood desire of having an opportunity of seeing in what respect his father's penis differs from his own and to find out how it behaves in copulating with his mother. He wants to become more adept and potent in sexual intercourse with his mother.[2]

---

castrate him as factors in homosexuality ('Ein Fall von multipler Perversion mit hysterischen Absenzen', 1910). Ferenczi has pointed out that homosexuals entertain cruel death-wishes against their father as well as lustful-cruel phantasies of attack upon their mother ('On the Nosology of Male Homosexuality', 1914). Ernest Jones showed that oral sadism is a fundamental factor in the development of homosexuality in women. ('The Early Development of Female Sexuality' (1927).)

[1] The disproportion between the huge penis and vast quantities of semen which he thinks are needed to satisfy his mother and the smallness of his own penis is one of the things that help to render him impotent in later life.

[2] Boehm refers (loc. cit.) to a patient who used, among other things, to find out in his homosexual affairs with men what their 'sexual technique' with women was.

Case Material — Mr B

I shall now proceed to give extracts from a case history in order to illustrate the significance of some of the above-discussed factors in the adoption of the homosexual position. Mr B, a man in his middle thirties, came to me for treatment on account of a severe inhibition in work and deep depression. His inhibition in work, which was a fairly long-standing one, had been increased to such a degree by a certain event in his life which I shall presently describe, that he had been obliged to give up the research work he was engaged in and to resign his post as a teacher. It appeared that although the development of his character and his ego had been perfectly successful and he was unusually gifted intellectually, he suffered from severe disturbances of mental health. His fits of depression went back to early childhood but had become so acute in recent years that they had brought on a general state of depression and had led him to cut himself off from other people to a great extent. He was afraid—quite without cause—that his external appearance was repulsive, and this added more and more to his dislike of society. He also suffered from a severe doubting-mania, which covered the field of his intellectual interests to an ever-widening extent and was particularly painful to him.

Behind these more manifest symptoms I was able to elicit the presence of a profound hypochondria[1] and strong ideas of persecution and reference, which at times took on the character of delusions but to which he seemed curiously indifferent. As an example, on a journey he spent some time at a boarding house where he felt that a woman who was one of the guests living in the same house was pursuing him sexually and even plotted against his life. An indisposition—slight in itself—caused him to believe that he had been poisoned by a loaf of bread which this woman had bought for him. As a result of this feeling Mr B left the boarding house at once; but the following year he returned to it, although he knew that he would meet this woman again as she was a permanent guest there. This was the case and an intense social relationship developed between the two and they became close friends. In spite of this, Mr B did not abandon his suspicion that the woman had tried to poison him the previous year. He persuaded himself that she would not repeat the attempt as they were now on such good terms. It was remarkable that he did not resent the alleged attempt at murder. This was due partly to his far-reaching displacement of affects, partly to his tolerance and

---

[1] B—'s continual worry and preoccupation about his appearance proved to be a displacement outwards of his worry about the interior of his body and of his hypochondriacal anxiety concerning it.

intuitive understanding of other people. Apart from these factors his extraordinary power of dissimulation contributed to the fact that his ideas of reference and persecution, his hypochondriacal anxiety and even, to some extent, his serious obsessional symptoms did not become apparent to the people close to him. This extraordinary power of dissimulation went along with his paranoid characteristics, which were very strong. Although he felt that he was being observed and spied upon by people and was very suspicious of them, his psychological understanding was so great that he knew how to hide his thoughts and feelings completely. But alongside this dissembling and calculating strain in him there was a great freshness and spontaneity of feeling which sprang from his positive object-relationship and went back to strong hopeful feelings which originally existed in the depths of his mind; these latter had also helped him to conceal his illness from view, but in the last few years they had almost entirely ceased to work.

Mr B was a true homosexual. While having good relations to woman (and to men) as human beings,[1] as sexual objects he rejected them so completely that he was quite unable to understand how they could be supposed to possess any attraction whatever.[2] From a physical point of view they were something strange, mysterious and uncanny to him. The shape of their bodies repelled him, especially their breast and buttocks and their lack of a penis.[3] His dislike of their breast and buttocks was based on intensely strong sadistic impulses. He had phantasies of beating those 'sticking out' parts of their body until they became, as it were, 'beaten in' and thus 'reduced', and then perhaps, he said, he would be able to love women. These phantasies were determined by his unconscious idea that the woman was so full of the father's penises and dangerous excrements equated to the penis, that they had burst her open and were protruding out of her body. Thus his hatred of her 'sticking out' parts was really aimed at his father's internalized and re-emerging penises.[4] In his imagination the interior of the woman's body was an infinite and unexplorable expanse where every kind of danger and death lurked, and she

[1] But this good object-relationship to men and women was from time to time subjected to grave disturbances. At those times Mr B withdrew from contact with people as far as possible.
[2] He had had sexual intercourse once or twice in his life with women but he had never had any real satisfaction from it. His chief motives for engaging in an ephemeral affair of this kind were curiosity, a wish to do what other, heterosexual, men did, and, in especial, a dislike of wounding the feelings of the other party, who had in each case been the more willing one.
[3] We shall see later on why this lack terrified him so much.
[4] Mr A's sadistic feelings against the women's buttocks too, were determined by similar phantasies. As has been said in Chapter IV, the head, arms,

herself appeared to him only as a kind of container for terrifying penises and dangerous excrements. Her delicate skin and all her other feminine attributes he regarded as a quite superficial cover for the destruction that was going on inside her, and, although in themselves they pleased him, he dreaded them all the more as being so many signs of her deceitful and treacherous nature.

By likening the penis to pieces of stool my patient extended his displacement of the fear excited by his father's penis on to his mother's body still further and applied it to her poisonous and dangerous excrements as well. In this way he somehow covered up and put away all the things that he hated and feared inside his mother's body. That this far-reaching process of displacement had failed can be inferred from the fact that Mr B became once more aware of his concealed anxiety-objects in the shape of the female breasts and buttocks. They symbolized persecutors who were looking out of the woman's body and watching him; and, as he told me with evident dislike and anxiety, he would never dare even to strike or attack them because he was too frightened of touching them.

At the same time as he had thus displaced on to his mother's body all those things which aroused his fear, so that it became an object of aversion to him, he had idealized the penis and the male sex in a very high degree. To him, only the male, in whom all was manifest and clearly visible and who concealed no secrets within himself, was the natural and beautiful object.[1] As he displaced all that was capable of arousing his fear from his father's body on to his mother's interior so he very strongly repressed everything concerning the inside of his own body and accentuated everything that was visible, in particular his penis. But how strong were his doubts about this could be seen from the fact that when he was about five years old he had asked his nurse which she thought was worst—'in front or behind' (meaning penis or anus) —and had been very much taken aback when she had answered 'in front'. He also remembered when he was about eight years old standing at the top of the stairs and looking down them and hating himself and the black stockings he had on.[2] His associations

---

hands and feet of the woman are often regarded in the unconscious as the father's internalized penis that has come out again; her limbs—the pair of legs, feet or arms or even fingers—often signify both internalized parents.

[1] Since the possession of a penis was so necessary to him for overcoming anxiety, all B—'s fears about the interior of the woman's body were increased by the fact of her having no such external organ.

[2] Looking down meant looking inside himself. In other cases I have been able to discover that looking into the distance stood for introspection. It would seem that for the unconscious nothing is more distant and more unfathomable than the inside of the mother's body and, still more, the inside of one's own body.

showed that the interior of his parents' house had always seemed specially gloomy to him—'dead', in fact—and that he held himself responsible for this gloominess—or rather for the destruction inside his mother's body and his own, symbolized by the gloomy house—which he had brought about by his dangerous excrements (the black stockings). In consequence of his extensive repression of his 'inside' and his displacement of it on to his 'outside', Mr B had come to hate and fear the latter, not only in regard to his personal appearance, though this was a continual source of worry and care to him, but to other allied matters. For instance, he had the same loathing for certain articles of dress, especially his underclothes, that he had had for his black stockings and felt as though they were his enemies and were hemming him in and weighing him down by clinging so closely to his body.[1] They represented his internalized objects and excrements which were persecuting him from within. In virtue of the displacement of his fears of internal dangers into the external world, his enemies inside him had been transformed into enemies outside him.

I shall now turn to a consideration of the structure of the case. The patient had been bottle-fed. Since his libidinal components had not been satisfied by his mother, his oral-sucking fixation on the breast had been prevented. Owing to this frustration, too, his destructive impulses against the breast had been increased and he had transformed that part of the body into dangerous beasts and monsters in his imagination. (In his unconscious he likened female breasts to harpies.) This process had been assisted by his equation of the breast with his father's dangerous penis, which, he thought, had been put inside her body and was re-emerging from it. He had, moreover, very soon begun to liken the pacifier and the mouthpiece of the bottle to a 'good' penis and, in consequence of his frustration in regard to the breast, to turn to it with special eagerness as an object of satisfaction for his oral-sucking desires. His adoption of a homosexual attitude had been very greatly helped on by the fact that he had been seduced very early in life—some time approximately in his second year—by his brother, Leslie, who was about two years his senior. Since the act of *fellatio* satisfied his hitherto starved oral-sucking desires, this event led him to become excessively fixated on the penis. Another factor was that his father, who had up till then been a monosyllabic and

[1] In other cases of adults and children too, I have found things on the outside of the body represent things inside it. My six-year-old patient, Gunther, used always to be making paper snakes, winding them round his neck and then tearing them up. He did this in order to master his fear not only of his father's penis which was strangling him from outside, but of his father's penis which was suffocating him and killing him from within.

very undemonstrative man, became more affectionate under the influence of his youngest son. The little boy had been determined to win his love and he had succeeded. Analysis showed that he regarded this victory as a proof that he was able to turn his father's 'bad' penis into a 'good' one. And his efforts to effect a transformation of this kind and thus dissipate a number of fears became in later years one of his motives for having affairs with men.

Mr B had two brothers. For Leslie, who was two years older than himself, he had had a great admiration and love even as a small boy, and he made him the representative of the 'good' penis—partly, no doubt, on account of the early satisfaction of his oral cravings which he had received from him through the sexual act. His greatest ambition was to be intellectually his equal and to become worthy of his friendship; and, in fact, he chose the same profession. To his older brother, David, who was older than himself by four years, he had quite a different attitude. This brother was his father's son by a former marriage, and Mr B felt, probably correctly, that his mother showed a preference for her own sons over him. He did not like this brother and had managed to get the upper hand of him as a small child in spite of the difference in their ages. This was partly due to David's masochistic attitude, partly to his own great mental superiority over him. He vented his sadistic impulses towards the 'bad' penis upon this brother, with whom he had also had sexual relations in early childhood,[1] and at the same time he regarded him as the dangerous mother in whom were contained his father's penises. His brothers, it will be seen, were substitutes for both parents, to be more precise for the phantastic parent-imagos and it was towards them that he activated his relations to those imagos; for whereas he was devoted to his mother in real life and loved her much more than his father, he was possessed in phantasy, as we know, by imagos of the magical 'good' penis (his father) and of the terrifying mother. He never got to like David even in later life, and this was partly because, as analysis showed, he felt so very guilty towards him.

While, therefore, a number of factors were present to encourage Mr B's adoption of a homosexual attitude, a number of other external ones were already working very early on against his establishment of a heterosexual position. His mother was very fond of him, but he soon found out that she was not really loving towards his father and had an aversion to the male genital in general. He was

---

[1] B—'s sexual relations with his brothers were discontinued after the first period of childhood; nor had he any conscious recollection of them. On the other hand, he remembered quite clearly and in great detail having tormented his brother David very much, and this cruel behaviour was closely related, as analysis showed, with the sexual activities he had forgotten about.

most likely right in his impression that she was frigid and disapproved of his own sexual desires, and her very marked love of order and cleanliness gave the same effect. The nurses he had had as a small child were also antipathetic towards anything that was sexual or instinctual. (This was also implied in his nurse's answer that 'in front' was worse than 'behind'.) Another thing which worked against the establishment of a heterosexual position was his having had no little girls to play with. There is no doubt that his fear of the mysterious interior of the woman's body would have been greatly lessened had he been brought up with a sister, for then he would have satisfied his sexual curiosity concerning the female genitals much earlier. As it was, it was not until he was about twenty years old that, on looking at a picture of a naked woman, he first consciously realized in what respect the female body differed from the male. It turned out in analysis that the voluminous and spreading skirts which women wore (at that time) increased a thousandfold his idea of the mysterious and perilous expanse of the interior of their bodies. His not knowing about these matters which sprang from his anxiety but which had been encouraged by the external factors described above had helped to make him reject the woman as a sexual object.

In my description of the development of the male individual I have shown that the centering of his sadistic omnipotence on his penis is an important step in the establishment of a heterosexual position, and that in order to effect such a step his ego must have acquired sufficient capacity to tolerate his sadism and anxiety in earlier stages of his development. In Mr B this capacity was small. His belief in the omnipotence of his excrements was stronger than is usual in boys.[1] His genital impulses and his feelings of guilt, on the other hand, had come to the fore very early and had soon brought with them a good relationship to his objects and a satisfactory adaptation to reality. His ego, strengthened early on as it was, had in consequence been enabled to repress his sadistic impulses violently, especially those directed against his mother, so that these could not get into sufficient contact with his real objects and remained for the most part — again, most of all as far as his mother was concerned — attached to his phantastic imagos. The result of this was that side by side with the good relation he had to his objects of both sexes[2] there still went a

[1] For the same reason he had fairly strong feminine characteristics and his sublimations were of a predominantly feminine cast. This point will receive notice later on.

[2] B—'s unsuccessful super-ego formation (i.e. the overstrong action of his earliest anxiety-formations) had not only led to severe disorders in his mental health, to an impairment of his sexual development and to an inhibition of his capacity to work, but was the reason why his object-relationships, while in themselves good, were at times subjected to grave disturbances.

profound and dominating fear of their bad and phantastic imagos, and these two attitudes towards his objects ran a parallel but separate course without ever being sufficiently interwoven.

Not only could Mr B not employ his penis as the executive organ of his sadism against his mother; he could not give effect to his desires to restore her by means of his 'good' penis in the sexual act.[1] As regards his father's penis his sadism was much less strongly repressed. Nevertheless, he could not give sufficient effect to his direct Oedipus trends because the factors discussed above worked too powerfully against the attainment of a heterosexual position. His hatred of his father's penis could thus not be modified in a normal way. It had to be in part over-compensated by a belief in the 'good' penis, and this formed the basis of his homosexual position.

In the course of his flight from all that was anal and all that had to do with the inside of the body, and assisted by his very strong oral-sucking fixation on the penis and by the factors already described, B had very early in life developed a great admiration for the penis of other boys—an admiration which in certain instances amounted almost to worship. But analysis showed that in consequence of his intense repression of anal matters the penis had taken on anal qualities in a high degree. He thought of his own penis as inferior and ugly (as 'dirty' through and through, it turned out), but even his admiration for the penis of other men and boys was subject to certain conditions. A penis which did not fulfil these conditions was repulsive to him, for it then took on all the characteristics of his father's dangerous penis and of 'bad' pieces of stool. In spite of this limitation, however, he had attained a fairly stable homosexual position. He had no conscious sense of guilt or inferiority about his homosexual activities, for in them his restitutive trends, which had not been able to come out in the heterosexual position, unfolded their capacity to the full.

Mr B's erotic life was dominated by two types of object. The first, to which he had turned again and again ever since his schooldays, consisted of boys, and later on men, who were not attractive and who felt with reason that they were unpopular. This type answered to his brother David. Mr B got no pleasure from having sexual relations with a person of this type because his sadistic impulses came into play too powerfully, and he was himself aware that he used to make the other feel his superiority and torment him in all sorts of ways. At the same time, however, he would be a good friend to his love object and would exert a favourable mental influence on him and help him in every way. The second type answered to his other brother, Leslie. He

---

[1] In the previous chapter mention has been made of one or two factors which enable the individual of either sex to restore his or her object by means of the sexual act.

used to fall very deeply in love with this kind of person and would have a real adoration for his penis.[1]

Both types served to satisfy Mr B's restitutive trends and to allay his anxiety. In his relations to the first type, copulating meant restoring his father's and his brother David's penis, which, on account of his powerful sadistic impulses against them, he imagined he had destroyed. At the same time he identified himself with his inferior and castrated object, so that his hatred of the object was also directed towards himself, and his restitution of the penis of that object implied a restitution of his own penis. But ultimately his restitutive trends towards the penis served the purpose of restoring his mother; for it transpired that his having castrated his father and brother meant having attacked the children inside his mother and that he felt deeply guilty towards her on account of this. In restoring his father's and his brother's penis he was endeavouring to give his mother back an unhurt father, unhurt children and an intact interior. The restoration of his own penis meant, furthermore, that he had a 'good' penis and could give his mother sexual satisfaction.

In Mr B's relations to the Leslie type his desires to make restitution came less into prominence, for in this case he was concerned with the 'perfect' penis. This admired penis stood for a whole number of magical counter-proofs against all his fears. And since he identified himself with his loved object in this case as well, the 'perfect' penis was a proof that his own penis was 'perfect' too; and it also showed that his father's penis and his brother's were intact and strengthened his belief in the 'good' penis in general and thus in the unharmed state of his mother's body. In this relation to the admired penis, too, his unconscious sadistic impulses found an outlet; for here as well his homosexual activities signified a castration of his loved object, partly on account of his jealousy of him and partly because he wanted to get hold of his partner's 'good' penis so as to be able in all respects to take his father's place with his mother.

Although Mr B's homosexual position had been established so early on and so strongly, and although he consciously rejected a heterosexual one, he had always unconsciously kept the heterosexual aims in view towards which, as a small boy, he had striven so ardently in his imagination, and as an adult never quite relinquished. To his unconscious his various homosexual activities represented so many bypaths leading to this unconsciously desired goal.

The standards imposed by his super-ego upon his sexual activities were very high. In copulation he had to make good every single thing

[1] On one occasion he had an affair with a third type of person who corresponded to his father. It happened against his will, but he could not avoid it and it aroused great anxiety in him.

he had destroyed inside his mother. His work of restoration began, for the reasons we have seen, with the penis, and there, too, it ended. It was as though a person wanted to put up a particularly fine house but was filled with doubts as to whether he had well and truly laid the foundations. He would keep on trying to make those foundations more solid and would never be able to leave off working at them.

Thus Mr B's belief in his ability to restore the penis was also the foundation of his mental stability, and when that belief was shattered he fell ill. This was what happened: Some years before, his beloved brother Leslie had lost his life on a journey of exploration. Although his death had affected Mr B very deeply, he did not break down mentally. He was able to bear the blow because it did not arouse his sense of guilt or undermine his belief in his constructive omnipotence to any great extent. Leslie had been for him the possessor of the magical 'good' penis, and Mr B could transfer his belief in him and love of him on to someone else as a substitute. But now his brother David fell ill. Mr B devoted himself to him during his illness and hoped to effect his cure by the exertion of a strong and favourable influence upon him. But his hopes were cheated and David died. It was this blow that shattered him and brought on his illness. Analysis showed that this second blow had hit him much harder than the first because he had a strong sense of guilt towards his eldest brother. Above all, his belief that he could restore the damaged penis had been undermined. This meant that he had to abandon hope about all the things which in his unconscious he was endeavouring to restore—in the last resort his mother and his own body. The severe inhibition in his work that overtook him was another consequence of his loss of hope.

I have emphasized the reasons why it was that his mother could not become the object of his restitutive trends, as carried out by copulation, and therefore could not be a sexual object to him. She could only be the object of his tender emotions. But even so his anxiety and sense of guilt were too great; and not only were his object-relations exposed to severe disturbances, but his sublimatory trends were much impeded. It turned out that Mr B, who was consciously a good deal preoccupied about his mother's health—although, as he said himself, she was not ill, but 'delicate'—was in his unconscious completely dominated by this worry. He gave expression to it in the transference-situation by being in continual fear, just before his analysis broke off for the holidays (and, as it turned out later, before every week-end, and even between one day and the next), that he would never see me again, as some fatal accident might have overtaken me in the meantime. This phantasy, which recurred again and again with all sorts of variations, had the same main theme running through it—that I should be knocked down and run over by a motor-car in a crowded street. This street was in fact a street in his home town in America and played a great part in his childhood memories. When he used to go out with his nurse he had always crossed it in the fear—as analysis showed—that he would never see his mother again. Whenever he was in a state of deep depression he used to say in his analysis that things could never be 'right again' and he would never be able to work any more unless certain things which had happened in the world since he was a small child could be made not to have happened—as, for instance, that all the traffic which had passed along that street should not have passed along it. To him, as to the children whose analyses I have reported in an earlier part of this book, the movement of cars represented the act of copulation between his parents, which in his early masturbation phantasies, he had transformed into an act fatal to both parties, so that he became a prey to the fear that his mother and (because of his introjection of the 'bad' penis) he, too, would be wrecked by his father's dangerous penis incorporated within her (run over by a car). Hence his manifest fear that she and he would be run over by a car. In contrast to his native town, which he thought of as a dark, lifeless and ruined place in spite of the fact—or because of the fact, as it became clear—that there was a lot of traffic there (i.e. continual copulation between his father and mother), he pictured an imaginary city full of life, light and beauty, and sometimes found his vision realized, though only for a short time, in the cities he visited in other countries.[1] This far-off visionary city represented his mother once more made whole and reawakened to a new life, and also his own restored body. But the excess of his anxiety made him feel that a restoration of this kind could not be accomplished. His inhibition in work sprang from the same source.

During the time when Mr B was still able to work he was engaged in writing a book in which he set down the results of his scientific researches. This book, which he had to give up writing when his inhibition in work grew too strong, had the same meaning for him as the beautiful city. Each separate bit of information, each single sentence, denoted his father's restored penis and wholesome children, and the book itself represented his internalized wholesome mother and his own restored body. It emerged in analysis that it was his fear of the 'bad' content of his own body which was the principal hindrance to his creative powers. One of his hypochondriacal symptoms was a feeling of immense emptiness inside. On the intellectual plane

[1] Here again every detail of his beautiful make-believe city pictured a restoration and further beautification and perfecting his mother's body and his own, which, as he imagined, had suffered damage and destruction.

it took the form of a complaint that things that were valuable and beautiful and interesting to him lost their value and were 'worn out' and taken away from him in some way. The deepest root of this complaint turned out to be his fear that in ejecting his bad imagos and dangerous excrements he might have lost those contents of his body which were 'good' and 'beautiful'.

The most powerful motive force of his creative work came from his feminine position. In his unconscious a certain condition was imposed: not unless his body was filled with good objects—actually with beautiful children[1]—could he create, i.e. bring children into the world. In order to obey this condition he had to get rid of the 'bad' objects inside him (but then he felt empty); or else he had to turn them into 'good' ones, just as he wanted to turn his father's penis and his brother's into 'good' penises. If he had been able to do this he would have gained the assurance that his mother's body and her children and his father's penis were all restored too; then his father and mother would have been able to live together in amity and to give each other complete sexual satisfaction, and he himself, in identification with his 'good' father, could have given his mother children and could have consolidated his heterosexual position

When my patient once more took up his book, after an analysis of fourteen months' duration, his identification with his mother came to the fore very clearly. It showed itself in the transference-situation in phantasies of being my daughter. He remembered that when he was a small boy he longed to be a girl consciously, because he knew that his mother preferred a daughter; but, unconsciously, he could then have loved her sexually as well. For he would not have had to be afraid of hurting her with his penis, which was hateful to her and which he himself felt to be dangerous.[2] But in spite of his strong identification with his mother and his markedly feminine characteristics—characteristics which came out in his book as well—he had not been able to maintain the feminine position. This was a fundamental stumbling-block in the way of his creative activities, which had always to some extent been inhibited.

As his identification with his mother and his desire to be a woman

---

[1] In the last chapter we have seen that the girl's belief in the omnipotence of excrements is more strongly developed than the boy's and that this factor has a specific influence on the character of her sublimations. I have shown the current of sublimation which flows from the 'bad' and ugly piece of stool to the 'beautiful' child. B—'s belief in the omnipotence of his penis as the executive organ of sadism was not adequately effective and his belief in the omnipotence of excrements was relatively stronger; consequently his sublimations were of a distinctly feminine type.

[2] B— recollected having repeatedly tried as a small boy to squeeze his penis between his thighs so as to make it vanish from view.

became more prominent in his analysis his inhibition in work gradually diminished. His wish to have children and, concurrently, his creative capacities had been checked by his fear of his internalized objects in the first instance. For his fear of his mother as a rival was directed first and foremost towards his internalized 'bad' mother who was united with his father. It was to those internalized objects, too, that his intense fear of being watched and observed referred. He had, as it were, to preserve every thought from them, for each thought represented a 'good' bit inside him—a child.[1] For this reason he would commit his thoughts to paper as rapidly as possible so as to protect them from the 'bad' objects which would get in his way in writing. He had to undertake a separation of 'good' objects from 'bad' ones inside his body and also to transform the 'bad' ones into 'good' ones. His work in writing his book and the whole process of mental production entailed by it were likened in his unconscious to restoring the inside of his body and creating children. These children were to be his mother's, and he restored his 'good' mother within himself by filling her with beautiful restored children and by carefully trying to preserve those re-created (i.e. restored) objects from the 'bad' objects inside him, which were his parents combined in copulation and his father's 'bad' penis. In this way he made his own body sound and beautiful as well, because his 'good' beautiful and wholesome mother would in her turn protect him from the 'bad' objects inside him. With this 'good' restored mother Mr B was able also to identify himself. The beautiful children (thoughts, discoveries) with which, in his imagination, he peopled his inside were the children which he had conceived in identification with his mother as well as the children which he had begot with her as the 'good' mother—that is, the mother who gave him wholesome milk and thus helped him to get a sound and potent penis. And it was not until he was able to adopt and sublimate this feminine position that his masculine components became more effective and fruitful in his work.

As his belief in his 'good' mother grew stronger and, in consequence, his paranoid and hypochondriacal anxiety and also his depressions became less intense, Mr B became proportionately more able to carry on his work, at first showing every sign of anxiety and compulsion but later doing it with much greater ease. Hand in hand with this there went a steady diminution of his homosexual impulses. His adoration of the penis grew less and his fear of the 'bad' penis, which

[1] His fear of his bad imagos, which made him endeavour to deny and subdue his unconscious to a more than ordinary degree, had a great deal to do with the inhibition of his productive powers. He could never abandon himself completely to his unconscious, and so an important source of creative energy was closed to him.

had hitherto been overlaid by his admiration for the 'good' (the beautiful) penis, came to light. In this phase we became acquainted with a particular fear, namely, that his father's 'bad' internalized penis had got possession of his own penis by thrusting its way inside it and controlling it from within.[1] Mr B felt that he had thus lost command over his own penis and could not use it in a 'good' and productive way. This fear had come up very strongly when he was in the age of puberty. At that time he was trying with all his might to keep himself from masturbating. In consequence he was having nocturnal emissions. This started a fear in him that he could not control his penis and that it was possessed by the devil. He also thought that it was because it was possessed by the devil that it could change its size and become larger or smaller, and he attributed all the changes it underwent in connection with his development to the same cause.

This fear had greatly contributed to his dislike of his own penis and to his feeling that it was inferior, in the sense of being anal, 'bad' and destructive. There arose in connection with it an important impediment, too, to his adoption of a heterosexual position. Since he must suppose that his father's penis would always be watching him while he had coitus with his mother and would force him to commit bad actions, he was obliged to keep away from women. It now became evident that the excessive emphasis he had put upon his penis as the representative of the conscious and the visible and, connected with this, his manifold repressions and denials regarding the inside of his body had failed in this point as well. As soon as this set of fears had been analysed, Mr B's capacity for work was still further increased and his heterosexual position reinforced.

At this point in the progress of his analysis my patient had to stop coming to me for some time for external reasons.[2] The results so far

[1] In my analyses of male patients of all ages I have more than once come across this special danger-situation in which the father's 'bad' penis fills up the subject's own penis from within and thus takes complete possession of it. For instance, a small patient of mine once put a pencil with a pencil-cap into the fire. He wanted to burn out of the pencil-cap something 'bad', something strong and hard, that was contained in it. The pencil-cap represented his own penis and the 'bad' thing (the pencil itself) that had to be burnt out of it was his father's penis. On another occasion he put a bit of wood in the fire and at the same time sharpened his pencil, explaining that he did this so that the 'bad' wood should burn better. It turned out that in his imagination the bit of wood and the pencil belonged together and stuck into each other and fought with one another. Upon being analysed, this danger-situation sets free anxiety of a specially intense kind and it is, I think, a serious obstacle to sexual potency in the man.

[2] For personal reasons Mr B was obliged to return to his home country. He intends to continue his analysis which has lasted 380 treatment sessions in two years.

were that his deep depressions and his inhibition in work had been almost completely removed and his obsessional symptoms and the paranoid and hypochondriacal anxiety considerably diminished. These results justify us, I think, in believing that a further period of treatment will enable him fully to establish a heterosexual position. But in order to bring this about it is clear from the analysis that has already been done that his fears of his unrealistic mother-imago will have to be still further reduced, so that his real objects and his imaginary ones, so widely separated in his mind, may come closer together, and his growing belief in his 'good' restored mother and in his possession of a 'good' penis, which has up till now for the most part been directed towards his internalized mother and helped to remove his inhibition in work, may have its full effect upon his relations to women as sexual objects. Furthermore, his fear of his father's 'bad' penis must be still further reduced so as to strengthen his identification with his 'good' father.

In the case under discussion it will be seen that the factors upon whose stronger operation depends the patient's complete change from homosexuality to heterosexuality are the same factors as those whose presence has been mentioned in the first part of this chapter as a necessary condition for the firm establishment of a heterosexual position. In tracing the development of the normal male individual I pointed out there that the foundation of a successful sexual development of the male is the supremacy of the 'good' mother-imago which assists the boy to overcome his sadism and works against all his fears. As in the case of his fears of the mother's body and his own interior, the boy's desire to restore his mother's body and his desire to restore his own interact, the fulfilment of the one being essential to the fulfilment of the other. In the genital stage they are a pre-condition for his attainment of sexual potency. An adequate belief in the 'good' contents of his body which neutralizes, or rather opposes, its 'bad' contents and excrement seems to be necessary in order that his penis, as the representative of his body as a whole, shall produce 'good' and wholesome semen. This belief, which coincides with his belief in his capacity to love, depends upon his having sufficient belief in his 'good' imagos, especially in his 'good' mother and in her intact and wholesome body.

When he has attained the full genital level the male individual returns in copulation to his original source of satisfaction, his bountiful mother, who now gives him genital pleasure as well; and, partly as a return gift, partly as a reparation for all the attacks he has made on her from the time he did injury to her breast, he gives her his 'wholesome' semen which shall endow her with children, restore her body and afford her oral satisfaction as well. The anxiety and sense of guilt that are still present in him have increased and deepened and lent shape to his primary libidinal impulses as an infant at the breast, giving his attitude towards his object all that wealth and fullness of feeling which we call love.

APPENDIX

The Scope and Limits of Child Analysis

IN regard to the adult the function of psycho-analysis is clear. It is to correct the unsuccessful course which his psychological development has taken. In order to do this it must aim at harmonizing his id with the demands of his super-ego. In effecting an adjustment of this kind it will also put his now strengthened ego in a position to satisfy the demands of reality as well.

But what about children? How does the analysis affect a life which is still in the process of development? In the first place, analysis resolves the sadistic fixations of the child and thus decreases the severity of its super-ego, at the same time lessening its anxiety and the pressure of its instinctual trends; and, as its sexual life and super-ego both reach a higher stage of development its ego expands and becomes able to reconcile the demands of its super-ego with those of reality as well, so that its new sublimations are more solidly founded and its old ones shed their erratic and obsessive character.

At the age of puberty the child's detachment from its objects, which should go along with a rising of its internal demands, can only take effect if its anxiety and sense of guilt do not overstep certain limits. Otherwise its behaviour will have the character of flight rather than of genuine detachment; or the detachment will break down and the adolescent will remain for ever fixated to his original objects.

If the child's development is to have a satisfactory outcome the severity of its super-ego must become mitigated. Greatly as the aims at each developmental period may differ from one another, the attainment of them depends in each case upon the same fundamental condition, namely, upon an adjustment between the super-ego and the id, and the consequent establishment of an adequately strong ego. Analysis, in helping to effect an adjustment of this kind, follows and supports the child's natural line of growth at every stage of its development. At the same time it regulates the child's sexual activities. By lessening the child's anxiety and feelings of guilt it restricts those activities in so far as they are compulsive and promotes them in so far as they have led to a fear of touching or being touched. In thus affecting the factors that underlie a faulty development as a whole, analysis also lays the foundations for the unimpeded development of the child's future sexual life and personality.

My observations during child analysis have shown that the further analysis penetrates into the underlying strata of the mind the more the pressure of the super-ego is relieved. But we must ask ourselves whether it is not possible that the analytic procedure may go too deep and greatly diminish the function of the super-ego or even abolish it altogether. As I see it, libido, super-ego and object-relationship interact in their development, and the libidinal and destructive impulses, besides being fused together, exert a reciprocal action upon each other; and we have also seen that when anxiety is aroused as a result of sadism the demands of those two sets of impulses are heightened.[1] Thus the anxiety which emanates from the earliest danger-situations not only exerts a great influence upon the libidinal fixation-points and sexual experiences of the child, but is actually bound up with them and has itself become an element of those libidinal fixations.

Psycho-analytic experience has shown that even a very thorough-going treatment will only lessen the strength of the child's pre-genital fixation-points and sadism, never remove them altogether. Only a portion of its pre-genital libido can be converted into genital libido. This familiar fact is equally true, in my opinion, of the super-ego. The anxiety which the child has as a result of its destructive impulses, and which answers both in quantity and quality to its sadistic phantasies, coincides with its fear of dangerous internalized objects[2] and leads to definite anxiety-situations; and these anxiety-situations are attached to its pre-genital impulses, and as I have endeavoured to show, can never be entirely done away with. Analysis can only weaken their power, in so far as it reduces the child's sadism and anxiety. Hence it follows that the super-ego belonging to the early stages of childhood never completely relinquishes its functions. All that analysis can do is to relax the pre-genital fixations and diminish anxiety and thus assist the super-ego to move forward from pre-genital stages to the genital stage. Every advance in this lessening of the severity of the super-ego is a further victory for the libidinal instinctual impulses over the destructive ones and signifies that the libido has attained the genital stage in a fuller measure.

The view that the early anxiety-situations never cease to operate completely also demarcates the limits of psycho-analysis, for it follows that a complete cure does not exist, and that psycho-analytic treatment—whether in the child or in the adult—cannot exclude the possibility of a future breakdown with absolute certainty. In this context I should like to consider the factors that bring on psycho-neurotic illness. I shall not discuss those very numerous cases in which the illness has gone back to the early childhood of the individual, sometimes changing its features in the course of his life, sometimes keeping to its original character, but shall confine myself to those cases in which the outbreak of the illness has apparently dated from a particular moment in his life. Here, too, analysis shows that the illness was there already in a latent form, but that, as a result of certain events, it entered upon an acute stage which made it an

[1] Whereas a certain modicum of anxiety in the child increases its need for love and shapes its capacity for loving, excess of anxiety has a paralysing effect on them.

[2] Cf. Chapter VIII.

illness from a practical point of view. One way in which this can happen is that the individual may meet with events in his life which confirm his predominating early anxiety-situations to such an extent that the quantity of anxiety present in him rises to a pitch which his ego cannot tolerate and becomes manifest as an illness. Or, again, external events of an unfavourable kind may receive their pathogenic effect by causing disturbances in the process of mastering anxiety, with the result that his ego is left helplessly exposed to the excessive pressure of anxiety. In this way, by shaking his belief in his helpful imagos and in his own constructive capacities[1] and thus disrupting his means of mastering anxiety, some disappointment, quite slight in itself, can precipitate an illness in him quite as well as an event which confirms his early fears in reality and increases his anxiety. These two factors go hand in hand to a certain extent; and any occurrence which acts in both ways at once is specially calculated to bring on mental illness.[2]

It will be seen from what I have said that the child's early anxiety-situations are the basis of all psycho-neurotic affections. And since, as we know, analysis can never stop the operation of those situations altogether, either in the treatment of adults or children, it cannot ever effect a complete cure nor entirely exclude the possibility that the individual will succumb to a psychological illness at some later date. But what it can do is to bring about a relative cure in the child and so greatly lessen the chances of a future illness—and this is of the greatest practical importance. The more analysis can do in the way of reducing the force of the child's early anxiety-situations and of strengthening its ego and the methods employed by its ego in mastering anxiety, the more successful will it be as a prophylactic measure.

I see another limitation of psycho-analysis in the fact that it has varying success with different individuals owing to the variations that exist, even in small children, in the mental composition of the individual in question. The extent to which analysis is able to resolve anxiety will depend very greatly upon how much anxiety is present, what anxiety-situations predominate, and which are the

[1] In the previous chapter I described a patient whose breakdown was precipitated by the unkind behaviour of his landlady who nursed him badly during an illness. In that patient every dominant anxiety-situation was activated by the dysentery from which he suffered; in addition, the landlady's attitude seemed to confirm that there was no 'good' mother and that his restitutive trends were fruitless, too.

[2] In his paper, 'The Problem of Paul Morphy' (1931), Ernest Jones has described an instance where the occasion of illness was based on different mechanisms. He has shown that the psychosis to which Morphy, the famous chess-player, succumbed had the following causes. His mental balance depended upon the fact that in playing chess he was able to express his aggression—directed towards his father-imagos—in an ego-syntonic manner. It so happened that the person whom he most wanted to meet as his opponent evaded his challenge and behaved in such a way as to arouse his sense of guilt; and this was the exciting cause of Morphy's illness.

principal defensive mechanisms which the ego has predominantly evolved in the early stages of his development—in other words, upon what the structure of his mental disturbance in childhood has been.[1]

In fairly severe cases I have found it necessary to carry on analysis for a long time—for children from five to thirteen years old, between eighteen and thirty-six working months, and in one case forty-five months, and for some adults longer still—before the anxiety had been sufficiently modified, both in quantity and quality, for me to feel justified in ending the treatment. On the other hand, the disadvantage of such a lengthy treatment is fully made up for by the more far-reaching and enduring results which a deep analysis achieves. And in many cases a much shorter time suffices—not more than from eight to ten working months—to obtain quite satisfactory results.[2]

Repeated attention has been drawn in these pages to the great possibilities offered by child analysis. Analysis can do for children, whether normal or neurotic, all that it can do for adults, and much more. It can spare the child the many miseries and painful experiences which the adult goes through before he comes to be analysed; and its therapeutic prospects go beyond those of adult analysis. The experience of the last few years has given me and other child-analysts good grounds for believing that psychoses and psychotic traits, malformations of character, asocial behaviour,[3] grave obsessional neuroses and inhibitions of development can be cured while the individual is still young. When he is grown up, these conditions, as we know, are inaccessible or only partly accessible to psycho-analytic treatment. What course an illness will take in future years often cannot, it is true, be foretold in childhood. It is impossible to know with certainty whether it will turn into a psychosis, criminal behaviour, malformation of character or severe inhibition. But successful analysis of abnormal children may prevent all these possibilities. If every child who shows disturbances that are at all severe were to be analysed in good time, a great number of those people who later end up in prisons or mental hospitals, or who go completely to pieces, would be saved from such a fate and be able to develop a normal life. If child analysis can accomplish a work of this kind—and there are many indications that it can—it would be the means not only of helping the individual but of doing incalculable service to society as a whole.

[1] It may be remarked that where intense anxiety and severe symptoms are exhibited in analysis the structure of the illness is often more favourable than where there are no symptoms at all.

[2] In Chapter V we have seen how in a number of instances in which treatment had to be broken off, even a few months' analysis brought about considerable improvement by diminishing anxiety in the deepest levels of the mind.

[3] Cf. in this connection Melitta Schmideberg's paper, 'The Psycho-Analytic Treatment of Asocial Children and Adolescents' (1932).

EXPLANATORY NOTE

The Psycho-Analysis of Children is the culmination of Melanie Klein's early work. Above all, it is a classic text of child analysis. It sets out the psycho-analytic play technique Melanie Klein pioneered in Berlin in the early 1920's, at about the time that Dr H. B. Hug-Hellmuth ('On the Technique of Child Analysis', 1921) and Anna Freud ('Introduction to the Technique of Child Analysis', 1927) founded a different line of development. These differences are discussed by Melanie Klein in 'Symposium on Child Analysis' (1927), and she gives the early history of her own technique in 'The Psycho-Analytic Play Technique' (1955).

Melanie Klein never altered the technical principles laid down in *The Psycho-Analysis of Children* which remains her foundation work on child analysis. She had already by this time developed her own distinctive general conception of mental functioning. The ego forms an inner world of internalized figures which by the processes of projection and introjection interact with real objects. As a result of sadism to its objects the ego suffers anxiety, and its chief early task is to work through its anxieties, which are psychotic in character, and which gradually, as development proceeds, give way to neurotic anxieties.

These ideas originated in earlier papers and are here fully and more systematically elaborated. Her general contention is that anxiety, provided it is not excessive, acts as a spur to development, and that the first anxieties normally overcome are psychotic, which are the source, if not modified, of both childhood psychoses and mental illness in adult life. The book also propounds her hypotheses about the early stages of the super-ego and the Oedipus complex, phenomena previously known to psychoanalysis only in their later manifestations. She describes the severe super-ego which precedes normal conscience and charts the jealousies and anxieties of the labile sexual relations in the pre-genital oedipal situation, including the child's sadistic phantasies about the mother's body, the feminine position of both sexes, and the truly feminine origins of female sexuality. Her general view is that the development of object relations, the ego, the super-ego, sexuality and the modification of imagos cannot be considered in isolation—each affects all of the others. The original presentation of these findings will be found in the series of papers from 1919 to 1939 in *The Writings of Melanie Klein* (Volume I).

In addition, the book contains new developments. Of major theoretical importance for the future is the fact that Melanie Klein here, for the first time, puts her work expressly on the foundation of the life and death instincts. This means that her thinking has now in it the theoretical means for two of her foremost discoveries—the depressive position and, later on, the paranoid-schizoid position—which conceptually rest, among other things, on the presence and interaction of the opposed impulses of love and hate. In this volume, however, Freud's older notion, as added to by

Abraham, of the progression of libido through psycho-sexual stages, is still a pivotal idea and apart from a general acceptance of the interaction of the life and death instincts as fundamental to mental functioning, only two concepts are explicitly, if briefly, put on a new basis. Anxiety, a phenomenon which had preoccupied Melanie Klein since 1923, is attributed (p. 126) to the death instinct: anxiety originates from the presence and danger of the death instinct in the self. Melanie Klein maintained this view of anxiety from now on; its fullest statement is in 'Notes on Some Schizoid Mechanisms' (1946). In the passage in which she connects anxiety and the death instinct she also links the origin of the super-ego to the death instinct: the super-ego comes from a division in the id which is used by the ego as a defence against that portion of the death instinct that remains within; as soon as the process of incorporation begins, the incorporated object assumes the function of the super-ego. However, elsewhere Melanie Klein still follows Freud in connecting super-ego formation to the introjection of oedipal objects. She also clarifies the functioning of the super-ego in the present work, distinguishing anxiety and guilt in its operation: the early super-ego is felt by the ego as anxiety, and only later as the super-ego develops does it give rise to a sense of guilt. For a general account of Melanie Klein's views on the super-ego the reader should consult the Explanatory Note to 'The Early Development of Conscience in the Child' (1933) in Volume III of her *Writings*.

In this work, too, for the first time, are Melanie Klein's views on feminine masochism, phobias, and the guilt and taboos surrounding masturbation and incest, and she gives a new and intricate account of the sexual development of the boy and the girl. She also puts forward a new conception of obsessional neurosis mentioned in a sentence in the paper which precedes this book 'A Contribution to the Theory of Intellectual Inhibition' (1931). In contra-distinction to Freud, who took obsessional neurosis to be a later regression to anal fixations, she sees obsessional neurosis as an attempt to bind early psychotic anxieties. The concept of reparation is not yet in Melanie Klein's thinking, and she here regards omnipotent restitutive impulses as the other main method of modifying early anxieties. And, notwithstanding a reference to the narcissistic phase, it is clear throughout that she conceives of very early object relations.

What is the place of *The Psycho-Analysis of Children* in the general compass of her work? It is the fullest account of her first series of findings and conceptions, but written at a moment of transition. It puts forward views that only partially accord with its main theoretical basis, which is soon to be much less relied on—Freud's and Abraham's theory of psycho-sexual stages of libido. This, together with a still limited use of Freud's theory of the interaction of the life and death instincts, leads to complexity and at times inconsistency. There is an over-emphasis, as in all Melanie Klein's work of this first period, on aggression, since much of her new work examines aggression in its own right. Furthermore, there is a rapid series of discoveries in this first period, and Melanie Klein when impelled by new facts is indifferent to considerations of theoretical consistency.

However, within three years she began to transform the descriptive ac-

count of development in the present volume into an integrated and powerful theory of the earliest months of life, the three main papers being 'A
Contribution to the Psychogenesis of Manic-Depressive States' (1935),
'Mourning and Its Relation to Manic-Depressive States' (1940) and
'Notes on Some Schizoid Mechanisms' (1946). These, as Melanie Klein
explains in the 1948 Preface to the third edition of the present work,
retrospectively alter some of her views; above all, love is given a greater
place than she accords it here.

Editorial Board
MELANIE KLEIN TRUST

BIBLIOGRAPHY

Abraham, K. (1917). 'Ejaculatio Praecox.' in: *Selected Papers on Psycho-Analysis* (London: Hogarth, 1927).

—— (1920). 'The Narcissistic Evaluation of Excretory Processes in Dreams and Neurosis.' *ibid.*

—— (1922). 'Manifestations of the Female Castration Complex.' *ibid.*

—— (1924a). 'The Influence of Oral Erotism on Character Formation.' *ibid.*

—— (1924b). 'A Short Study of the Development of the Libido, Viewed in the Light of Mental Disorders.' *ibid.*

—— (1921–5). 'Psycho-Analytic Studies on Character Formation.' *ibid.*

Alexander, F. (1927). *The Psychoanalysis of the Total Personality: The Application of Freud's Theory of the Ego to the Neuroses* (New York & Washington: Nerv. & Ment. Dis. Pub. Co., 1930).

Benedek, T. (1931). 'Todestrieb und Angst.' *Int. Z. f. Psychoanal.*, **17.**

Boehm, F. (1920). 'Homosexualität und Polygamie.' *Int. Z. f. Psychoanal.*, **6.**

—— (1926). 'Homosexualität und Ödipuskomplex.' *Int. Z. f. Psychoanal.*, **12.**

—— (1930). 'The Femininity Complex in Men.' *Int. J. Psycho-Anal.*, **11.**

Chadwick, M. (1925). 'Uber die Wurzel der Wissbegierde.' *Int. Z. f. Psychoanal.*, **11,** Abstract in *Int. J. Psycho-Anal.*, **6.**

Deutsch, H. (1925). *Psychoanalyse der weiblichen Sexualfunktionen.* (Vienna: Int. Psychoanal. Vlg.) English Review: *Int. J. Psycho-Anal.*, **7.**

—— (1928). 'The Genesis of Agoraphobia.' *Int. J. Psycho-Anal.*, **10.**

—— (1930a). 'The Significance of Masochism in the Mental Life of Women.' *Int. J. Psycho-Anal.*, **11.**

—— (1930b). *Psychoanalysis of the Neuroses* (London; Hogarth, 1932).

Federn, P. (1913). 'Beiträge zur Analyse des Sadismus und Masochismus.' *Int. Z. f. Psychoanal.*, **1.**

Fenichel, O. (1926). 'Identification.' In: *Collected Papers of Otto Fenichel* 1st series. (New York: Norton, 1953).

—— (1928). 'Some Infantile Sexual Theories not Hitherto Described.' *Int. J. Psycho-Anal.*, **9.**

—— (1930). 'Pregenital Antecedents of the Oedipus Complex.' *Int. J. Psycho-Anal.*, 1931, **12.**

—— (1931). 'Respiratory Introjection.' In: *Collected Papers of Otto Fenichel* 1st series. (New York: Norton, 1953).

Ferenczi, S. (1913). 'Stages in the Development of the Sense of Reality.' In: *First Contributions to Psycho-Analysis* (London: Hogarth, 1952).

—— (1914a). 'The Origin of Interest in Money.' *ibid.*

—— (1914b). 'On the Nosology of Male Homosexuality.' *ibid.*

—— (1919). 'Psycho-Analytic Observations on Tic.' In: *Further Contributions to Psycho-Analysis* (London: Hogarth, 1926).

—— (1922). *Thalassa: Theory of Genitality* (New York: Psychoanal. Quart. Inc.).

—— (1924). 'On Forced Phantasies.' In: *Further Contributions.*

—— (1925). 'The Psycho-Analysis of Sexual Habits.' *ibid.*

—— (1926). 'The Problem of the Acceptance of Unpleasant Ideas.' *ibid.*

Flugel, J. C. (1930). *The Psychology of Clothes* (London: Hogarth).

Freud, A. (1927). *The Psychoanalytical Treatment of Children* (London: Imago, 1946).

Freud, S. (1900). *The Interpretation of Dreams. S.E.* **4–5.**

—— (1905a). *Three Essays on the Theory of Sexuality. S.E.* **7.**

—— (1905b). 'Fragment of an Analysis of a Case of Hysteria.' *S.E.* **7.**

—— (1909a). 'Analysis of a Phobia in a Five-Year-Old Boy.' *S.E.* **10.**

—— (1909b). 'Notes upon a Case of Obsessional Neurosis.' *S.E.* **10.**

—— (1910). *Leonardo da Vinci and a Memory of his Childhood. S.E.* **11.**

—— (1913a). The 'Predisposition to Obsessional Neurosis.' *S.E.* **12.**

—— (1913b). *Totem and Taboo. S.E.* **13.**

—— (1914). 'On Narcissism: an Introduction.' *S.E.* **14.**

—— (1915). 'Instincts and Their Vicissitudes.' *S.E.* **14.**

—— (1916–17). *Introductory Lectures on Psycho-Analysis. S.E.* **15–16.**

—— (1918). 'From the History of an Infantile Neurosis.' *S.E.* **17.**

—— (1920). *Beyond the Pleasure Principle. S.E.* **18.**

—— (1922). 'Some Neurotic Mechanisms in Jealousy, Paranoia and Homosexuality'. *S.E.* **18.**

—— (1923). *The Ego and the Id. S.E.* **19.**

—— (1924a). 'The Economic Problem in Masochism.' *S.E.* **19.**

—— (1924b). 'The Dissolution of the Oedipus Complex.' *S.E.* **19.**

—— (1925). 'Some Psychical Consequences of the Anatomical Distinction between the Sexes.' *S.E.* **19.**

—— (1926a). *Inhibitions, Symptoms and Anxiety. S.E.* **20.**

—— (1926b). *The Question of Lay Analysis. S.E.* **20.**

—— (1927). 'Humour.' *S.E.* **21.**

—— (1930). *Civilization and its Discontents. S.E.* **21.**

—— (1931). 'Female Sexuality.' *S.E.* **21.**

Glover, E. (1924). 'The Significance of the Mouth in Psycho-Analysis.' *Brit. J. med. Psychol.,* **4.**

—— (1925). 'Notes on Oral Character-Formation.' *Int. J. Psycho-Anal.,* **6.**

—— (1927). 'Symposium on Child Analysis.' *Int. J. Psycho-Anal.,* **8.**

Horney, K. (1924). 'On the Genesis of the Castration Complex in Women.' *Int. J. Psycho-Anal.*, **5.**

—— (1926). 'The Flight from Womanhood.' *Int. J. Psycho-Anal.*, **7.**

Hug-Hellmuth, H. v. (1921). 'On the Technique of Child Analysis.' *Int. J. Psycho-Anal.*, **2.**

Isaacs, S. (1929). 'Privation and Guilt.' *Int. J. Psycho-Anal.*, **10.**

Jekels, L. (1930). 'The Psychology of Pity.' In: *Selected Papers* (New York: Int. Univ. Press).

Jones, E. (1916). 'The Theory of Symbolism.' In: *Papers on Psycho-Analysis* (London: Baillière) 2nd and 5th edns.

—— (1923a). 'The Madonna's Conception through the Ear.' In: *Essays in Applied Psycho-Analysis* (London: Hogarth).

—— (1923b). 'The Nature of Auto-Suggestion.' In: *Papers on Psycho-Analysis* 3rd and 5th edns.

—— (1926). 'The Origin and Structure of the Superego.' *ibid.*, 4th edn.

—— (1927a). Symposium on Child Analysis.' *Int. J. Psycho-Anal.*, **8.**

—— (1927b). 'The Early Development of Female Sexuality.' *Papers on Psycho-Analysis*, 4th and 5th edns.

—— (1929). 'Fear, Guilt and Hate.' *ibid.*, 4th and 5th edns.

—— (1931). 'The Problem of Paul Morphy.' In: *Essays in Applied Psycho-Analysis.*

Klein, M. [details of first publication of each paperbook are given here; the volume number in which they appear in *The Writings of Melanie Klein* is indicated in square brackets].

—— (1921). 'The Development of a Child.' *Imago*, **7** [1].

—— (1922). 'Inhibitions and Difficulties in Puberty.' *Die neue Erzichung*, **4** [1].

—— (1923a). 'The Role of the School in the Libidinal Development of the Child.' *Int. Z. f. Psychoanal.*, **9** [1].

—— (1923b). 'Early Analysis.' *Imago*, **9** [1].

—— (1925). 'A Contribution to the Psychogenesis of Tics.' *Int. Z. f. Psychoanal.*, **11** [1].

—— (1926). 'The Psychological Principles of Early Analysis.' *Int. J. Psycho-Anal.*, **7** [1].

—— (1927a). 'Symposium on Child Analysis.' *Int. J. Psycho-Anal.*, **8** [1].

—— (1927b). 'Criminal Tendencies in Normal Children.' *Brit. J. med. Psychol.*, **7** [1].

—— (1928). 'Early Stages of the Oedipus Conflict.' *Int. J. Psycho-Anal.*, **9** [1].

—— (1929a). 'Personification in the Play of Children.' *Int. J. Psycho-Anal.*, **10** [1].

—— (1929b). 'Infantile Anxiety Situations Reflected in a Work of Art and in the Creative Impulse.' *Int. J. Psycho-Anal.*, **10** [1].

—— (1930a). 'The Importance of Symbol-Formation in the Development of the Ego.' *Int. J. Psycho-Anal.*, **11** [1].

BIBLIOGRAPHY

—— (1930b). 'The Psychotherapy of the Psychoses.' *Brit. J. med. Psychol.*, **10** [1].

—— (1931). 'A Contribution to the Theory of Intellectual Inhibition. *Int. J. Psycho-Anal.*, **12** [1].

—— (1932). *The Psycho-Analysis of Children* (London: Hogarth) [2].

—— (1933). 'The Early Development of Conscience in the Child.' In: *Psychoanalysis Today* ed. Lorand (New York: Covici-Friede) [1].

—— (1934). 'On Criminality.' *Brit. J. med. Psychol.*, **14** [1].

—— (1935). 'A Contribution to the Psychogenesis of Manic-Depressive States.' *Int. J. Psycho-Anal.*, **16** [1].

—— (1936). 'Weaning.' In: *On the Bringing Up of Children* ed. Rickman (London: Kegan Paul) [1].

—— (1937). 'Love, Guilt and Reparation.' In: *Love, Hate and Reparation*, with Riviere (London: Hogarth) [**1**].

—— (1940). 'Mourning and its Relation to Manic-Depressive States.' *Int. J. Psycho-Anal.*, **21** [1].

—— (1945). 'The Oedipus Complex in the Light of Early Anxieties.' *Int. J. Psycho-Anal.*, **26** [1].

—— (1946). 'Notes on some Schizoid Mechanisms.' *Int. J. Psycho-Anal.*, **27** [3].

—— (1948a). *Contributions to Psycho-Analysis 1921-1945* (London: Hogarth) [1].

—— (1948b). 'On the Theory of Anxiety and Guilt.' *Int. J. Psycho-Anal.*, **29** [3].

—— (1950). 'On the Criteria for the Termination of a Psycho-Analysis.' *Int. J. Psycho-Anal.*, **31** [3].

—— (1952a). 'The Origins of Transference.' *Int. J. Psycho-Anal.*, **33** [3].

—— (1952b). 'The Mutual Influences in the Development of Ego and Id.' *Psychoanal. Study Child*, **7** [3].

—— (1952c). 'Some Theoretical Conclusions regarding the Emotional Life of the Infant.' In: *Developments in Psycho-Analysis* with Heimann, Isaacs and Riviere (London: Hogarth) [3].

—— (1952d). 'On Observing the Behaviour of Young Infants.' *ibid.* [3].

—— (1955a). 'The Psycho-Analytic Play Technique: Its History and Significance.' In: *New Directions in Psycho-Analysis* (London: Tavistock) [3].

—— (1955b). 'On Identification.' *ibid.* [3].

—— (1957). *Envy and Gratitude* (London: Tavistock) [3].

—— (1958). 'On the Development of Mental Functioning.' *Int. J. Psycho-Anal.*, **29** [3].

—— (1959). 'Our Adult World and its Roots in Infancy.' *Hum. Relations*, **12** [3].

—— (1960a). 'A Note on Depression in the Schizophrenic.' *Int. J. Psycho-Anal.*, **41** [3].

—— (1960b). 'On Mental Health.' *Brit. J. med. Psychol.*, **33** [3].

—— (1961). *Narrative of a Child Psycho-Analysis* (London: Hogarth) [4].

—— (1963a). 'Some Reflections on *The Oresteia.*' In: *Our Adult World and Other Essays* (London: Heinemann Medical) [3].

—— (1963b). 'On the Sense of Loneliness.' *ibid.* [3].

Laforgue, R. (1926). 'Scotomisation in Schizophrenia.' *Int. J. Psycho-Anal.*, **8.**

Lewin, B. D. (1930). 'Kotschmieren, Menses und weibliches Über-Ich.' *Int. Z. f. Psychoanal.*, **16.**

Mack-Brunswick, R. (1928). 'A Supplement to Freud's "History of an Infantile Neurosis".' *Int. J. Psycho-Anal.*, **9.**

Ophuijsen, J. H. W. v. (1920). 'On the Origin of the Feeling of Persecution.' *ibid.*, **1.**

Radó, S. (1926, 1928). 'The Psychic Effects of Intoxicants: An Attempt at a Psychoanalytic Theory of Drug Addiction.' *ibid.*, **7, 9.**

—— (1928). 'The Problem of Melancholia.' *ibid.*, **9**, pp. 420–38. Also in: *Psychoanalysis of Behavior: Collected Papers* (New York: Grune & Stratton).

Rank, O. (1915). 'Das Schauspiel im Hamlet.' *Imago*, **4.**

—— (1919). *Psychoanalytische Beiträge zur Mythenforschung* (Vienna : Int. Psychoanal. Vlg., 1922).

Reich, W. (1925). *Der Triebhafte Charakter* (Vienna: Int. Psychoanal. Vlg.).

—— (1927). *The Function of the Orgasm* (Vienna: Int. Psychoanal. Vlg.; London: Panther Books, 1968).

—— (1931). 'Character Formation and the Phobias of Childhood.' *Int. J. Psycho-Anal.*, **12.** Also in: *The Psychoanalytic Reader*, ed. Fliess. (New York: Int. Univ. Press, 1948; London: Hogarth Press, 1950.)

Reik, T. (1929). 'Angst und Hass', 'Libido und Schuldgefühle' both in *Der Schrecken* (Vienna: Int. Psychoanal. Vlg.).

Riviere, J. (1927). 'Symposium on Child Analysis.' *Int. J. Psycho-Anal.*, **8.**

—— (1929). 'Womanliness as a Masquerade.' *ibid.*, **10.**

Róheim, G. (1922). 'Das volkerpsychologische in Freud's Massenpsychologie und Ichanalyse.' *Int. Z. f. Psychoanal.*, **8.**

—— (1923). 'Nach dem Tode des Urvaters.' *Imago*, **9.**

Sachs, H. (1920). 'Gemeinsame Tagträume.' *Int. Z. f. Psychoanal.*, **6.** (Also: Vienna: Int. Psychoanal. Vlg., 1924.)

—— (1929). 'One of the Motive Factors in the Formation of the Super-Ego in Women.' *Int. J. Psycho-Anal.*, **10.**

—— (1937). 'Zur Theorie der Psychoanalytischen Technik.' *Int. Z. f. Psychoanal.*, **23.**

Sadger, J. (1910a). 'Ein Fall von multipler Perversion mit hysterischen Absenzen.' *Jahrb. f. Psychanal. Forsch.*, **2.**

—— (1910b). 'Über Urethralerotik.' *ibid.*

Schmideberg, M. (1930). 'The Role of Psychotic Mechanisms in Cultural Development.' *Int. J. Psycho-Anal.*, **11.**

—— (1931a). 'A Contribution to the Psychology of Persecutory Ideas and Delusions.' *ibid.*, **12.**

—— (1931b). 'Psychoanalytisches zur Menstruation.' *Z. f. Psychoanal. Päd.*, **5.**

—— (1932a). 'Some Unconscious Mechanisms in Pathological Sexuality and their Relation to Normal Sexual Activity.' *Int. J. Psycho-Anal.*, **14.**

—— (1932b). 'The Psychoanalytic Treatment of Asocial Children and Adolescents.' *ibid.*, **16.**

Searl, M. N. (1927). 'Symposium on Child Analysis.' *ibid.*, **8.**

—— (1928). 'A Paranoiac Mechanism as Seen in the Analysis of a Child.' *Int. Z. f. Psychoanal.*, **16.** Abstract in *ibid.*, **9.**

—— (1929). 'The Flight to Reality.' *ibid.*, **10.**

—— (1930). 'The Roles of Ego and Libido in Development.' *ibid.*, **11.**

'Sexual Enlightenment.' *Zeitschrift für Psychoanalytischer Pädagogik*, 1 Jahrgang. October 1926–September 1927. Published in Vienna, 1927. Contains a number of papers on 'Sexuelle Aufklarung'.

Sharpe, E. F. (1929). 'History as Phantasy.' *Int. J. Psycho-Anal.*, **10.**

—— (1930). 'Certain Aspects of Sublimations and Delusions.' *Collected Papers on Psycho-Analysis* (London: Hogarth, 1950).

Simmel, E. (1926). 'The "Doctor-Game", Illness and the Profession of Medicine.' *Int. J. Psycho-Anal.*, **7.**

Stärcke, A. (1920). 'The Reversal of the Libido-Sign in Delusions of Persecution.' *ibid.*, **1.**

—— (1921). 'Psycho-Analysis and Psychiatry.' *ibid.*, **2.**

Strachey, J. (1930). 'Some Unconscious Factors in Reading.' *ibid.*, **11.**

Weiss, E. (1925). 'Über eine noch unbeschriebene Phase der Entwicklung zur homosexuellen Liebe.' *Int. Z. f. Psychoanal.*, **11.**

LIST OF PATIENTS

INDEX

INDEX

Compiled by Barbara Forryan

defensive mechanisms of ego against anxiety, *see* anxiety *s.v.* ego
defiance 68, 89, 92, 97; in transference, *see* transference
defloration 210
delusions of persecution 264, 265; in adult, and child's paranoid phantasies 44; cause of 45, 146 & *n*, 261 (*see also* watched, being);
delusions of poisoning 261, 264
delusions of reference 146 & *n*, 261, 264, 265; *see also* paranoia
demon of illness 115*n*, 216*n*; *see also* devils
dentist, analyst identified with 80
depression 43, 48, 51, 61*n*, 84*n*, 87, 110*n*, 156, 264, 273, 277; during play 43–4; following anal phantasies 45, 46*n*; melancholic 3; in normal child 104; 'there's something I don't like about life' (Erna) 35, 50*n*
depressive feelings and Oedipus complex, impetus towards xiv
depressive position xiii, xiv, 283
deprivation, as punishment 62 & *n*, *see also* frustration
destruction, pleasure in 20
destructive impulses/instincts 114*n*, 249; directed against the self 126 & *n*, 127 & *n*, 202–3; ego's defences against 5*n*, 127, 134*n*, 137*n*, 139; —, premature/excessive 244 & *n*; and libidinal instincts (fusion) 126, 130, 134, 150, 201, 280 (*see also* death-instinct and life-instinct); in paranoid position xiii; and reparation xiv; and restoration 170; as source of anxiety, *see* anxiety; turned outwards to objects 126, 137, 177, 202; *see also* aggression; sadism
detachment from incestuous/libidinal/love-objects *see* object(s) *s.v.* love-
detective stories 81*n*
Deutsch, Helene 29*n*, 196*n*, 202*n*, 209*n*, 210, 211*n*, 213*n*, 217*n*, 218*n*, 224–5, 227
devil(s) 156; penis possessed by 276; *see also* demon
devouring phantasies 129, 238; and breast, *see* breast *s.v.* sucking etc.;

and father's penis, *see* penis, father's *s.v.* oral-sadistic attacks; and super-ego, *see* super-ego *s.v.* biting
dirty, fear of being 109
dirtying/soiling 5, 20, 41; 'Miss Dirt Parade', 41, 48*n*
discipline, as sadistic act 40
disease, primitive method of expelling 115*n*; *see also* illness
dislikes, *see* aversion(s)
disobedience 97
displacement 82, 153, 158, 166, 192, 246, 255*n*, 264*n*; of affects 91, 264; of anxiety, *see* anxiety; of boy's hatred of father/father's penis onto mother 130*n*, 131, 132, 254, 255*n*, 260, 266; onto external world 177; of fear of 'bad' parents to stranger 24; 'from above downwards' 196*n*–197*n*; onto something very small' 172, 173
dissimulation 265
distrust 113; in latency period, *see* latency; and negative transference 21
docility: excessive 87, 188*n*; and rejection of reality 12; *see also* 'good' children; obedience
dog, fear of 19, *see also* animal phobias
doll(s): boy's play with 106*n*; as helpful object 223*n*; many different meanings of 8; play 182, 184, 190, 208
doubting-mania 264
drawer of toys 209 & *n*
drawing 34, 58–9, 66, 67, 74; compulsive 87, 88, monotonous 74, 75, 82
dream(s) anxiety 64; associations to, in child's play 8; —, and uncovering of latent content 18; —, verbal 23; language of 7; and play, relationship 8, 105, 177*n*; punishment- 11*n*; in traumatic neurosis 177 & *n*; wish-, and sense of guilt in 11*n*; -work, mechanisms of 8; dream-world, protected from reality 43–4; *Instances* 11, 23, 64, 65, 66
drowning with urine, phantasies of 128, 169

sadism 160; ambivalence and 135*n*; and death-instinct 128; deepest layers of, and inhibition 57; diminution of 109, 152, 279; —, essential 47, 52, 57; girl's against mother, 91 (*see also* mother *s.v.* girl's hatred/aggression); as internal enemy 127*n*; libidinal frustration and heightening of 126, 130; means of 146*n*; muscular 127*n*, 129; overcoming of 140; physical sources of 127*n*; and presents 99; primal 202; primary 172; quantitative and qualitative changes in 132; and sexual relations between brothers 114; urethral, *see* urethral;

sadism, phase/stage of 143; in boy 241; earliest 144;

sadism, phase of, maximal/at its height ix, 150, 151, 159, 240; and attacks on mother's body 130, 164; dating of xiii, xiv, 130, 146*n*; in girl 206; and knowledge, desire for 173, 174; and Oedipus trends/ genital impulses 134–5, 150, 173, 201; and paranoia/psychosis 146 & *n*, 155; and parents' coitus 132, 200; and (persecutory) anxiety xiii, 140, 142; and super-ego formation, *see* super-ego formation

sadistic/impulses/trends/instincts 126, 137*n*, 140; towards analyst 54; and cutting out paper 37; making fun of 13 & *n*; in male sexuality 246–7; and masochism 114; and object relations 142, 152–3; sublimation of 13; and super-ego 169

sadistic phantasies 140, 142, 166; anal, *see* anal; analysis of 46; and anxiety 280; of attacks on mother 29–30; against brother 85, 113–14; brother as substitute for parents in 113, 115; details of, and hypochondria 258*n*; —, and restitution, *see* restitution; masturbation, *see* masturbation; oral, *see* oral; against parents 85, 115; —, in coitus, *see* coitus *s.v.* child's (sadistic) attacks; and reaction-formations, in water games 33–4; of stealing from mother 39; urethral, *see* urethral; *see also* aggression;

destructive impulses

sadness, in children 155–6

Salzburg Congress (1924) 9

schizoid features in child 86

schizophrenia 68, 143, 144 & *n*

Schmideberg, Melitta xii, 71*n*, 115*n*, 144*n*, 146*n*, 206*n*, 215*n*, 219*n*, 225*n*, 257*n*, 282*n*

school: and adaptation to schoolfellows 36; anxiety in 66*n*; boarding- 78, 87; failure 61 & *n*, 62, 63, 185*n*; in games of pretence 34, 61; girl's reports on 86, 89; tasks 89, 90 (*see also* homework; writing); work, compulsive, *see* compulsive; *see also* learning

schoolmaster, adolescent's scorn for 82, 189

scoptophilia 212*n*, 217

scotomization 144*n*, 152, 177*n*

scribbling 72*n*

scybalum 145 & *n*

Searl, M. Nina xi, xii, 30, 103*n*, 116*n*, 131*n*, 138*n*, 172*n*

secretiveness 113, 156, 205*n*

seduction: by adult 224*n*; cleansing of genitals and anus as 48; by elder brother 113, 114, 267; by nurse (Mary) 64–6; by older friend 85; by sister 159, 160; wish for/accusation of 48–9

self-preservation 203, *see also* life-instinct

self-reliance 91

semen 38, 40, 251*n*, 263 & *n*, 277; *see also* coitus *s.v.* fluids

sexual activities: and analysis 279; compulsive 279; —, and super-ego 115; perverse, in criminals 114

sexual curiosity, linked with anxiety and guilt 59*n*

sexual development: of adult, disturbances in, *see below* sexual life of adult; of boy, *see* boy; of girl, *see* girl; and interests in play 105

sexual differences: brooding on 59 & *n*; curiosity about 75, 88; uncertainty about 69; *see also* anatomical differences

sexual enlightenment 59*n*, 60*n*; child's resistance to 60*n*, 98; as consequence of analysis 12

sexual impulses: experienced by

urine:—*contd.*
99, 213; and milk, 213 & *n*, 232*n*;
from mother's body 167; in
sadistic phantasies 128–9, 145 & *n*,
205, 213, 243, 248, 258*n*; stream of,
as penis 244*n*

vagina: and anus 218; *dentata* 136*n*;
and infantile sexual development
210–12, 217; in masturbation
50; mother's: father's penis
retained in, in phantasy 131*n*,
(*see also* mother *s.v.* father's penis);
—, as death-trap/dangerous
opening 132, 136, 204, 210; —,
in restoration 220; and mouth
196*n*, 210, 211*n*; penis concealed in
246*n*; sucking activity of 196*n*, 217*n*
vaginal phase 211 & *n*
vampire-like behaviour 128*n*
Van Ophuijsen, *see* Ophuijsen
verbal associations, *see* associations;
see also language; speech; words

walks, aversion to 96
watched, being 266, 275; by mother
44
watchfulness, suspicious 44, 146, 205*n*
water: games with, in analysis 33,
38, 41; in latency 60; water-tap as
'milk-tap' or 'whipped cream tap'
10, 33*n*, 38
water, passing, *see* urination; wetting
weaning 48; and Oedipus conflict
55; trauma 259; *see also* breast *s.v.*
child's pain at withdrawal
Weiss, Edoardo 250*n*
Werner, *see* List of Patients, p. 292
wetting 65, 213, 248; as attack upon
parents' copulation 5, 134; bed-
wetting 13, 30*n*, 129, 134; and
burning, connection 34*n*;
incontinence during analytic

session 5, 19*n*, 30; and masculine
position 213, 214; *see also*
enuresis; urination
whooping-cough 100*n*
wish-fulfilment in game, *see* game(s)
witches 156
withdrawn character 67, 70, 84*n*
woefulness 3; *see also* plaintiveness
wolf/wolves, 159–60; as faeces 127*n*
Wolf Man, *see* Freud, S.: CASES
woman: and child, comparison 236;
'deceitful and treacherous' 266;
and desire for new clothes 98;
ego development of 232–6; man's
aversion to 255, 265–6; own child
of, *see* child *s.v.* adult woman's;
'pure' 251*n*; super-ego in 232–6;
'with a penis', *see* mother *s.v.*
'woman . . .'
womb, mother's, child's phantasy of
coitus/father's penis in 131*n*
words: analyst's, patient's aversion to
258–9; assessed pictorially by
children 32*n*; child's own, used in
interpretations 32 & *n*; child's
special, for genitals etc. 17*n*;
difficulty in using 88; of grownups,
child's inability to understand 174;
obscene 64; *see also* language; speech
work, inhibitions in, *see* inhibition(s)
working over: of anxiety 102; of
interpretation/knowledge, conscious 12; —, unconscious 13
working through: and early deep
interpretations 23–4; in phantasy
18
writing: inhibition in 61, 72*n*;
symbolism of 57, 184 & *n*
Würzburg, First Conference of
German Psycho-Analysts (1924)
xi, 35*n*

youngest child 62